Persons with Disabilities

D1522408

Brookings Dialogues on Public Policy

The presentations and discussions at Brookings conferences and seminars often deserve wide circulation as contributions to public understanding of issues of national importance. The Brookings Dialogues on Public Policy series is intended to make such papers and commentary available to a broad and general audience. The series supplements the Institution's research publications by reflecting the contrasting, often lively, and sometimes conflicting views of elected and appointed government officials, other leaders in public and private life, and scholars. In keeping with their origin and purpose, the Dialogues are not subjected to the same formal review procedures established for the Institution's research publications. Brookings publishes the contributions to the Dialogues in the belief that they are worthy of public consideration but does not assume responsibility for their objectivity and for the accuracy of every factual statement. And, as in all Brookings publications, the judgments, conclusions, and recommendations presented in the Dialogues should not be ascribed to the trustees, officers, or other staff members of the Brookings Institution.

Persons with Disabilities
Issues in Health Care Financing and Service Delivery

Edited by

JOSHUA M. WIENER

STEVEN B. CLAUSER

DAVID L. KENNELL

THE BROOKINGS INSTITUTION / Washington, D.C.

Copyright © 1995 by

THE BROOKINGS INSTITUTION

1775 Massachusetts Avenue, N.W.

Washington, D.C. 20036

Library of Congress Cataloging-in-Publication Data
Persons with disabilities : issues in health care financing and
    service delivery / Joshua M. Wiener, Steven B. Clauser,
    David L. Kennell, eds.
        p.   cm.
    Includes bibliographical references.
    ISBN 0-8157-9379-0 (pbk.: alk. paper)
        1. Chronically ill—Medical care—United States—Finance.
    2. Physically handicapped—Medical care—United States—Finance.
    3. Long-term care of the sick—United States—Finance.
    4. Insurance, long-term care—United States.   I. Wiener,
    Joshua M. II. Clauser, Steven Boyd. III. Kennell, David L.
    RA395.A3P473 1995   95-37969
    338.4'33621—dc20   CIP

9 8 7 6 5 4 3 2 1

Typeset in Palatino

Composition by Linda Humphrey
Arlington, Virginia

Printed by Kirby Lithographic Company, Inc.
Arlington, Virginia

343344

Preface

An increasing number of Americans are disabled. Extraordinary growth in the elderly population is projected for the next century, and the number of Americans age 85 and older—those most in need of long-term care services—is expected to grow even faster than the overall elderly population. In addition, younger persons with disabilities account for a substantial portion of persons needing long-term care. Government programs, principally medicare and medicaid, are major sources of funding for nursing homes, intermediate care facilities for mentally retarded persons, psychiatric hospitals, and a wide range of home and community-based services. These programs are also major sources of financing of acute care services for persons with disabilities. The chapters in this book add to the policy debate about how to finance and deliver acute and long-term care services for persons with disabilities by addressing three important areas of concern—the interaction between public and private financing, the use of and expenditures for acute and long-term care services by persons with disabilities, and home and community-based services.

This book is the capstone of five years of research sponsored by the Health Care Financing Administration's Office of Research and Demonstrations. The project sponsored a consortium of research organizations led by Lewin-VHI, Inc. In addition to Lewin-VHI, Inc., the consortium included the Brookings Institution, Duke University, Mathematica Policy Research, Inc., the Johns Hopkins University, the Urban Institute, DataChron, and the MEDSTAT Group. The studies presented here are a sampling of the analyses done for the project; earlier versions of these chapters were presented at a conference at the Brookings Institution on November 3, 1994.

We acknowledge with thanks the financial support of the conference and this volume by the Health Care Financing Administration, HCFA Contract No. 500-89-0047, Long-Term Care Studies. Marvin Feurerberg, Judith Sangl, and Carolyn Rimes, the project officers at the Health Care Financing Administration, provided invaluable advice and assistance in all aspects of the project. Lisa Alecxih, Tim Dall, and Kevin Coleman of Lewin-VHI, Inc., provided useful comments on several chapters. Colette Solpietro of the Brookings Institution was instrumental in the success of the conference and provided excellent staff assistance. The book also benefited greatly from the editorial expertise of Debbie Styles, Steph Selice, Theresa Walker, and Colleen McGuiness.

The views expressed in this book are those of the authors and should not be attributed to the institutions or persons acknowledged or to the trustees, officers, or staff members of the Brookings Institution. No endorsement of the views in this volume by the Health Care Financing Administration or the U.S. Department of Health and Human Services is intended or implied.

Joshua M. Wiener
Steven B. Clauser
David L. Kennell

Contents

Part 4   Home and Community-Based Care

Contributors

Lisa Maria B. Alecxih is a senior manager at Lewin-VHI, Inc.

Brian Burwell is director of health care organization and economics at the MEDSTAT Group.

Steven B. Clauser is director of the Office of Beneficiary and Program Research and Demonstrations at the Health Care Financing Administration.

John Corea is an analyst at Lewin-VHI, Inc.

Teresa Coughlin is a senior research associate at the Urban Institute.

William H. Crown is a senior project leader at the MEDSTAT Group.

Jean Hanson is a research assistant at Resources for the Future.

Judith D. Kasper is an associate professor in the Department of Health Policy and Management, School of Hygiene and Public Health, at the Johns Hopkins University.

David L. Kennell is a vice president at Lewin-VHI, Inc.

Korbin Liu is a senior research associate at the Urban Institute.

Sharon K. Long is a senior research associate at the Urban Institute.

Steven Lutzky is an associate at Lewin-VHI, Inc.

Kenneth C. Manton is a research professor and acting director of the Center for Demographic Studies at Duke University.

Jennifer Schore is a senior researcher at Mathematica Policy Research, Inc.

Eric Stallard is an associate research professor at the Center for Demographic Studies at Duke University.

Catherine M. Sullivan is a senior research analyst in the Brookings Economic Studies program.

Bruce C. Vladeck is administrator of the Health Care Financing Administration.

Joshua M. Wiener is a senior fellow in the Brookings Economic Studies program.

Chapter 1

JOSHUA M. WIENER, STEVEN B. CLAUSER, AND
DAVID L. KENNELL

Introduction

With the success health care providers have had in preventing and
treating acute illnesses, the leading causes of morbidity and mortality
are now almost all related to chronic illnesses.[1] Although elderly
persons predominate among those with severe disabilities, younger
persons account for a substantial portion of persons needing long-
term care.

Chronically disabled people often require a broad array of both
acute and long-term care services. It is commonly recognized that the
disabled population needs nursing home, home care, and other long-
term care services, but it is less widely appreciated that they also use
physician services and hospital care extensively.[2]

Most long-term care services are provided by the disabled person's
family members and friends. But in all industrialized countries, government is a major source of financing for paid long-term care services.
In the United States, government spending—primarily medicare,
medicaid, and state-funded programs—accounted for more than two-
thirds of total long-term care expenditures for elderly persons, physically disabled younger persons, and mentally retarded or developmentally disabled individuals in 1993.[3] An estimated 61 percent of
elderly nursing home residents depend on medicaid to help pay for
their care.[4] From a program perspective, long-term care accounted for
about 36 percent of medicaid expenditures and skilled nursing facility
and home health care for about 10 percent of medicare spending.[5]

Medicare and medicaid play even more important roles in financing acute care for disabled people than they do in financing long-term
care. Virtually all elderly persons and a substantial number of
younger people with disabilities have medicare coverage, which
covers an array of acute, postacute, and rehabilitation services.
Lower-income elderly people are also eligible for medicaid, which
fills in the gaps of medicare. For this population, medicaid pays the

part B premium, deductibles, and coinsurance, and provides coverage for additional services, such as prescription drugs. These services accounted for slightly less than 10 percent of medicaid expenditures in 1992.[6] Similarly, medicaid provides acute care coverage for lower-income disabled persons, accounting for 20 percent of medicaid expenditures in 1992.[7]

Given the importance of persons with disabilities to health policy in general and to government programs in particular, this book adds to the debate by presenting research on the acute and long-term care needs of disabled Americans. The chapters explore three broad areas: interaction of public and private financing, use of and expenditures for acute and long-term care services by disabled people, and home and community-based services.

PERSPECTIVES ON LONG-TERM CARE

Setting the policy context for research on long-term care, in chapter 2 Bruce Vladeck, administrator of the Health Care Financing Administration (HCFA), reviews some of the progress made in the last ten years and presents an agenda for future action. In assessing the recent past, he notes improvement in three areas. Quality of care in nursing homes has substantially improved; use of noninstitutional long-term care services (especially financed by medicaid) has increased considerably; and mechanisms to evaluate the performance of providers have been developed and, in some cases, implemented.

Against this backdrop, Vladeck suggests that the deeply ingrained culture of HCFA is changing in ways that will have a positive effect on long-term care. As part of that change, the agency is thinking strategically about how to achieve its main goal: making sure that beneficiaries have access to high-quality health care services when they need them. Vladeck articulates three basic principles for long-term care. First, to build a client-focused, beneficiary-oriented, long-term care system, financing of services should follow the client rather than be locked into certain settings or services. Second, quality needs to be redefined from a client perspective. And finally, clients must play a larger role in choosing and directing the services they receive.

PUBLIC/PRIVATE INTERACTIONS

The first theme recognizes that financing of long-term care involves both public and private funds. In this context, recent developments in private long-term care insurance and state efforts to stop patients from transferring assets in order to qualify for medicaid are assessed in the following chapters.

Private Long-Term Care Insurance

In chapter 3, Lisa Alecxih and Steven Lutzky analyze the rapidly growing market for private long-term care insurance, focusing on whether government should play a greater role in regulating such insurance and educating the public about it. Despite dramatic improvements in the quality of products in recent years, few Americans have actually purchased private long-term care insurance. In addition, although no one knows the reasons for it, many people who buy policies drop them within a few years.

Several broad barriers deter the purchase and retention of long-term care insurance policies. First, consumers lack information about their risk of needing long-term care or about the coverage provided by medicare and their supplemental private insurance policies. This is complicated by the fact that insurance agents, who want to sell policies and are often misinformed themselves, are the principal sources of information about private long-term care insurance. Second, many consumers cannot afford policies. Third, some characteristics of insurance policies make it less desirable for consumers to purchase and retain them. These include the lack of a formal mechanism for policies to adapt to changes in consumer circumstances or for benefits to adjust to the changing delivery system. The possibility that premiums may increase can also pose problems for consumers.

To address these problems, Alecxih and Lutzky review a number of proposals to change how long-term care insurance is sold and regulated. These include having states provide consumer education, requiring special training and certification for agents selling private long-term care insurance, altering the agent commission structure to give more weight to renewals, standardizing definitions of benefits and benefit triggers to facilitate price comparisons, establishing regulatory standards defining those for whom this product may be inappropriate, and monitoring sales practices more aggressively.

In addition, the authors analyze proposals to address concerns about the policies themselves. These proposals include providing tax breaks to those who buy insurance to make it more affordable, incorporating provisions into policies that allow consumers to change their coverage without penalty, monitoring long-term care pricing better, limiting the extent to which insurance companies can raise premiums, and including features that provide a residual benefit to people who purchase policies and then drop them after a number of years.

Medicaid Estate Planning

Brian Burwell and William Crown focus on medicaid estate planning in chapter 4. Such planning refers to the efforts of elderly people who purposefully divest and shelter their assets or income to appear poor enough to qualify for medicaid nursing home benefits. For this study, the authors interviewed state medicaid officials and eligibility workers in Massachusetts, California, New York, and Florida.

One objective of their study was to qualitatively assess the magnitude of medicaid estate planning. Although there was evidence of such planning in all four states, it appears that the vast majority of people who apply for medicaid long-term care benefits do not purposefully divest or shelter their assets before applying. Overall, eligibility workers consistently reported that married applicants engage in estate planning more often than unmarried applicants, but married persons do not constitute a large number of medicaid nursing home patients.

The second objective of Burwell and Crown's study was to identify the most commonly used medicaid estate planning techniques, which tended to vary by marital status. One common tactic used by married couples is the "just say no" strategy, in which the spouse who is a community resident "refuses" to help pay for care of the institutionalized spouse. Another practice involves using court orders to increase the amount of income and assets the noninstitutionalized spouse can receive from the spouse who is receiving long-term care. In contrast, single persons generally rely on knowing how the medicaid ineligibility penalty periods are calculated and manipulating assets accordingly, and on financial instruments such as trusts and annuities that shelter income and assets. The prevalence of each of these strategies varies by state.

Assessing the impact of legislative changes enacted under the Omnibus Budget Reconciliation Act of 1993, Burwell and Crown conclude that many aspects of medicaid estate planning remain unaffected and then discuss possible ways to further curtail such activity. Finally, they argue that policymakers must also address the issues of fairness and equity. Medicaid estate planning is often rationalized on the basis that current eligibility criteria are unreasonably strict. The more medicaid is perceived as unfair, the more willing people will be to circumvent the system.

USE AND EXPENDITURES FOR PAID SERVICES

Persons with disabilities need both acute and long-term care services. Chapters 5, 6, and 7 provide quantitative estimates of the use of and expenditures for these services by persons with disabilities in the United States. They also assess whether elderly persons with cognitive impairment have reduced access to physician and hospital services, and examine the extent to which nursing home patients incur catastrophic out-of-pocket costs.

Health Care Use and Expenditures for the Noninstitutionalized Population

Using the 1987 National Medical Expenditure survey, in chapter 5 Lisa Alecxih, John Corea, and David Kennell examine health care expenditures for those with and without disabilities among people who are not institutionalized. Consistent with other research, they find that both elderly people and younger persons with disabilities have far higher average expenditures than do those without disabilities. Persons with disabilities also have far higher out-of-pocket costs, largely attributable to expenditures for home and community-based services.

The authors draw four main implications from their findings. First, they underline the need to risk-adjust capitated payments to compensate health maintenance organizations and other managed care entities fairly and to reduce the incentive to avoid enrolling disabled people. Second, though health care costs are high for persons with disabilities, these individuals are a very small percentage of the population. Thus, if it had been possible to equitably distribute coverage for younger people with disabilities across all private health insurance plans, the cost of private health insurance would have increased by only $78 in 1987. The cost impact of including persons with disabilities in community rated plans is therefore small. Third, the high cost and use of health care services by persons with disabilities (especially for hospital care) suggest that there may be opportunities for managed care plans to cut costs. Finally, Alecxih, Corea, and Kennell note that proposals to increase cost sharing in medicare and private insurance fall particularly heavily on people with disabilities. The high out-of-pocket costs for home and community-based services underscore the lack of widespread public or private financing of these services.

Program Payment and Utilization Trends
for Medicare Beneficiaries with Disabilities

In chapter 6 Kenneth Manton and Eric Stallard use the National Long-Term Care Survey to examine how changes in medicare service use from 1982 to 1990 differed among disabled and nondisabled beneficiaries. Overall, during that period, use of home health agencies, skilled nursing facilities, hospital outpatient services, and physician services increased, while inpatient hospital services decreased. For this study, the authors used a statistical technique called grade of membership (GOM) to create eight pure type groups of medicare beneficiaries, differing by health, disability, and residential status. Hospital care, physician services, outpatient hospital services, skilled nursing facility care, home health care, durable medical equipment, and other services are analyzed separately.

The study clearly demonstrates that changes in use of services and expenditures varied substantially by health status and disability characteristics of medicare enrollees. Overall, the average increase in expenditures for all services was 58 percent in constant dollars. While the group with one instrumental activity of daily living (IADL) impairment had a 12 percent decrease in service payments, the institutionalized group had a 95 percent increase. The only other groups with above average increases were the active and healthy group and the circulatory problem group. The three groups in frail or poor health all had increases of 20 to 28 percent, substantially below the average. These findings imply that policymakers should be sensitive to the impact of possible changes in medicare on different subgroups of people with and without disabilities.

Cognitive Impairment and Use of Acute Care Services

Cognitive impairment is a potential barrier to appropriate care of elderly people for a number of reasons, including its interference with an individual's ability to recognize and communicate health problems and the difficulty it causes in diagnosing and treating illness in this population. Given that patients are sometimes hostile and abusive, doctors and hospitals may also resist serving these patients. In chapter 7, Judith Kasper examines the effect of cognitive impairment among elderly Americans—principally those diagnosed with Alzheimer's disease—on access to physician care and use of hospital services using the community resident component of the 1989 National Long-Term Care Survey. Almost 29 percent of the survey sample have some cognitive impairment.

Ambulatory care access was measured using three indicators: having a physician visit in the past month, reporting a regular source of care, and using an emergency room visit without a hospital admission in the past month. For the first two measures, Kasper found that elderly persons with moderate or severe cognitive impairment had lower use of services than disabled persons with only mild or no cognitive impairment. For emergency room visits, there was no clear trend by cognitive status.

Hospital care access was also measured using three indicators: a hospital admission within the last year, admission rate per 1,000 disabled persons, and average length of stay. In contrast to the findings on physician use, on all three measures persons with moderate or severe cognitive impairment were more likely to use hospital services than disabled elderly individuals with only mild cognitive impairment or none at all. These results on hospital use are particularly striking given the less frequent use of physician services. It is possible that medical conditions are left untreated until they require hospitalization or that hospital care is substituting for physician services. Based on these findings, Kasper concludes that moderate or severe cognitive impairment appears to be a barrier to use of physician services, but she cautions that additional research is needed.

Catastrophic Costs of Long-Term Care for Elderly Americans

Concern about the financial hardship high out-of-pocket costs for long-term care impose on elderly people in the United States has been a long-standing health policy issue and a major rationale behind many proposals for reform. In chapter 8 Joshua Wiener, Catherine Sullivan, and Lisa Alecxih use the Brookings–ICF Long-Term Care Financing Model to estimate current and future financial burdens on nursing home patients.

The three measures of catastrophic out-of-pocket expenses used in this chapter suggest that the proportion of elderly nursing home patients who face catastrophic out-of-pocket expenses will remain fairly stable from 1993 to 2018. First, the proportion of nursing home patients who depend on medicaid to finance their care will decline only slightly and will still include more than half of all patients. Second, about one-third of elderly nursing home admissions will incur out-of-pocket costs of $20,000 or more (in 1993 dollars) per stay. And third, approximately 40 percent of elderly persons admitted to nursing homes will have out-of-pocket expenses that equal or exceed 40 percent of their combined income and nonhousing assets. Not surprisingly, lower-income elderly persons shoulder a disproportionate share of catastrophic expenses compared with their wealthier counterparts.

In discussing the policy implications of their analysis, the authors note that the desire to shield elderly Americans from impoverishment resulting from high out-of-pocket spending for long-term care is tempered by concerns about the use of public funds to protect private assets. At the center of the debate is the question of how to achieve a balance between what elderly people can reasonably be expected to pay either out of pocket or through private insurance, and what portion should be considered a public responsibility.

HOME AND COMMUNITY-BASED CARE

The current system of long-term care leans heavily toward institutional rather than home and community-based services. Over the last decade, public policy has sought to expand noninstitutional long-term care services. The chapters in this section address such questions as why some disabled persons do not participate in home care programs, the extent to which paid care might supplant informal care, regional variation in the medicare home health benefit, and new directions in the organization and financing of long-term care for younger persons with disabilities.

Persons Screened into Connecticut's Home and Community-Based Waiver Program

In chapter 9, Korbin Liu, Jean Hanson, and Teresa Coughlin examine the cases of disabled elderly people who met the eligibility requirements for Connecticut's medicaid home and community-based waiver program. The goal of the program is to reduce nursing home use by providing home and community-based services to persons at high risk of institutionalization.

Not all persons eligible for the Connecticut program ended up receiving services. The authors divide nonparticipants into four distinct groups: those who exceeded the program's allowable cost caps, those who withdrew from the assessment process or refused care plans, those who were expected to be placed in institutions, and those who died shortly after the assessment.

Of greatest interest from a public policy standpoint are those disabled elderly persons whose care plans cost too much. In Connecticut, individuals who are otherwise eligible may not participate in the home and community-based waiver program if the cost of their non-institutional services would exceed the state's costs of nursing home care. A substantial number of persons who met the eligibility criteria were prevented from receiving services because their plan of care was too expensive. Ironically, those who exceeded the cost caps tended to be substantially more disabled and to have far fewer informal supports—strong indicators of high risk of institutionalization—than did persons who were allowed to participate in the program.

In discussing the implications of their findings, Liu, Hanson, and Coughlin note a conflict between targeting the most severely disabled individuals at risk of institutionalization and controlling program costs. From a state medicaid perspective, it may cost too much to keep some severely disabled elderly people in the community. For many of them, nursing home placement may well be an appropriate, cost-effective option. As a result, the waiver programs may end up serving a population that is less at risk of entering a nursing home than those who are excluded.

Combining Formal and Informal Care

The fear that a government program of paid home care would reduce unpaid family care has left government funding with a strong institutional bias. In chapter 10 Sharon Long examines whether paid home care displaces unpaid informal care, using a sample of low-income, frail elderly persons who enrolled in the Connecticut Community Care, Inc., program. Participants in Connecticut's home and community-based medicaid waiver program are a subset of this sample.

Most previous studies have not detected substitution effects, but Long finds a relatively small but statistically significant displacement of informal care by paid care. For an individual receiving average levels of formal and informal care, a two-hour increase in formal care would result in a reduction of about one-half hour of informal care. However, this finding must be interpreted with caution. It may be an artifact of the appropriate decision by case managers to allocate less paid care to those disabled elderly persons who receive a substantial amount of unpaid care and more paid care to those individuals with weak family supports.

When the analysis is limited to the most impaired elderly population, who have been the focus of most proposals for additional aid (elderly persons with three or more activity of daily living [ADL] limitations), Long finds an increase in formal care is associated with an increase in informal care. For the most impaired elderly individuals, formal care entirely supplements informal care. Most of the displacement of informal care by paid care is for the less disabled persons in the study.

In discussing the policy implications of her findings, Long notes that the increase in the clients' total quantity of care (even with some displacement of informal care) seems consistent with program goals to address both the unmet needs of disabled elderly persons and to reduce the burden on informal caregivers. Under such programs, a partial offset in informal care as a result of an increase in paid care is a desirable and intended outcome.

Regional Variation in the Use of Medicare Home Health Services

Use of the medicare home health care benefit has grown very rapidly in recent years. Substantial regional variation in levels of home health care received by medicare beneficiaries have raised policy concerns about equity and efficiency across geographic areas. For example, for home health episodes that started in 1990 and 1991, the mean number of home visits per episode varied from twenty-five in western states to approximately fifty in southern and southwestern states. In chapter 11 Jennifer Schore investigates why the use of medicare home health care varies so widely by region and whether the corresponding variation across regions leads to differences in outcomes. These questions are important—if this variation is due to unnecessary care in some regions, there are potential savings to the medicare program if such care can be identified. However, if the variation results from necessary care being withheld, which then leads to adverse patient outcomes, savings may be achieved by providing more home health care.

Schore's study found that characteristics of patients clearly differ between the regions with the highest and lowest use of medicare home health services. Home health agencies in the high-use regions (the East and the West South Central) seem to be providing levels of care consistent with the needs of their relatively frail and chronically ill patients. In addition, alternative home and community-based services may be in relatively short supply in these high-use regions. Low-use regions (the Pacific and the Middle Atlantic) served medicare beneficiaries who were much less frail and chronically ill, and agencies serving people within these regions tended to be located in relatively more populated, higher-income areas. In addition, alternatives to home health care may be more widely available in low-use regions, decreasing reliance on the medicare home health benefit.

Although the data on patient outcomes are weak, Schore tentatively concludes that low levels of home health care use do not lead to poorer patient outcomes. For example, home health patients in the low-use Pacific region had some of the lowest rates of home health readmission, inpatient admission, and mortality in the periods immediately after episodes, while patients in the high-use East South Central region had some of the highest rates.

Long-Term Care for the Younger Disabled Population:
A Policy Synthesis

Although attention to the deficiencies of the current system of financing and organizing long-term care for disabled elderly

Americans is increasing, similar problems facing persons under age 65 have been almost totally ignored by policymakers until recently. Moreover, although 40 percent or more of the disabled population is not elderly, little is known about how this group finances and uses long-term care. Chapter 12 by Joshua Wiener and Catherine Sullivan synthesizes what is and is not known about younger disabled people and long-term care.

The authors make four main points. First, for a variety of conceptual and methodological reasons, good data on younger disabled Americans are lacking. To a substantial extent, the data gap exists because few surveys include more than a small number of nonelderly disabled persons.

Second, the philosophical underpinnings of the disability movement have forced a general rethinking of the goals of long-term care for both elderly people and their younger counterparts. Traditionally, the goals of long-term care have been minimal—to keep the disabled person safe, clean, and reasonably well fed. Younger disabled people reject these goals as far too limited. They insist on maximizing independence and self-sufficiency and providing access to the same freedoms and life-style enjoyed by nondisabled citizens, including the right to live independently and to realize their full potential as human beings.

Third, this philosophy has a profound impact on the desired delivery system. In the view of advocates for younger disabled people, home and community-based services should be at the center of the service system, and institutions should play little if any role. Additionally, because every disabled person is an individual with different needs, the range of services available should be extremely broad, with few services prohibited. Moreover, advocates for younger disabled individuals believe that the disabled person, rather than agencies, should have the ability to hire, train, direct, and fire the people who provide services. This vision of the service system raises issues of cost containment, entitlements versus capped programs, accountability and use of public funds, quality of care, and employer responsibilities such as social security and income tax withholding.

Finally, the current system of financing creates a strong incentive toward dependency. A dilemma in current public programs is that medicare and medicaid eligibility for persons with disabilities is contingent on being unable to work. This creates a catch-22. If a set of services enable the disabled person to work, then that person is no longer eligible for the services; if a person is no longer eligible for the services, then he or she can no longer work.

RESEARCH AGENDA FOR THE FUTURE

The chapters in this book highlight the complex interrelationship between disability, use of acute and long-term care services, and the health care financing system. Future research on people with disabilities should reflect those relationships in at least three different ways.

First, although policymakers tend to view the population of persons with disabilities as monolithic, it is in fact highly diverse. These populations include (among others) younger and older persons with physical disabilities, mentally retarded and developmentally disabled people, mentally ill people, and persons with Alzheimer's disease. More research that disaggregates data on disabled populations by age and type of disability is needed. In addition, these studies should examine how racial, cultural, financial and insurance coverage, and other socioeconomic differences might present special barriers to receiving acute and long-term care services quickly and effectively.

Second, medicare and medicaid finance most health care for disabled Americans. For medicare, the traditional focus on acute care is becoming increasingly difficult to maintain. Growing numbers of beneficiaries have chronic illnesses, and expenditures for home health and skilled nursing facility services have risen rapidly. Potential increased state control of medicaid and reductions in the growth of expenditures could also have significant effects on persons with disabilities.

New initiatives for managed care offer the potential for better service to the disabled population as well as potentially significant cost savings. New approaches that combine both acute and long-term care could provide a seamless system that would meet the total needs of each individual. However, with their emphasis on reducing use of services, limiting the choice of providers, and cutting back on use of specialists, managed care organizations possibly threaten the provision of high-quality care to disabled persons. It is therefore critical to evaluate the impact of managed care on medicare and medicaid beneficiaries with disabilities. Of particular interest is how the use and outcomes of medicare postacute care services differ in managed care and fee-for-service settings.

Because of its central role in financing long-term care, additional research on medicaid is critical. In particular, research efforts that combine programmatic and person-based data could contribute significantly to our understanding of how federal and state policy affects use of services and expenditures by disabled beneficiaries.

The 12 percent of medicare beneficiaries who are also eligible for medicaid are particularly important and have not been researched sufficiently. These individuals with dual eligibility have a high prevalence of disability and are very costly users of both programs. Studies of service use and expenditures could give insight on how to improve coordination of services between the two programs.

Examining the interactions between public and private financing also raises several new research issues. For example, with regard to private financing, research should continue to analyze the changing marketplace for long-term care insurance and explore options for reconciling the need for regulation with the industry's desire to keep insurance products affordable. The impact of medicaid estate planning on the sale of long-term care insurance also merits further examination.

Third, the growth in expenditures for home and community-based care has outpaced our understanding of these services. Availability of home health care and other services varies widely by state and within each state by disability group. In addition, research should focus on cost and quality issues related to providing home and community-based services to severely disabled Americans. Finally, inspired by demands of younger people with disabilities, studies are needed on how to develop a beneficiary-centered system of long-term care. Research on financing and delivery arrangements that empower persons with disabilities (and their caregivers) in care planning and service delivery is central to this line of inquiry.

NOTES

1. Gregory L. Pawlson, "Chronic Illness: Implications of a New Paradigm for Health Care," *Journal of Quality Improvement*, vol. 20 (January 1994), pp. 33–39.

2. Mark Freiman and Christopher Murtaugh, "Interactions Between Hospital and Nursing Home Use" (Rockville, Md.: Agency for Health Care Policy and Research, October 1994).

3. Office of the Assistant Secretary for Planning and Evaluation, *Cost Estimates for the Long-Term Care Provisions Under the Health Security Act* (Department of Health and Human Services, 1994).

4. Pamela Short and others, "Public and Private Responsibility for Financing Nursing Home Care," *Milbank Quarterly*, vol. 70, no. 2 (1992), pp. 277–98.

5. Kaiser Commission on the Future of Medicaid, "The Impact of a Five Percent Medicaid Expenditure Growth Cap: A State Level Analysis," Policy Brief (Washington, 1994); and "Medicare and Medicaid Statistical Supplement," *Health Care Financing Review* (February 1995), figure 10, p. 31.

6. "Medicare and Medicaid Statistical Supplement," tables 114 and 117, pp. 361, 367–68.

7. Ibid., tables 114 and 118, pp. 361, 369, and 370.

PART 1
Overall Perspectives

Chapter 2

BRUCE C. VLADECK

Long-Term Care: The View from the Health Care Financing Administration

The long-term care system is a rapidly expanding and evolving part of the health care service system in America. Estimates for 1993 indicate that almost 12 percent ($108 billion) of all national health care expenditures were spent on long-term care services. Expenditures on nursing home and home health care, two principal components of long-term care expenditures, increased significantly over the past decade. In 1980, approximately $20 billion was spent on nursing home care, compared with $70 billion in 1993. Home health expenditures have risen even more dramatically, from $2 billion in 1980 to $25 billion in 1993. Although expenditures for nursing home services continue to be almost triple those for home health services, national expenditures for home health care grew faster than any other category of personal health care in four out of the past five years.

Medicare and medicaid play a major role in the financing of long-term care, accounting for more than half of all such spending. Medicare, however, has not typically been associated with the delivery of long-term care services. Yet even though medicare was designed to be an acute care benefit, its services have evolved. Changes in technology, consumer preferences, the structure of the postacute care industry, and medicare policy have altered the role that medicare benefits (such as skilled nursing facility services, home health services, rehabilitative therapy, hospice care, and durable medical equipment) play in serving a growing number of beneficiaries who need both acute and long-term care. For example, when the number of home health visits exceeds one hundred fifty per year, or when an in-

This chapter is an edited transcript of the administrator's remarks at the Conference on Long-Term Care: Current Issues in Financing and Delivery, November 3, 1994.

dividual receiving durable medical equipment is significantly functionally disabled, the traditional distinction of the medicare program between acute and long-term care is blurred.

Medicaid is the primary source of public funding for long-term care; more than one-third of all state medicaid budgets were devoted to long-term care spending in 1993. Medicaid finances a wide variety of long-term care services, including nursing home care, intermediate care facilities for mentally retarded persons (ICF/MRs), home health care, personal care, and home and community-based services. It also finances long-term care for persons with a wide range of disabilities. In 1992, for example, 59 percent of medicaid long-term care spending was for elderly patients, 36 percent for younger adults, and 5 percent for children. Medicaid has historically had a bias toward financing institutional long-term care services; in 1993, almost 80 percent of such medicaid expenditures were for institutional care in either nursing homes or ICF/MRs. However, several states have developed innovative programs for providing home and community-based services. Medicaid spending on home health care and home and community-based services exceeded $4.5 billion in 1993, a more than tenfold increase in home care spending since 1980.

What follows is an historical perspective on how far we have come in long-term care policy and how far we still have to go, and a discussion of an important shift in the worldview of the Health Care Financing Administration (HCFA) regarding the relationship between medicare and long-term care. I conclude with a look at the future of medicare and medicaid long-term care programs and the kinds of initiatives HCFA is considering to improve quality of care for beneficiaries who need long-term care.

PROGRESS

There has been progress in the quality of health care, the availability of home and community-based services, and the assessment of patient needs.

First, remarkable improvement has been made in long-term care quality. In the near future, HCFA will publish the survey and enforcement regulations (final rules) to implement portions of the

Omnibus Budget Reconciliation Act of 1987 (OBRA 87). This is the last in the trilogy of major regulatory initiatives to implement OBRA 87, the most important legislation affecting quality of long-term care services since the enactment of medicare and medicaid.

Indeed, by taking a close look at the initial Institute of Medicine research that resulted in OBRA 87 and examining HCFA's current activities in this area, it is easy to gain a sense of the enormous progress that has already been achieved.

Patterns of service in nursing homes have changed significantly. Without question, the quality of care in American nursing homes is substantially better now than it was ten years ago. For example, the use of physical and chemical restraints has been dramatically reduced. In addition, qualitative indicators are being used to assess the quality of service provided to nursing home residents.

Patient-centered care, quality of life, and quality of care are increasingly dominant forces affecting patterns of care in nursing homes. There has been significant improvement in the quality of professional services in nursing homes—in skills and job definitions, roles and number of registered nurses, and requirements for medical directors.

In the course of this, the characteristics of nursing home patients have changed remarkably. It is time to begin thinking about what this means both for long-term care policy and providers. Much has improved, but the challenges ahead are great.

Second, there has been significant progress in noninstitutional long-term care. Ten years ago, considerable discussion centered on the need to develop and expand community-based services so that the growing demand for long-term care would not be filled solely by institutions. Last year, HCFA had an average daily census in medicaid Home and Community-Based Services Waiver (HCBSW) programs of almost a quarter of a million people—a fraction of the number of people residing in nursing homes on any given day, but an increase of almost exactly 250,000 in average daily census of such programs over the last decade. Furthermore, more than 400,000 individuals received services over the course of the year from these programs. This growth is very rewarding, but there are ongoing concerns about quality standards, roles of various professions, mix of services, and financing.

The medicaid HCBSW program is a long-term care success story, yet one that has not been adequately understood. Indeed, medicaid

HCBSWs have done much to lay the groundwork for the more difficult stage of making these services available to everyone in need of long-term care who wishes to live in the community.

Finally, great progress has been made in the long-term care infrastructure. A uniform needs assessment instrument for hospital discharge planning is being field tested. This assessment tool will serve as the prototype for more standardized assessment instruments for intake as well as discharge and for a range of community services.

The Minimum Data Set (MDS) is well into its second generation of use as a tool for patient assessment and care planning for nursing home patients. The MDS has worked much better than expected, both for clinical purposes and for evaluating quality of care for nursing home residents. Thanks to the work of Peter Shaughnessey and his colleagues at the University of Colorado, HCFA is also much further along in developing outcome-quality indicators for home health care services.

HCFA is facing the future of long-term care with increasing sophistication, with more knowledge and information about the characteristics of the beneficiaries being served by medicare and medicaid.

THE FUTURE: HCFA'S PERSPECTIVE

HCFA must think strategically about how the future of long-term care fits into agency programs and responsibilities. The agency is in the process of significantly changing its overall orientation and attitude. In the past HCFA's culture seemed conducive to obstructionism and inflexibility. The basic tenets of the old HCFA belief system revolved around three fundamental principles.

The first principle was that medicare reimbursement was based on reasonable cost for services provided to beneficiaries. HCFA has moved very far from this principle. Today, a smaller and smaller portion of all medicare payments involve any definition of current or even prior year costs.

The second basic principle of the old belief system was that HCFA was responsible for medicare and medicaid, but medicare was much more important. It was always best summarized in the notion that there were medicare beneficiaries and medicaid recipients. Today, the term "recipient" is no longer used at HCFA. Medicaid beneficiaries are citizens with significant health care needs who are entitled to the highest quality health care services, just as medicare beneficiaries are. HCFA has 70 million beneficiaries, and for about half of them the agency works in a special partnership with the states to assure they get the health care they need.

The third basic principle in the old belief system was that medicare did not pay for long-term care. In the past, HCFA officials consistently defined medicare as an acute care program. The coverage of extended care, skilled nursing facilities, and home health services was provided as postacute rather than long-term care. Medicare was an acute care and not a long-term care program.

As discussed earlier, this part of the old belief system has run into increasing difficulty in recent years. The fact is that in FY93, between home health services and skilled nursing facility services, medicare paid in excess of $13 billion—just under 10 percent of total medicare outlays—for these postacute services. Looking at who is using these services and how they are being used, it is hard to distinguish postacute care from long-term care. In fact, the average home care beneficiary now receives about fifty-five to sixty visits, which is a long acute care process.

HCFA has also come to recognize that the expenditures for home health care and skilled nursing facilities are just the tip of the iceberg. For example, a significant fraction of medicare beneficiaries are also admitted to the hospital from nursing homes. These beneficiaries are as much a part of the long-term care system as of the acute care system.

Increasingly, HCFA has realized that although medicare benefits have not fundamentally changed since the statute was written, there have been significant changes in demographics, the nation's overall health care system, and the realities under which the agency must operate. Today, medicare is deeply involved in the long-term care system, and HCFA must recognize this and figure out how to do a better job.

DIRECTIONS

HCFA has a clear sense of exactly how to improve. Its reevaluation of itself, combined with its formal strategic planning and goal setting, has clarified HCFA's basic operating principle. That is, HCFA exists to make sure beneficiaries have access to high-quality health care services when they need them. This leads to a number of preliminary issues that help focus the future of long-term care policy.

The first and most difficult issue is that to build a client-centered, beneficiary-oriented, long-term care system, the dollars should follow the clients. Funding should probably not be limited to a particular kind of provider or service, or to a particular bureaucratic category, such as "skilled" level of care.

A mechanism is needed to tie an assessment of client needs, preferences, and choices to the way services are purchased. This probably should be done by an intermediary organization. This organization would help determine client needs and eligibility (including level of support needed) and provide a range of services particularly tailored to the client's needs and preferences. Instead of refining or recreating a whole set of definitions and then shoehorning clients into one or the other because that is the only way services are financed, the focus should be on the needs, characteristics, and idiosyncrasies of individual beneficiaries.

The second issue is an area where HCFA has made significant progress. More specifically, the quality of services must be redefined from a client's prospective. OBRA 87 achieved a great breakthrough in this area by requiring that the nursing home survey process include interviews with clients and questions about their perception of the quality of care and the kinds of services they receive.

As a result of the recommendations of the Institute of Medicine Committee on Nursing Homes, regulations were developed and implemented. For years there was skepticism about the usefulness of the information in these patient surveys; in fact, this information has been enormously useful. Indeed, it makes good sense that to assess the quality of care being provided to someone, it is important to ask that person what he or she thinks.

The assessment of the quality of care provided to hospital inpatients is experiencing a similar revolution through the work of the Boston-based Commonwealth-Picker program and other institutions around the country. The growth of a more competitive managed care marketplace in private insurance has attracted a number of experts who understand how to measure consumer preferences and consumer satisfaction. Unfortunately, most of them are reluctant to share this information, a necessary step for developing community-wide quality standards.

But as a matter of principle, it can be said that henceforth every time HCFA revises conditions of participation or quality standards, customer perceptions of quality and satisfaction with care will be reviewed and given much attention. Today, of the roughly 1.25 million beneficiaries who receive long-term care services financed wholly or in part by medicare or medicaid, the only ones HCFA systematically asks those questions of are nursing home residents. These practices have not yet been incorporated in home care, home and community-based services, or the other faster-growing parts of the long-term care system. This must be done—and soon.

The third area that must be addressed with a greater client focus is the extent to which clients direct and configure the services they will receive. This includes everything from the fundamental choice of a site of care to the difficult question of the extent to which clients should assume responsibilities such as supervising caregivers.

Many questions are raised by these issues, particularly in terms of the responsibility of public programs and custody of public funds. But they cannot be avoided. It emerges logically as HCFA tries to design systems responsive to the needs and concerns of clients, and clients are going to demand that it be done.

Historically, nonelderly disabled people have been much more vocal on these issues than the elders in the chronic care system. It is, however, just a matter of time before that changes. The design and conceptual problems associated with this almost 180-degree reversal in the decisionmaking process about what services the client receives from whom and when means that there is a lot of work and a lot of thinking to do. This issue calls for considerable experimentation before we can draw any further conclusions.

CONCLUSION

I have discussed some broad and general directions that HCFA can take. There is so much that needs to be done before greater clarity about program directions can be achieved. But there is a growing body of information and expertise to help us make good decisions about long-term care.

PART 2
Public-Private Interactions

Chapter 3

LISA MARIA B. ALECXIH AND STEVEN LUTZKY

Private Long-Term Care Insurance: Barriers to Purchase and Retention

Private long-term care insurance provides one of the few available mechanisms for elderly persons to protect themselves against the catastrophic costs of long-term care. However, few older persons have purchased this insurance, and those who have often failed to retain their policies. For example, less than 1 percent of expenditures for nursing facility and home and community-based services were paid by long-term care insurance in the mid-1990s.[1] Most long-term care is financed either by medicaid, which requires those in need of long-term care to deplete almost all of their financial assets and nursing home residents to contribute most of their income to the cost of their care, or by out-of-pocket payments by recipients and their families. The limited likelihood that a significant public social insurance program for long-term care will be enacted in the near future may encourage individuals to examine private long-term care insurance as a way to protect themselves against the high costs of this care, ensure their independence, and prevent themselves from being a burden to their families. However, some argue that private long-term care insurance is feasible only for a small portion of relatively well-off elderly persons, and only a public social insurance model can offer broad coverage for the cost of long-term care.[2]

Whether the government should be more involved in the private long-term care insurance market is an important public policy concern. Some argue that the federal government should regulate the market more aggressively because consumers do not have sufficient information about long-term care insurance for the market to function properly. Opposing this view, others believe that current regulation is sufficient and that most problems with the market stem from its newness. Moreover, they contend that further regulation would stifle innovation and limit the growth of the market; in the long run, such growth would be beneficial to consumers. Beyond consumer protection, some analysts believe that the possibility of medicaid savings gives the government an interest in having more people purchase long-term care insurance. Others argue that the possibility of medicaid savings is slight and that depending on private insurance to reform the financing and delivery system will not work.[3]

We examine the barriers related to individuals purchasing and retaining long-term care insurance policies and the options available to deal with them. Our research illuminates the problems individuals have in deciding whether to purchase a policy that will meet their needs and circumstances and how government involvement could affect the purchase and retention of policies.

BACKGROUND

The long-term care insurance market has emerged from the period during which companies were testing the feasibility of this new product. In the 1980s, companies offering long-term care insurance were unsure of the liabilities that would be associated with this type of insurance. To reduce their risks, they limited coverage and priced the policies conservatively, which resulted in high premiums. In recent years companies determined that long-term care insurance is viable. They have begun to liberalize requirements for the receipt of benefits, broaden coverage, and reduce prices. The market may be in a new phase in which companies are aggressively attempting to increase market share and the size of the market as a whole.

Recent Changes

The long-term care insurance market has grown rapidly since the mid-1980s. By the end of 1984, insurance companies had sold fewer than 50,000 policies.[4] By 1993 between 2 and 3 million policies were in force.[5] A small number of companies dominated the $1.6 billion market; ten companies accounted for 64 percent of the premiums.[6]

Long-term care insurance is a unique, new form of insurance incorporating aspects of health, disability, and life insurance. Like health insurance, it offers coverage for health-related needs typically on a fee-for-service basis. Like disability insurance, some policies provide cash to cover a wide array of services that are necessitated by a long-term disabling functional or cognitive impairment. And, like whole life insurance, long-term care insurance depends on prefunding a benefit that would typically be needed many years in the future.

Consumers purchase long-term care insurance to hedge against the risk, usually ten to twenty years in the future, of needing long-term care services. Prefunding sharply differentiates long-term care insurance from acute care health insurance policies. Consumers with long-term care insurance generally pay a level premium over the life of the policy. Purchasers pay more than the amount necessary to cover claims during the early years of the policy (when use of nursing home care and home care is lower) and less than the amount necessary to pay benefits during the later years of the policy (when service use is high). Without this feature, policies would be much more expensive at age 75 or 80.

According to profiles developed from policies gathered for this study, insurance plans sold in 1995 typically used indemnity-based reimbursement for nursing home care and offered home care coverage for an additional charge, giving the purchaser the option of buying a daily benefit of one-half the nursing home daily rate. Purchasers usually chose the level of daily indemnity benefit and whether that benefit level would increase over time to attempt to keep pace with inflation. Benefit periods ranged from one year to unlimited length, and deductible periods ranged from zero up to 365 days (table 3-1). Long-term care insurance premiums are age rated (that is, they depend on the age of initial purchase), vary with the benefits chosen, and are designed to be level over time.

According to a market review conducted by the Health Insurance Association of America (HIAA) at the end of 1993, insurance companies had sold 80 percent of long-term care insurance policies directly to individuals through an agent, mass marketing, or a group association. Purchasers obtained the remaining 20 percent of long-term care insurance policies through employers (12 percent) or as part of a life insurance policy (8 percent).[7] A study by LifePlans, Inc., found the typical individual policy purchased in 1990 covered only nursing home care, had a benefit duration of between five and six years after a twenty-day deductible, and paid $72 per day in the nursing home, for an annual premium of $1,071 per year (table 3-2).[8] About four out of ten purchasers selected home care benefits; these benefits averaged

TABLE 3-1. *Coverage Offered by Sample of Eighteen Insurance Companies, 1995*

Types of services covered	
Service covered	Skilled, intermediate, and custodial nursing home care
	Home health care
	Adult day care
	Alternate care facility
	Respite care
	Hospice care
	Ambulance service
	Assisted care
Additional benefits	Alternative plan of care
	Bed reservation
	Prevention service
	Caregiver training
Benefit structures	
Daily benefit	$25–$300/day nursing home
	$20–$200/day home health care
Monthly cash benefit	$1,000–$3,000 nursing home
	$500–$1,000 home health care
Benefit period	1 year to lifetime coverage
Elimination periods	0–365 days
Inflation protection option	Future purchase option
	Compound inflation
	Simple inflation
Restoration of benefits	Available in some products
Underwriting	
Preexisting condition exclusion	Six months or less
Issue age	19–84
Premiums	
Spouse discounts	5% to 25% for both spouses or one spouse
Benefit triggers	
Benefit eligibility	Medical necessity *or* needing assistance with activities of daily living (ADLs) *or* cognitive impairment (or one of these or a combination of two)
Consumer protection features	
Nonforfeiture benefit	Return of premium
	Reduced paid-up
	Shortened benefit period
	Extended term
Waiver of premium	Available for all
Free-look period	30 days
Guaranteed renewable	All include
Reinstatement	Policy coverage
	Functional impairment
	Cognitive impairment

Source: Lewin-VHI, Inc.
Note: These features are present in some but not all policies. Data are based on eighteen companies representing 52.5 percent of earned premiums in 1993. Policies were received between May 1994 and May 1995.

TABLE 3-2. *Characteristics of Individual Long-Term Care Insurance Policies Purchased, 1990*

Policy characteristic	Average
Policy type	
Nursing home only	63%
Nursing home and home care	37%
Daily benefit amount of nursing home care	$72
Deductible period	20 days
Benefit duration[a]	5.6 years
Individuals choosing inflation protection	40%
Annual premium	$1,071

Source: Health Insurance Association of America, *Who Buys Long-Term Care Insurance?*, prepared by LifePlans Inc. (Washington, 1992).

Note: Based on an analysis of 14,400 individual long-term care insurance policies. Only one company provided information on the value of the home health benefit. The majority of policies paid a home health benefit equal to 50 percent of the nursing home daily benefit amount.

a. Lifetime policies were assumed to provide benefits for ten years in calculating average benefit duration.

50 percent of the selected nursing home indemnity amount. Because of changes in the features of policies offered since 1990, the typical policy subsequently purchased could be somewhat different. Among the sample of persons age 55 and older interviewed by LifePlans, the purchasers were age 68 on average. The average age of purchase could decline if more policies were to be sold through employers.

Long-term care insurance benefits changed frequently and dramatically between the mid-1980s and the mid-1990s. These changes were principally driven by consumer demands, insurer competition, and regulatory requirements. One major change in all policies was the elimination of the requirement that a person be hospitalized before being placed in a nursing home. All but a handful of states explicitly prohibit prior hospitalization requirements, and none of the major companies include this requirement in their policies.[9]

A second major change is that policies now offer consumers the option to purchase home care benefits. Few of the initial policies offered home care coverage. For those that did, companies based the benefits on the number of days a purchaser had been in a nursing home and limited services to skilled care provided by a registered nurse (RN) or licensed practical nurse (LPN).[10] By the mid-1990s, most policies offered a home care rider that covered custodial care services (such as those provided by home health aides and homemakers) for purchasers who met specified functional limitation criteria (such as needing assistance with activities of daily living [ADLs]—for example, bathing, dressing, and eating).

A third change is that policies offer consumers the option to purchase inflation protection. In the past, most policies did not offer inflation protection or, if they did, they generally limited the indexing of the benefits to simple indexing (for example, the benefit level would be increased each year by 5 percent of the original daily benefit amount) that would be suspended once a policyholder reached a specific age. Most policies now at least offer the option of purchasing inflation protection in which the indemnity level would be compounded at 5 percent annually.

Finally, insurers are offering new features that permit greater flexibility in the types of benefits covered. For example, some insurers provide cash payments to consumers who have a specified level of disability, regardless of whether they use paid services. These policies are similar to a cash disability policy and were generally more expensive than service-based policies. Although these policies only accounted for a small portion of the market in 1995, one of the larger companies sold cash disability-like policies in all fifty states. Other policies allow for an "alternate plan of care," which permits payments on a case-by-case basis for items not otherwise covered, such as durable medical equipment (DME) or home modifications.

Regulation

As with other insurance products, states assume responsibility for the regulation and monitoring of the long-term care insurance market. The goal is twofold: ensuring that companies have sufficient funds to pay claims in the future (solvency), and providing protection for consumers. To address these goals, state insurance commissioners and their staffs assume five primary responsibilities: (1) establishing long-term care insurance regulations and statutes, (2) determining whether policies meet minimum statutory requirements; (3) reviewing the premium rates; (4) ensuring the solvency of companies selling long-

term care insurance; and (5) monitoring marketing and business practices (for example, responding to complaints and approving advertis-
ing materials).

Most states base their regulation of long-term care insurance on
model standards developed by the National Association of Insurance
Commissioners (NAIC), which in 1995 addresses four main areas: (1)
minimum benefit requirements, such as stipulating that policies
include at least one year of nursing home coverage and offer inflation
protection; (2) prohibitions against some policy restrictions, such as
three-day prior hospitalization and requiring that skilled care be provided before intermediate or custodial care; (3) marketing practices,
including prohibitions against knowingly misrepresenting benefit
features, high-pressure sales tactics, and marketing in a way that
hides the fact that the company is selling insurance; and (4) loss ratios
(a minimum of 60 percent for individual policies) that measure the
return of premiums in the form of claims paid—the higher the loss
ratio, the larger the share of premiums purchasers receive as benefits.

Members of Congress and others have criticized states for not in-
stituting the most recent NAIC long-term care model act and regulation.[11] As of October 1994, only the District of Columbia had not
adopted insurance regulation specific to long-term care insurance. A
handful of states were in the process of drafting or had legislation
pending, based in part on the NAIC model; all but three of the remaining states based their regulations in part on the NAIC models.[12]
No state has adopted all of the most recent model provisions, which
were issued in April 1995, and many have not updated their regulations in several years. Adherence to the NAIC models is voluntary,
and states do not necessarily amend their regulations as often as
NAIC updates the model because changes often have to be made
through legislation. The NAIC long-term care regulations have
changed almost every six months since they were introduced in 1986.
Many states delay updating long-term care insurance regulations
until NAIC resolves all pending issues. Some states actively choose
not to adopt certain portions of the NAIC model because they do not
agree with the provisions or believe that unique circumstances in the
state call for alternative regulation. Consumer groups worry that
states may be slow to adopt some NAIC regulations because they are
overly influenced by the lobbying efforts of insurance companies.

METHODOLOGY

We assessed long-term care insurance products, the market, regulatory issues, and enforcement through extensive interviews with state regulatory agencies, insurance companies, agents, consumer groups, industry representatives, congressional staff, and other experts. The purpose was to understand the product, market, enforcement, and beneficiary issues related to long-term care insurance from a variety of perspectives. Specifically, we addressed the possible impact of proposed regulation on the quality of products and the growth of the market and explored issues related to an increased government role in the long-term care insurance market.

Interviews were conducted with more than one hundred people involved with long-term care insurance, including representatives from eighteen insurers representing both large and small shares of the market and five state agencies responsible for regulating insurance. The interviews with a broad scope of groups interested in long-term care insurance make this study unique. Representatives from interested parties assessed the current state of the market and regulation, special problem areas, emerging issues, and suggestions for improving the product and its regulation. Site visits to states provided the opportunity for in-depth discussion of innovations in enforcement, market monitoring, and consumer education. We visited Arizona, Indiana, North Dakota, Oregon, and Wisconsin.

Insurance policies were also collected from May 1994 to May 1995 from the insurers participating in the study. The eighteen insurers represented 52.5 percent of private long-term care insurance premiums in 1993.

BARRIERS TO PURCHASE AND RETENTION

Individuals with long-term care needs can be faced with catastrophic costs that they may be unable to finance. For example, the average annual cost of private pay nursing facility care exceeded $40,000 in 1995. Thus even a short stay in a nursing home could be catastrophic, given that in 1993 elderly Americans had median family income of only $15,500 and median financial assets of $19,350.[13] Despite evidence that nearly one-quarter of persons turning age 65 are expected to require a year or more of care in a nursing home over the remainder of their lives and that nursing homes stays are very expensive, a relatively small percentage of elderly persons have long-term care insurance.[14] Assuming that 90 percent of the policies in force are held by persons age 65 or older, less than 5 percent of elderly persons have private long-term care insurance.[15] In contrast, approximately 75 percent of elderly medicare beneficiaries have some form of individually purchased or employer-provided medicare supplemental coverage.[16]

The lack of coverage is attributable not only to consumers' reluctance to purchase long-term care insurance policies, but also to their failure to retain them. Consumer groups express concern about persons who discontinue paying premiums for long-term care insurance policies because those whose policies lapse for nonpayment also forfeit their prefunded reserves and thus overpay for the period during which they had protection. High lapse rates mean that individuals could spend substantial amounts of money on premiums without receiving benefits when they need them. Based on data from ten companies, the Society of Actuaries estimated that more than half of purchasers allowed their policies to lapse over a four-year period (between 1986 and 1990).[17] However, the industry claims that lapse rates are much lower than previously thought and are steadily decreasing. They also point out that many lapses are the result of factors such as death or replacement of older policies with newer, more appropriate policies. In these cases, purchasers would not be without coverage when they require it. Companies also point out that individuals who let their policies lapse did have coverage while they were paying premiums.

The barriers to purchase and retention of long-term care insurance policies can be grouped into three general categories: insufficient information about long-term care insurance (which reduce demand for policies), affordability of the premiums, and characteristics of policies that make them less desirable for consumers to purchase and retain.

Insufficient Information

Some people do not consider purchasing long-term care insurance because they lack knowledge about the need for protection against catastrophic long-term care expenses. Others do not purchase policies because they do not have adequate information about long-term care insurance itself. Still others may be reluctant to purchase a policy because they do not know anyone who benefited from long-term care insurance and they are distrustful of it.

Lack of perceived need for the product. Many potential purchasers do not understand the need for long-term care insurance. Although lack of perceived need is primarily a barrier to purchase, individuals who do not strongly believe that they need the product may be more likely to let it lapse.

Surveys indicate that a significant portion of elderly Americans underestimate the likelihood of requiring long-term care services and the potential cost of those services.[18] Individuals discount their need for long-term care for a variety of reasons, such as their age ("I'm too young to worry about it"), their good health status ("I've always been healthy"), or denial ("It won't happen to me").

Many elderly persons believe that the medicare program or medigap policies will cover extended long-term care services. Individuals may also not understand the difference between medicare and medicaid. One survey indicated that only 51 percent of adults knew that medicare does not pay for long-term care for elderly persons.[19] This confusion arises because medicare and medigap provide limited coverage of skilled nursing facility care and home health visits. Some argue that medicaid gives elderly persons a sense that the government will take care of their long-term care needs.[20] According to this perspective, individuals do not think they need to protect themselves against the cost of long-term care because they believe that medicaid will provide coverage for their care. This argument is supported by the finding in one survey that nonpurchasers of long-term care insurance were more likely to view government as a primary payer of long-term care costs than were purchasers.[21]

Others simply are not aware of the availability of private long-term care insurance. One industry representative noted that the vast majority of elderly Americans have not had any direct contact with someone selling long-term care insurance.

Even if an individual were given information about the costs associated with long-term care and the ability of insurance to protect against those costs, she or he may still decide not to buy the product for several reasons. For example, individuals could have confidence that their family would take care of them. People prefer that family members provide long-term care, rather than formal service providers.[22] Many individuals make arrangements with family members to provide needed care and thus do not need a financial mechanism to fund long-term care services.[23] In contrast, preserving independence and choice and assuring the affordability of services are the chief reasons for purchasing long-term care insurance.[24]

In addition, some people do not purchase long-term care insurance because they think that the government will adopt social insurance coverage for long-term care. Individuals may be reluctant to invest sizable amounts of money in long-term care insurance when the government may implement a program that would make such coverage unnecessary. Many agents and company representatives cited the prospect of health reform as a reason for slow sales of long-term care insurance from 1993 to the fall of 1994 and identified the belief that the government would eventually provide coverage for long-term care a major barrier to sales. Many insurance company representatives have said that their records showed that sales increased dramatically since the demise of federal health reform. Each of these reasons for choosing not to purchase long-term care insurance may be rational given an individual's circumstances.

Lack of experience. In addition to the lack of information about the need for long-term care insurance, many individuals may be distrustful of this new form of insurance because they personally have not known anyone who has this insurance and received benefits from it. Many agents mentioned that another reason for not purchasing long-term care insurance was discomfort with insurance companies and insurance products in general. This discomfort could also make individuals less likely to keep a long-term care insurance policy once they purchased one. Unlike home, auto, and health insurance, long-term care insurance typically is not provided for or required by an employer, state government, or lending institution. Also, in contrast to these other types of insurance, long-term care insurance provides coverage for a distant event and the purchaser must place a fair amount of faith in the company's stability. Because few people with this insurance have filed a claim, few potential purchasers of long-term care insurance know of someone who has benefited from long-term care insurance. This deprives consumers of a sense of security they would have if they had personally observed a company following through on their promise of coverage. Thus many people view long-term care insurance as something untrustworthy. Evidence from a LifePlans study done for HIAA suggested that those who purchased long-term care insurance had a more favorable view of insurance companies than those who did not.[25]

Unfamiliarity with product features. Consumers could fail to buy or keep a long-term care insurance policy because they do not know enough about the features of the policies or do not understand these features well enough to find a policy that meets their needs. Many experts we interviewed emphasized that the long-term care policy a consumer most likely would buy and keep is one tailored to the particular needs and resources of that individual. Whether a consumer purchases an appropriate policy is based in part on the knowledge about long-term care and long-term care insurance of both consumers and agents. Although some experts interviewed, especially agents, emphasized that some consumers spend a great deal of time educating themselves about long-term care insurance, almost all experts said that a large portion of consumers had a poor understanding of their potential long-term care needs and the particulars of long-term care insurance. Consistent themes included the difficulty many people had understanding and comparing policies that used different definitions and language, and the importance of agents in matching the needs of a person to the provisions of a policy.

Agents play a crucial role in providing consumers with information about the features of long-term care insurance policies. The quality of the information provided by agents depends on the agents' personal knowledge of long-term care issues, financing, and long-term care insurance policies available and how motivated they are to meet the needs of their individual customers (as opposed to maximizing commissions). Several agents stated that one of their goals was to tailor a policy to the individual consumer. Thus the agent must determine if long-term care insurance is appropriate for the individual at all and if so, work with the individual to determine what type of coverage he or she needs, wants, and can afford. For example, an agent could persuade a client who lives alone without any immediate family to reduce his or her premiums by not buying home care coverage, because the level of coverage offered would only keep the client out of an institution if it were used together with an informal caregiver. Long-term care insurance has been described as a difficult sale that typically requires an agent to explain the need for and the features of a policy over two to three sessions with the potential purchaser. The difficult sale argument was used to justify the high proportion of first-year premiums paid to agents as commissions relative to the proportion for renewal years.

Several consumer advocacy groups expressed concern about the quality of the information provided by agents and the influence of agents' financial incentives on that advice. Charismatic agents may persuade some consumers to purchase a product that they do not understand and that may not be suited to them. These consumers may eventually allow their policies to lapse because they discover that they cannot afford the premiums and do not need the coverage the policies offer, or that the policies do not offer the coverage they thought they did.

A number of agents, company representatives, and consumer groups thought that many agents were not well informed about long-term care needs and products and could be providing bad advice to potential purchasers. This finding is consistent with investigations concluding that agents misrepresented policies and were misinformed about long-term care.[26] Agents and insurance company representatives interviewed in this study noted, however, that the percentage of sales these agents represented was relatively small.[27] Respondents also identified a small group of problem agents motivated by the high first-year commissions (as much as 70 percent of the first-year premiums) who were more concerned about completing a sale than determining whether the product purchased was appropriate and the purchaser could afford the premiums over time. Agents, other industry representatives, and some experts argued that well-informed agents appear to be, along with individualized counseling from state insurance programs, the best mechanisms currently available for gaining information and advice about the purchase of the product. Independent agents who work with a variety of insurers may have an advantage over captive agents who work for one insurance company only.

Affordability

Even if people have a clear understanding of the need for coverage offered by long-term care insurance, they could fail to purchase and retain a policy because the premiums are too expensive. For someone age 50 in 1993, an average policy with inflation protection but no non-forfeiture benefits (provisions that allow consumers to receive some value for their policy if they lapse) cost $630 annually; at age 65, the same policy cost $1,452, and at age 79, $5,076.[28] Most elderly persons have modest financial resources.[29] For some individuals, particularly those with meager financial resources, purchasing long-term care insurance could be inappropriate, particularly if they would quickly qualify for medicaid coverage. Others who would not spend down to medicaid coverage quickly still could find the premiums for long-term care insurance too high. Most people who sought information on long-term care insurance and then declined to purchase it cited cost as the major reason for their inaction.[30] Most studies that used minimum income and financial asset criteria to estimate the proportion able to afford long-term care insurance concluded that 10 to 20 percent of the current elderly population met the specified criteria.[31] Using alternative assumptions (including policies with limited coverage and assuming the use of assets to pay for premiums), other research found the percentage of elderly Americans who could afford private insurance to be higher.[32]

Several experts interviewed in this study argued that affordability is not a black-and-white issue of the ability to pay, but an individual's perception of the value of the product relative to its cost. Affordability is therefore not only an issue of premium cost relative to financial resources, but also involves what level of risk consumers are comfortable with, what they think of the insurance company and the features of the policy, what level of coverage they want, and whether other family members would assist with paying premiums.

Although long-term care insurance premiums are expensive, the policies may be priced fairly. The state regulators interviewed in this study saw overpricing of policies as a major consumer protection issue because, if consumers pay too much for the benefits covered, insurance companies will make high profits. However, many industry representatives said that overpricing was not a major issue because market competition prevents companies from pricing their policies too high. Given the newness of the product, the extent to which premiums increase depending on the age at which an individual purchases the product, and the major focus of marketing to older consumers, the problem of affordability is not surprising. Affordability of long-term care insurance could change over time as individuals have a greater opportunity to buy products at younger ages, possibly through their employers.

Policy Characteristics

In addition to insufficient information reducing demand for long-term care insurance, consumers could have a number of concerns about current policies that prevent them from purchasing and keeping a policy. Experts interviewed in this study identified three additional barriers to purchase and retention of long-term care insurance policies: inability of policies to adapt to changes in the consumer's circumstances; inability of policies to adapt to changes in the service delivery system; and the possibility that premiums would increase over time.

Changes in the consumer's circumstances. Individuals may choose not to purchase a long-term care insurance policy or may let that policy lapse because policies cannot adapt to changes in their circumstances. The purchase of a long-term care insurance policy is an extended commitment that a person cannot change or withdraw from without losing their built-up equity. Lack of flexibility may prevent individuals from purchasing and could cause those who purchased a policy to let that policy lapse. Many people may find that they no longer can afford the premiums for a policy. For example, a man could purchase a policy during his last years of employment. After a few years, when he retires, he could realize that he overestimated his postretirement income. His long-term care insurance policy premium, which was not a financial burden when he was employed, could then become a major hardship. At this point, he would not have the option of buying a less expensive policy with less coverage without sacrificing the equity in his current policy. To buy a new policy, he would also have to meet certain medical criteria (which he may no longer be able to do), and he may have to pay higher premiums because of his older age. Faced with these problems, the consumer might decide to let his current policy lapse and not replace it.

Individuals could also let their policies lapse because their service needs change. For example, a man could buy a policy with a modest amount of home care benefits that will be adequate to meet his potential needs when combined with care from his wife. However, if she becomes impaired or dies before him, the home care benefit will not be adequate.

Changes in the service delivery system. The lack of flexibility in covered services could make long-term care insurance policies less desirable because consumers cannot be assured that they will have coverage for innovative services available in the future. Since the mid-1980s, several new long-term care services have emerged, including adult day care centers and assisted living facilities. Consumers who bought policies five years ago that only covered nursing home care in facilities certified by the medicare program do not have coverage for these newer forms of care. This concern argues for products that provide sufficient flexibility to respond to the changing environment. The addition of the "alternative plan of care" options that permit mutually agreed-upon substitutes for the policy-specified benefits potentially provide increased flexibility. However, some states have disallowed the inclusion of this provision because it suggests that additional services *will* be covered; in fact, it only states that the insurer *may* provide additional coverage.

Premium increases over time. Policyholders may be reluctant to purchase a policy or may let a policy lapse because the price of their premiums cannot be guaranteed. Although most products are priced to have level premiums, insurance companies can request rate increases if benefit payments that are higher than expected. Most states require long-term care insurance companies to increase prices for all purchasers of a particular policy. Insurers cannot single out individual purchasers for price increases. To date, most companies have not increased their premiums on existing products, and AMEX, the largest seller of long-term care insurance, has never increased premiums on existing products in twenty years in the market.

For long-term care insurance, underpriced policies present a more serious threat to consumers than overpriced policies. Consumers who purchase an underpriced policy may face unanticipated premium increases that could create financial hardship and lead to policy lapses, especially for older persons on fixed incomes. Consumer groups and regulators are concerned that the following scenario could play out: A disreputable company enters the long-term care insurance market with products that are priced significantly lower than the rest of the industry. The company sells a fair number of policies because it has lower premiums than its competitors. When the amount of benefits paid becomes high in comparison to premiums received, the company requests and receives rate increases, which cause a high percentage of purchasers to allow their coverage to lapse because they can no longer afford it. Eventually, the company abandons the sale of long-term care insurance but pockets the equity that has built up from premiums that have been paid. Several of the people interviewed mentioned one company that had significantly underpriced its product and managed to obtain a large share of the market in the early 1990s. This company subsequently filed for large rate increases, which could force many of its policyholders to let their policies lapse.

Underpricing of policies could be caused by faulty assumptions. For example, companies could miscalculate the amount of long-term care use among purchasers by either underestimating the number of policyholders who will meet eligibility criteria and who will use services or by overestimating lapse rates. Underpricing could also result from changes in the nature of long-term care services (for example, states certifying facilities providing a wider range of care). Although forbidden by actuarial standards of conduct, intentional underpricing could provide a competitive price advantage to gain market share because an insurer would offer lower premiums than its competitors. A more subtle cause of underpricing could result from market pressures to set premiums on the low side of a range of possible prices given by actuaries. HIAA data indicate that the premium for a four-year policy for a person age 65 steadily declined from $1,135 in 1990 to $898 a year in 1993, despite no significant additional information on the amount of benefit payments.[33] Although this does not mean that policies are currently underpriced, it does suggest that market forces can induce companies to be less conservative about pricing policies.

GOVERNMENT OPTIONS

Federal or state government could intervene in the long-term care insurance market in several ways to help the market grow and to ensure consumer protection. These goals, however, often conflict. Interventions aimed at protecting consumers, such as mandating nonforfeiture benefits, could limit the growth of the market by raising the price of policies and reducing demand.

The government could try to improve the level of information people selling and buying long-term care insurance have and foster more appropriate sales, make policies more affordable, and address the concerns consumers have about policies. Governmental action could come through nonregulatory mechanisms, such as providing and distributing accurate information; tax incentives; and regulatory mechanisms such as mandating agent training and requiring the inclusion of certain provisions in policies.

A consistent split on which direction the government should take existed among those interviewed. Industry representatives generally argued that market forces are creating policies that could provide broad protection for a substantial number of (but not all) individuals. They welcome government efforts that would encourage the growth of the market but oppose regulations that could drive up the cost of policies. Although conceding that long-term care insurance policies have improved dramatically, consumer groups generally argued that long-term care insurance policies are only viable for a small segment of the population. They contend that all people who purchase a long-term care insurance policy should receive adequate protection, even if the market would be significantly smaller. They would welcome the regulatory involvement of the federal government because they think that many states are too slow in addressing long-term care insurance consumer protection issues.

Improving the level of information. Our interviews strongly suggest that the long-term care insurance market suffers from a lack of accurate information. For individuals to purchase and keep a long-term care insurance policy, two conditions need to be met: The person must think that he or she needs long-term care protection and believe that long-term care insurance could provide that protection, and agents must have the knowledge and incentives to carry out the sale. If both components are in place, an agent can match a person with a policy that meets his or her needs and circumstances. Thus the government could encourage the purchase and retention of long-term care insurance coverage by doing the following:

— Educating consumers;

— Improving information consumers obtain from agents by requiring that agents receive training or be certified;

— Altering agents' incentives so that they are more motivated to supply consumers with accurate information;

— Standardizing definitions so that policies could be more easily understood and compared;

— Establishing suitability standards that would allow the consumer to understand if the policy is appropriate for her or him; and

— Monitoring sales practices to ensure that agents supply accurate information.

Providing consumer education. Consumers may feel more comfortable buying a policy and may purchase a policy that is better suited to their needs and circumstances if they had a fuller understanding of their need for coverage and the types of protection that different long-term care insurance policies offer. Currently, elderly Americans can learn about the risks and costs of long-term care from the mass media, personal experiences with someone close to them requiring long-term care, financial planners, insurance agents, state counseling programs, or other sources. Typically, individuals must be proactive in gathering information about long-term care needs and long-term care insurance. The available sources of information are often biased or have only a limited understanding of the complex issues surrounding the decision to purchase long-term care insurance.

This situation could be improved if consumers were provided with information from sources other than agents, possibly by expanding the role of state counseling programs or developing tools to aid individuals in deciding whether they should purchase long-term care insurance and assist them in comparing policy features and likely coverage under different circumstances.[34] State counseling programs have started to provide information about long-term care insurance, and some states provide consumers with guides describing available policies. One examination of the medigap market suggested that the price comparison documents developed by states helped consumers to evaluate the features of products more easily.[35] Information dissemination might best be accomplished at the state level because states could better tailor information to local circumstances and distribute this information more efficiently.

Training or certification of agents. In addition to ensuring that the consumer understands long-term care needs and long-term care insurance, the sale of policies could be improved if agents had more substantial knowledge of these issues. For most consumers, the agent is the expert who shapes their understanding of whether they need long-term care insurance coverage and what type of coverage is best. For an agent to do that job effectively, she or he must have a strong understanding of the complexities of protecting consumers against the costs associated with long-term care.

The knowledge of agents could be improved by requiring certification and continuing education to sell the product. Alternatively, agents could be required to work with an agent who has expertise in long-term care insurance. Few experts interviewed objected to certifying agents. Although some expressed concern that this additional hurdle would drive some agents out of the market, it was generally felt that agents who would leave were less committed to the market, and hence less likely to make sales or to sell appropriately.

Altering agents' incentives. Agents could be induced to make appropriate sales by changing their incentives. Ideally, agents' incentives should be constructed so that it is in their interest to convey accurate and complete information to the consumer and make sure that the consumer purchases a policy that meets his or her needs. Currently, agents receive first-year commissions as high as 70 percent and renewal commissions as low as 2 percent of the premiums. Reducing the differential between the first-year and renewal commissions could change the agents' incentives from trying to sell as many policies as possible with little concern over how long people held them to trying to sell policies to people who were likely to keep them over time. Agents interviewed were generally opposed to this option. They argued that because long-term care insurance is so difficult to sell, agents need high first-year commissions to compensate for their time. If they were deprived of these commissions, many good agents might leave the market and sell other forms of insurance that are more profitable.

Sales practices also could be improved through companies assuming greater responsibility for the actions of their agents. Companies could build incentives into the financial reward and recognition structures for their sales forces by paying bonuses to agents who score well on a test of long-term care knowledge and have low lapse

rates among their clients. This "carrot" approach might be more effective than the "stick" approach of requiring agent certification and
changing commission structures, but it would also probably mean
less consistent compliance.

Standardizing definitions. Consumers may be more inclined to purchase long-term care insurance policies if they were better able to
make comparisons across policies. This could be facilitated by standardizing components of the policies. Standardization done at a national level might be more appealing to all parties because it would
reduce the confusion and cost associated with adapting policies to the
requirements of each state. Some observers argue only for standardized definitions and minimum policy features.[36] Others argue that
long-term care insurance should be limited to a set number of fully
standardized plans, similar to what is done for medigap policies.[37] A
rigid standardization of plans trades diversity in products and choice
for reduced confusion.[38] The majority of those interviewed warned
against such standardization of long-term care insurance products at
this stage of the market because it could stifle innovation, but many
supported more uniform definitions of benefit eligibility criteria and
covered services to aid in comparison shopping.

Setting suitability standards. In addition to clarifying the product, the
purchase of long-term care insurance could be improved by providing
consumers with information about who is an appropriate purchaser of
the product. Inappropriate sales could be reduced by setting standards
to define a suitable purchaser of long-term care insurance. Many consumer groups and regulators argue that long-term care insurance
should not be sold to certain people, particularly those who would
quickly qualify for medicaid if they needed long-term care. However,
industry representatives argue that the group for whom long-term care
insurance is appropriate is unclear and that, while some general guidelines could be helpful, everyone should be able to purchase long-term
care insurance if they choose to do so. If the children of an individual
with meager financial resources choose to pay his or her premiums or
a couple wishes to pay for long-term care insurance premiums out of
their assets, suitability standards should not necessarily preclude such
a purchase. Intertwined with this issue is the right to privacy. Many
agents and insurance company representatives say that consumers

view having to disclose information about their income and assets as an invasion of privacy, and consumer groups are concerned about agents having access to this information. Some consumer advocates believe that state insurance counseling programs should help consumers decide if long-term care insurance is for them.

Thus, although the vast majority of the people interviewed agreed that some sort of suitability judgment should be made, no consensus emerged on how to determine who is suitable. Government action could vary from providing financial worksheets or general guidelines about appropriate consumers of long-term care insurance, to mandating that the agent demonstrate that the consumer has a certain level of assets and income before a sale could be made. NAIC has proposed that companies develop their own income and asset suitability standards, inform applicants who do not meet the standard, and provide them with an opportunity to refuse coverage.

Monitoring sales practices. Sales agents who use abusive and aggressive tactics to sell long-term care insurance may taint the image of the market, making people more reluctant to buy, and may sell inappropriate policies, which are later lapsed or replaced. The likelihood of purchase and retention could be improved if questionable sales tactics were curbed.

In the mid-1990s, most sales of long-term care insurance take place in the purchaser's home based on one-on-one conversations with an agent. Regulating and monitoring this transaction is difficult. The states we examined took a reactive approach by responding to complaints. State regulators expressed frustration that consumers do not follow through on complaints. Many state insurance departments require consumers to submit written complaints before they will take any action. Some consumers are reluctant to file grievances because they do not want to get involved or because they worry about getting an agent into trouble. Even if a consumer files a complaint, obtaining the documentation to substantiate that claim is often not easy.

Despite these difficulties, investing more resources into investigating abusive sales agents could help the market by improving the quality of information consumers receive and by enhancing the reputation of long-term care insurance. Regulators in one state thought that after an effort to prosecute problem agents, other agents curbed their abusive sales techniques.

Making Policies More Affordable

The federal government could provide tax incentives to make long-term care insurance policies more affordable, thus encouraging more people to buy and keep them. Tax incentives would allow the individual buying the policy to deduct the premium from his or her gross income or to receive a tax credit against the amount of taxes owed. Tax deductions could also be offered to employers who pay for long-term care insurance policies. Almost all the industry representatives interviewed thought that tax incentives would result in increased sales because policies would be more affordable. Many of these industry experts thought that the message that the government would be sending—that the individual and not the government is responsible for covering the costs of long-term care—would have a powerful effect on demand for policies.

Consumer groups were generally opposed to tax incentives because they thought that the product did not merit spending limited government resources. They argued that these resources could be used in more productive ways, such as changing medicare coverage to include more long-term care services. Some experts stated that they could accept limited tax incentives for the purchase of long-term care insurance provided that these incentives were tied to minimum federal government standards ensuring that policies provide adequate protection. Consumer groups also were concerned that tax credits would benefit only relatively well-off elderly persons who were paying substantial amounts of taxes. These tax breaks probably cannot be justified using the argument that they will save the government money, because the people who are most likely to receive tax breaks are those least likely to rely on medicaid if they needed long-term care. One study estimated that the tax loss would be four times the medicaid savings.[39]

Addressing Concerns about Current Policies

Even if a consumer is matched with the best long-term care insurance policy available, he or she may have concerns that prevent purchase or retention of the policy. If the government wishes to encourage people to buy and keep long-term care insurance policies, it should consider steps to make policies more flexible and to ensure that premiums remain level. Incorporating upgrade and downgrade options in policies, improving the monitoring of long-term care insurance pricing, limiting the extent to which insurance companies can raise premiums, and incorporating nonforfeiture provisions into policies could help achieve those goals.

Upgrades and downgrades. The ability of long-term care policies to adapt to changes in an individual's circumstances or the service delivery system could be improved by including standard provisions in policies that allow consumers to alter the terms of their coverage. Consumers then could be less hesitant to commit themselves to a long-term care insurance policy, and lapses could be discouraged by allowing consumers to upgrade to newer policies as they become available or downgrade to less expensive policies that they could continue to afford if their ability to pay decreases. Being able to upgrade or downgrade a policy would mean that the consumer could change the policy without losing the equity already established. These provisions would make the inclusion of nonforfeiture benefits less necessary, because consumers would be less likely to lose established policy equity. In the case of downgrades, the consumer could lower his or her premiums by reducing coverage without proof of insurability. For upgrades, consumers probably would pay higher premiums. However, the premiums would be lower than those for new policies bought by consumers of the same age, because those seeking upgrades would get credit for the payment of past premiums. Those wishing to upgrade would likely have to demonstrate that they meet certain underwriting criteria to prevent poor risks from disproportionately taking advantage of this option and exposing companies to unacceptably high risk (adverse selection). NAIC did not have provisions regarding upgrades and downgrades as of April 1995.

Consumer groups and regulators strongly supported the idea of including upgrade and downgrade provisions. One of the states that had a Robert Wood Johnson Partnership Program, a joint effort by the public and private sectors to increase the quality and quantity of long-term care insurance sales, mandated that companies include upgrade and downgrade provisions in the policies offered under the program.

Insurance company representatives did not have a strong reaction to this issue. Some companies offer upgrade options to holders of older policies on an ad hoc basis, at the companies' discretion. Formally establishing an upgrade or downgrade policy would involve numerous administrative complexities, including calculating policy equity. In addition, an upgrade option has the potential for older policies to be left with individuals who were not able to upgrade their policies because of medical conditions, thus necessitating premium increases.

From our interviews, we conclude that the inclusion of upgrade and downgrade options would have the most unambiguously positive effect on the desirability and quality of long-term care insurance policies of all the interventions reviewed. When consumers purchase a long-term care insurance policy, they lock themselves into a long-term commitment. Permitting consumers to upgrade their policy to cover new services or to downgrade to make premiums more affordable without loss of equity could reduce lapses and ensure that consumers have access to services when needed. Building flexibility into policies would make sense given the quickly changing nature of these policies and the uncertainty surrounding the long-term care insurance market. This option would put insurance companies at less risk than rate stabilization and would increase consumer choice instead of decreasing it as would mandating nonforfeiture benefits.

The government could facilitate the process of incorporating upgrade and downgrade provisions in all long-term care insurance policies in a number of ways. First, the government could reduce some of the technical difficulties of including these provisions by developing models for how these provisions can be written. Second, the government could educate consumers and companies about the value of these provisions and, thereby, create consumer demand. Third, the government could provide incentives for companies to include upgrade and downgrade provisions in their policies, such as making them part of the requirement for receiving tax benefits. Finally, the government could mandate that all policies include these provisions.

Rate monitoring. Enhancing the ability of regulators to deal with pricing issues at the time policies are initially filed could prevent price increases in the future. It could also take the place of proposals to limit the amount by which companies could increase premiums. However, states may be limited by resource constraints and a lack of consistency in product definitions and information on benefit payments (claims experience) on which to base pricing benchmarks.

Calculating premiums for long-term care insurance involves a number of assumptions, including the effect of underwriting, benefit design, lapse rates, number of purchasers expected to use services and for how long, the cost of services in the future, and investment income from premiums. Actuaries must base many of these assumptions on limited claims experience and national data for the general population. In most states, the insurance department requires companies selling long-term care insurance to file their rate requests and justification material for review. A congressional report on state regulation of insurance and a report for the American Association of Retired Persons (AARP) on long-term care insurance question the ability of state insurance departments to monitor insurance pricing because of inadequate staffing and resources.[40] The prefunded nature of the product increases the importance of pricing, which in part determines the fate of the company (viability) and whether it has sufficient funds available to pay claims (solvency). The combination of limited staff and expertise in state insurance departments and limited claims experience data hinder their ability to regulate overpricing and underpricing, either of which would have adverse effects on consumers. The bigger danger would likely be in underpricing policies, which few state insurance departments monitor.

Rate stabilization. If the government does not believe that it can adequately monitor long-term care insurance rates, it may wish to reassure potential purchasers and prevent lapses by not allowing insurance companies to increase rates dramatically. Rate stabilization limits the extent to which insurers can raise rates over time. NAIC adopted a model for rate stabilization that would limit the percentage increase in premiums depending on the age of the purchaser. Rate stabilization should make retaining policies easier for consumers and discourage companies from lowballing prices and subsequently raising rates dramatically. Rate stabilization does not mean an absolute ban on premium increases. State regulators could allow companies to raise rates if it became necessary to stay in business and to provide benefits.

Two viewpoints emerged on rate stabilization. Consumer groups and many regulators argue that companies should know enough about pricing long-term care insurance to be able to adjust to a moderately flexible form of rate stabilization. They believe that this would prevent lowball pricing. Industry representatives argue that rate stabilization would put the insurance company at risk instead of spreading the risk across consumers. They contend that rate stabilization would force insurers to increase rates as a precautionary measure; drive many insurers out of the market (although consumer groups and some industry representatives indicated that this may not be a bad outcome); and cause some companies with bad experience to become insolvent, thereby potentially providing the consumer with no protection. They add that the long-term care insurance market is relatively new, and they do not have the actuarial experience necessary to price policies with complete accuracy, particularly policies with coverage of home and community-based services.

Nonforfeiture. Instead of trying to prevent lapses, nonforfeiture benefits seek to ensure that people receive some value for the equity they have built up in their policies. Nonforfeiture benefits allow policyholders to receive some value for their policy, either in the form of a cash refund or a reduced benefit if they discontinue paying premiums. Nonforfeiture benefits are a hotly contested issue. Consumer groups argue that the inclusion of nonforfeiture benefits makes a policy more attractive for a consumer to purchase. However, industry representatives said that very few consumers choose to buy nonforfeiture benefits when they are offered and not mandated. Consumer groups contend that nonforfeiture helps ensure that consumers receive value for their premiums and eliminates insurance companies' incentives to have high lapse rates. Meanwhile, industry representatives and agents insist that mandating nonforfeiture benefits forces consumers to purchase a feature that they generally do not want and raises the price of policies so much that many people would be priced out of the market. Industry representatives were not opposed to mandating that an offer of nonforfeiture protection be made. This issue thus creates a tension among consumer protection, consumer choice, and affordability of the product.

If all states mandated nonforfeiture benefits, one aspect of the uncertainty of future premium increases and variation in premiums would be reduced and purchasers who let their policies lapse would receive a return on their premium equity. Inclusion of nonforfeiture benefits will raise premiums. Analyses prepared for NAIC and AARP found that adding nonforfeiture benefits could increase premiums by 15 percent to 132 percent at age 65, depending on the type of nonforfeiture benefit offered.[41] The NAIC model regulations recently required a shortened benefit period nonforfeiture benefit for long-term care insurance equal to the value of premiums paid up to the time of lapse. Thus, if states adopt this provision, consumers who allow their policies to lapse and subsequently need long-term care will receive the same level of daily coverage they would have otherwise received. However, the length of time they receive coverage would be determined by the dollar amount of premiums they paid before their policies lapsed. This form of nonforfeiture benefit provides consumers with a limited return on the premiums paid, because they receive no credit for accrued interest, which could be substantial if the policy was held for any length of time. As of April 1995, only two states had adopted the mandated nonforfeiture benefit regulation, and two states had stipulated that it must be offered as an option to consumers.

CONCLUSION

The long-term care insurance market has grown dramatically between the mid-1980s and the mid-1990s. Although significantly higher quality policies are available at lower prices, the penetration of the total senior market remains extremely low, especially when compared to the medicare supplemental insurance market. Market penetration remains low because consumers are not purchasing long-term care insurance and, when they do purchase it, are likely to let it lapse. Barriers to purchase and retention of policies include lack of perceived need for the product, distrust of insurance, difficulty matching the policy to an individual's needs, premiums that consumers cannot afford, inflexible products that make upgrades and downgrades difficult, and potential future premium increases that may make the policies unaffordable.

Our review of the potential barriers to the purchase and retention of long-term care insurance highlights at least three areas of concern. First, long-term care insurance is difficult to understand, varies from company to company in ways that are not always obvious, and is being sold to consumers who often have limited knowledge and understanding by agents who sometimes also know little about the product. Second, policies lock individuals into provisions that may not make sense for them at some point in the future and into a delivery system that may change. Third, market competition may lead to underpricing that, in turn, could someday result in premium increases.

Whether market forces will correct for these concerns or whether further regulation would be necessary remains unclear. Most experts agree that the government could assist the market by intervening in several ways. First, greater effort could be made to educate consumers about the existence and details of long-term care insurance. Consumers need to be made aware that they may have to bear potentially catastrophic long-term care expenses and that long-term care insurance is an option for protecting themselves against those expenses. In addition, consumers need accessible information that would educate them about what to look for and questions to ask when considering a policy. The appropriateness of the policies purchased could be improved by requiring that agents disclose key pieces of information. This would involve developing clear and easy-to-understand materials demonstrating the value of features such as inflation protection and nonforfeiture benefits that the agent would be required to give consumers. If consumers buy policies they can afford and that provide the coverage they want, they will be more likely to hold on to those policies.

Second, the training of agents needs to be more consistent and rigorous. The agent is the primary source of information about long-term care insurance. Agent certification that requires continuing education could eliminate some problem agents from the market. In addition, continuing education programs must be made available and their quality monitored.

Third, the vast majority of the experts interviewed in this study supported standardized definitions and benefit triggers. They would eliminate much of the difficulty in comparing products and could allow consumers to more easily pick and choose between products. Empowerment of consumers could result in market competition that rewards good quality products.

Despite the dramatic improvement in long-term care insurance policies, several concerns about the ability of the market to provide protection against the catastrophic costs of long-term care remain. Although the government could consider regulations that would increase the price of the products and limit the market, it could intervene in a number of other ways that would be beneficial to both consumers and the long-term care insurance industry.

NOTES

1. Office of the Assistant Secretary for Planning and Evaluation, *Cost Estimates for the Long-Term Care Provisions of the Health Security Act* (Washington: Department of Health and Human Services, March 1994).
2. Joshua Wiener, Laurel Hixon Illston, and Raymond Hanley, *Sharing the Burden: Strategies for Public and Private Long-Term Care Insurance* (Brookings, 1994).
3. Ibid.
4. ICF Incorporated, *Private Financing of Long-Term Care: Current Methods and Resources*, submitted to the Office of the Assistant Secretary of Planning and Evaluation (Department of Health and Human Services, 1995).
5. Authors' calculations based on the National Association of Insurance Commissioners, *1992 and 1993 Long-Term Care Insurance Experience Reports* (Kansas City, Mo., 1994). As of the end of 1993, the number of policies ever sold had increased to more than 3.4 million and more than 115 companies sold long-term care insurance; see Susan Coronel and Diane Fulton, *Long-Term Care Insurance in 1993* (Washington: Health Insurance Association of America, 1995). The number of policies sold was significantly higher than the number of policies in force because a large number of people dropped their coverage or died.
6. National Association of Insurance Commissioners, *1992 Long-Term Care Insurance Experience Reports.*
7. Ibid.
8. Health Insurance Association of America, *Who Buys Long-Term Care Insurance?* report prepared by LifePlans, Inc. (Washington, 1992).
9. National Association of Insurance Commissioners, unpublished table of state adoptions of long-term care insurance regulation provisions (Kansas City, Mo., October 1994).
10. ICF Incorporated, *Private Financing of Long-Term Care.*
11. General Accounting Office, *Long-Term Care Insurance: State Regulatory Requirements Provide Inconsistent Consumer Protection*, report to the Chairman, Subcommittee on Health and Long-Term Care of the House Select Committee on Aging, HRD-89-67 (1989).
12. National Association of Insurance Commissioners, unpublished table of state adoptions of long-term care insurance regulation provisions.
13. Wiener and others, *Sharing the Burden.*
14. Peter Kemper and Christopher Murtaugh, "Lifetime Use of Nursing Home Care," *New England Journal of Medicine*, vol. 324, no. 9 (1991), p. 597.
15. Assuming 90 percent of persons with long-term care insurance policies in force are age 65 and over could overestimate the proportion that were elderly. Data from an HIAA study of purchasers indicated that 75 percent of purchasers were age 65 or older and that the average age of purchase was 68

in 1990; see HIAA, *Who Buys Long-Term Care Insurance?* We would expect the proportion age 65 or older among policyholders to be somewhat higher than purchasers because many will have bought their policy earlier.

16. George S. Chulis and others, "Health Insurance and the Elderly," *Health Affairs,* vol. 12, no. 1 (1993), pp. 111–18.

17. Gary Corliss and others, *Society of Actuaries Long-Term Care Experience Committee, Intercompany Study: 1984–1991 Experience* (Schaumburg, Ill.: Society of Actuaries, January 1995). Some of these lapses could be the result of death or upgrades.

18. R. L. Associates, *American Public Views Long-Term Care* (Washington: American Association of Retired Persons and Villers Foundation, 1987); and HIAA, *Who Buys Long-Term Care Insurance?*

19. Employee Benefits Research Institute, *Public Attitudes on Long-Term Care, 1993: Summary Report* (Washington, 1993).

20. Stephen Moses, "Health and Long-Term Care Insurance," in Louis Mezzullo and Mark Woolpert, eds., *Advising the Elderly Client* (New York: Clark, Boardman, Calaghan, 1992), chapter 24.

21. HIAA, *Who Buys Long-Term Care Insurance?*

22. Margaret K. Straw, *Home Care: Attitudes and Knowledge of Middle-Aged and Older Americans* (Washington: American Association of Retired Persons, 1991).

23. Mark V. Pauly, "The Rational Nonpurchase of Long-Term Care Insurance," *Journal of Political Economy,* vol. 98, no. 1 (1990), pp. 153–68.

24. HIAA, *Who Buys Long-Term Care Insurance?*

25. Ibid.

26. "Gotcha! The Traps in Long-Term Care Insurance," *Consumer Reports,* July 1991, pp. 419–30; and City of New York Department of Consumer Affairs, *Promise Them Anything: The Selling of Long-Term Care Insurance for the Elderly* (April 1993).

27. These groups contend that the number of policies sold by uninformed agents is small because of the importance of being able to provide accurate and complete information to maintain a client's confidence and complete a sale. However, all fourteen of the agents in the *Consumer Reports* and all eight of the agents in the City of New York Consumer Affairs studies misrepresented either the risk of needing long-term care or the coverage offered by the policies they were selling.

28. Coronel and Fulton, *Long-Term Care Insurance in 1993.*

29. Wiener and others, *Sharing the Burden.*

30. HIAA, *Who Buys Long-Term Care Insurance?*

31. Robert Friedland, *Financing the Costs of Long-Term Care* (Washington: Employee Benefits Research Institute, 1990); Families USA Foundation, *Nursing Home Insurance: Who Can Afford It?* (Washington, February 1993);

Alice Rivlin and Joshua Wiener, with Raymond Hanley and Denise Spence, *Caring for the Disabled Elderly: Who Will Pay?* (Brookings, 1988); Wiener and others, *Sharing the Burden.*

32. Marc Cohen and others, "The Financial Capacity of the Elderly to Insure for Long-Term Care," *Gerontologist*, vol. 27 (August 1987), pp. 494–502; and Marc Cohen and others, "Financing Long-Term Care: A Practical Mix of Public and Private," *Journal of Health Politics, Policy and Law*, vol. 17 (Fall 1992), pp. 403–23.

33. Coronel and Fulton, *Long-Term Care Insurance in 1993.*

34. Shoshanna Sofaer, Erin Kenney, and Bruce Davidson, "The Effect of the Illness Episode Approach on Medicare Beneficiaries' Health Insurance Decisions," *Health Services Research*, vol. 27, no. 5 (1992), pp. 671–93; and Shoshanna Sofaer, Robert Wyn, and Diane Mellon-Lacey, *The California Consumers' Guide to Long-Term Care Insurance* (University of California at Los Angeles School of Public Health, 1990).

35. Lisa Maria B. Alecxih and others, "Can Regulation Improve Long-Term Care Insurance?: Lessons from the Medigap Experience," *Journal of Aging and Social Policy* (forthcoming).

36. Joshua Wiener and Katherine Harris, "Regulation of Private Long-Term Care Insurance," *Caring Magazine* (May 1991), pp. 36–42; and Office of the Inspector General, *State Regulation of Long-Term Care Insurance* (Department of Health and Human Services, 1991).

37. Gail Shearer, *Statement of the Consumers Union on the Private Long-Term Care Insurance Market*, Testimony before the Subcommittee on Health, U.S. House of Representatives Committee on Ways and Means, 102 Cong. 1 sess. (Government Printing Office, 1991).

38. Peter D. Fox, Thomas Rice, and Lisa Alecxih, "Medigap Regulation: Lessons for Health Care Reform," *Journal of Health Politics, Policy and Law* (1995), pp. 31–47.

39. Joshua Wiener, *Clarifying the Tax Status of Long-Term Care Insurance*, testimony before the Subcommittee on Health, U.S. House of Representatives Committee on Ways and Means, 104 Cong. 1 sess. (GPO, 1995).

40. Robyn I. Stone and others, *State Variation in the Regulation of Long-Term Care Insurance Products* (Washington: American Association of Retired Persons, 1992); and *Wishful Thinking: A World View of Insurance Solvency Regulation*, Committee Print, Subcommittee on Oversight and Investigations, House Committee on Energy and Commerce, 103 Cong. 2 sess. (GPO, October 1994).

41. American Association for Retired Persons, *Inflation Protection and Nonforfeiture Benefits in Long-Term Care Insurance Policies: New Data for Decision Making* (Washington, June 1992); and National Association of Insurance Commissioners, Long-Term Care Actuarial Task Force, *Inflation Protection and Nonforfeiture Benefits in Long-Term Care Insurance Policies* (Kansas City, Mo., 1991).

Chapter 4

BRIAN BURWELL AND WILLIAM H. CROWN

Medicaid Estate Planning: Case Studies of Four States

Medicaid is a health insurance program for poor Americans.[1] It is a means-tested program; applicants must have incomes and assets below certain financial criteria to qualify for medicaid benefits. Means-testing ensures that public resources are used to provide medical assistance to people who cannot afford to provide for their own health care.

Medicaid estate planning is a process by which elderly people purposefully divest their assets and income to qualify for medicaid benefits, particularly coverage for nursing home care. The goal of medicaid estate planning is to preserve assets for family and heirs, by avoiding a depletion of assets on the private cost of staying in a nursing home. Because private nursing home costs typically average more than $3,000 per month, individuals who pay privately for their nursing home care, and do not engage in medicaid estate planning, can easily use their entire life savings over an extended stay.

Medicaid estate planning has several variations. For married couples, it generally takes the form of ensuring that the spouse remaining in the community (the noninstitutionalized spouse) retains as much of the married couple's combined income and assets as possible, so that he or she can continue to maintain the same life-style and remain financially secure after the institutionalized spouse dies. For single persons, the goal of medicaid estate planning is generally to preserve inheritances for heirs, usually the nursing home resident's children. Medicaid estate planning also aims to protect estates (largely the family home) from recovery efforts by state medicaid programs acting as creditors against a deceased medicaid recipient's estate.

Although many people believe that medicaid estate planning is unethical, it is not illegal. The rules that determine whether individuals applying for medicaid coverage meet the program's financial eligibility criteria are complex and provide opportunities for savvy individuals to divest or shelter their assets without penalty. And because the rules are complex, individuals who participate in medicaid estate planning often seek the counsel of people who have special expertise in these matters, generally elder law attorneys. Since the mid-1980s elder law has been a rapidly growing specialty in the legal profession, and within the practice of elder law, medicaid estate planning represents a significant proportion of the business conducted.

OMNIBUS BUDGET RECONCILIATION ACT OF 1993

Medicaid estate planning has been an issue for many years in the medicaid program, and Congress has periodically moved to restrict its practice. In 1980 Congress passed legislation to deny medicaid eligibility to persons who purposefully transferred assets to obtain medicaid coverage. In 1982 transfer of asset restrictions was expanded to encompass certain excluded assets, such as the home. The Medicare Catastrophic Coverage Act (MCCA) of 1988 made a number of further amendments, including requiring all states to adopt transfer of asset restrictions, instead of having these restrictions be optional.

On August 10, 1993, President Bill Clinton signed into law the Omnibus Budget Reconciliation Act of 1993 (OBRA 93—P.L. 103-66), which included a number of changes to the medicaid statute that reflected Congress's latest attempt to address medicaid estate planning as a policy issue. Specific provisions of OBRA 93 included the following:

—The look-back period for asset transfers was extended from thirty months to thirty-six months. The look-back period defines the time before medicaid application in which asset transfers may be subject to a penalty period.[2] Transfers made before the look-back period are not subject to penalty.

—The cap on the asset transfer penalty period was eliminated. The asset transfer penalty period had been subject to a thirty-month cap. Under OBRA 93, no cap was placed on the penalty, so that if someone transfers a very large amount of assets, the penalty period could extend for many years.

—Multiple transfers over a period of time were treated as a single transfer. Before enactment of OBRA 93, some applicants and their attorneys were gaming the system by making multiple transfers of assets over several months and then arguing that each transfer had to be treated as a separate transfer subject to its own penalty period. By having penalty periods run concurrently, applicants could greatly reduce the amount of time they had to wait between transferring their assets and becoming eligible for medicaid. OBRA 93 clarified that penalty periods for multiple transfers were to run consecutively, not concurrently.

—Transfers of jointly held assets were considered illegal transfers subject to a penalty period. When transfers were made from joint accounts that reduced the applicant's control or ownership of the asset, the transfer would be subject to a penalty period. Before OBRA 93, some states believed that they could not treat withdrawals from joint accounts by nonapplicants as illegal transfers because the applicants had not made the transfer themselves.

—Transfers made by applicants and recipients of noninstitutional long-term care services were also subject to penalty, at the option of the state. Under this provision, states could, but were not required to, impose transfer of asset penalties on persons who had applied for or who were receiving noninstitutional long-term care services.

—Lengthy clarifications were made of how assets transferred by the applicant, the applicant's spouse, or someone acting on behalf of the applicant into a trust would be treated in the medicaid eligibility process. In most circumstances, the entire corpus of a trust was considered a countable asset. If not, the transfer of assets into the trust was subject to a penalty period with a sixty-month look-back period. Transfers into a trust—because they were more likely to have taken place for medicaid planning purposes—were treated more severely than other types of transfers.

—Certain kinds of trusts for disabled persons under age 65 were exempted from transfer of asset penalties. Most trusts created for the benefit of disabled persons under age 65 were not counted in the medicaid eligibility process, and distributions from these kinds of trusts could be used to purchase supplemental services, equipment, and so on for disabled medicaid recipients without affecting their medicaid eligibility.

—Trusts established with only the income of applicants in so-called income cap states were not considered an available resource. This provision essentially enabled individuals who were denied medicaid eligibility because they had incomes over medicaid eligibility limits in income cap states to become eligible by temporarily transferring their income into an income trust. Unlike other language in OBRA 93, this provision expanded medicaid eligibility to certain individuals who would otherwise not be able to obtain medicaid coverage for nursing home care in the fifteen states that used income caps.[3]

—States were required to specify procedures and policies for administering hardship rules. Hardship rules spelled out the circumstances under which states would waive transfer of asset penalties, trust rules, and estate recovery rules in cases where the application of these provisions would cause undue hardship on the applicant, recipient, or surviving family members.

—All states were required to implement estate recovery programs. Before OBRA 93, only about half the states operated estate recovery programs that sought to recover from the estates of deceased medicaid recipients costs that these recipients incurred under the medicaid program before they died. In addition, OBRA 93 expanded the definition of the term *estate* to include resources that passed to heirs outside of probate, such as through joint tenancy arrangements, tenancy in common, rights of survivorship, life estates, living trusts, and other arrangements. By expanding the definition, OBRA 93 widened the scope of assets that could be subject to state recovery efforts.

GROWTH IN MEDICAID ESTATE PLANNING

A number of factors have contributed to the growth in medicaid estate planning. First, older individuals have become increasingly aware that nursing home care is not covered by medicare. The debate surrounding the repeal of MCCA played an important role in this growing awareness, as did discussions of the need for public long-term care insurance in the 1993–94 congressional debate over President Clinton's proposed Health Security Act.

Second, the complexity of the spousal impoverishment provisions of MCCA, in combination with the rising economic status of the older population, has spurred many older persons to seek professional advice in planning for long-term care. Median net worth (in constant

TABLE 4-1. *Trends in Median Household Net Worth by Age of Household Head*

1991 Constant dollars

Age	1984	1988	1991
65 to 69			
Total net worth	88,151	96,834	104,354
Excluding home equity	28,718	31,879	33,345
70 to 74			
Total net worth	79,476	95,249	92,793
Excluding home equity	24,732	32,679	25,943
75 and over			
Total net worth	72,920	71,330	76,541
Excluding home equity	22,584	21,830	22,866
All elderly households (65 and over)			
Total net worth	79,576	85,226	88,192
Excluding home equity	25,006	27,673	26,442

Sources: T. J. Eller, "Household Wealth and Asset Ownership: 1991," *Current Population Reports*, P-20-34 (Washington: Bureau of the Census, 1994); and J. Eargle, "Household Wealth and Asset Ownership: 1988," *Current Population Reports*, P-70-22 (Washington: Bureau of the Census, 1989).

dollars) for persons age 65 and over has increased significantly in recent years (table 4-1).[4] However, most of this net worth was concentrated in home equity. Excluding home equity, the median asset level of elderly persons' households would finance less than a year of nursing home care in most locations.

Third, the increased demand for medicaid estate planning services has been met with increased supply. One indicator of supply, the membership level of the National Association of Elder Law Attorneys (NAELA), went from eighty members in 1987 (the year NAELA was founded) to about three thousand in 1994. Not only has the number of elder law attorneys been growing, but so too has the level of expertise among medicaid estate planning attorneys. This expertise is routinely shared through conferences and newsletters that keep elder law attorneys abreast of the latest medicaid planning techniques.[5]

Fourth, the cost of a nursing home stay has been rising. In the mid-1990s, the private pay rate for nursing home care averaged $3,000 to $4,000 per month and was substantially higher in some areas (for example, $5,000 to $6,000 per month on Long Island).

Finally, recent research has highlighted the substantial lifetime risk of a nursing home stay.[6] Although, at any one time, only about 5 percent of the population age 65 and over was in a nursing home, estimates of the lifetime risk of institutionalization exceed 40 percent.

In short, the confluence of the rising economic status of elderly persons, the rising costs of nursing home care, and the considerable lifetime risk of needing nursing home care has raised the financial consequences associated with needing long-term care. This growing risk, in combination with the shrinking numbers of elderly persons who mistakenly think that medicare covers long-term care, and the growth in the elder law industry itself, has contributed to the growth in the practice of medicaid estate planning.

RESEARCH ON MEDICAID ESTATE PLANNING

The policy debate over medicaid estate planning is full of rhetoric and strong emotion, but lacking in reliable and detailed information. Heated arguments frequently take place on the issue of how extensive medicaid estate planning activity is, as well as on its ethics. Some believe that medicaid estate planning is a major policy problem in the medicaid program and that many elderly individuals who qualify for medicaid coverage in nursing homes retain or divest significant assets that could be used to pay for their care privately.[7] Others argue that the vast majority of disabled elderly persons have no or few financial assets and that concerns over the magnitude of medicaid estate planning as a policy problem are vastly overblown.[8] The polemics over medicaid estate planning are also often made in the context of the unfairness of public policy regarding the lack of public insurance for nursing home care and the draconian nature of medicaid's means-tested benefits.[9]

Medicaid estate planning is complicated and not particularly amenable to quantitative measurement. Empirical studies of medicaid estate planning activity are few. In October 1992 the General Accounting Office (GAO) conducted a review of 403 applications for medicaid long-term care coverage in one of Massachusetts's three long-term care eligibility offices. The purpose of the review was to identify assets that had been converted from countable assets to excluded assets, as well as assets that had been transferred. GAO found that more than half the applicants had converted assets, although the vast majority of these cases involved applicants setting aside funds in burial accounts that were excluded in determining medicaid eligibility. In addition, in about 10 percent of the cases, applicants had transferred assets in the thirty-month period before making application, and the average amount of the transfer was about $46,000.[10]

To help fill the information gap, we conducted this study. The objectives of the study were to assess the magnitude of medicaid estate planning in selected states; identify the most commonly used medicaid estate planning techniques in the selected states and the variation in the use of techniques across states; assess the relationship between medicaid estate planning activities and (1) state medicaid eligibility practices and (2) state administrative practices in the eligibility determination process; and assess the impact of OBRA 93 on medicaid estate planning.

We used a case study methodology, focusing on four states: California, Florida, Massachusetts, and New York (table 4-2). California and New York were selected because they represented the two largest medicaid programs in the country. New York and Massachusetts had experienced the rapid growth in the medicaid planning industry, relative to other states. Florida was an income cap state, which has a definite relationship to medicaid estate planning techniques.[11]

The primary data collection approach used in the study was a one-week site visit to each state. Generally, on the first day of the site visit, we met with state medicaid eligibility staff to discuss long-term care eligibility policies, perceptions about the magnitude of medicaid estate planning activity, and state policy responses to medicaid estate planning. We then met with staff from the state's estate recovery program to discuss the organizational and administrative structure of medicaid estate recovery, recent developments in estate recovery efforts, and state implementation of OBRA 1993 mandates related to estate recovery.

During the remaining days of the site visit, we conducted interviews with frontline medicaid eligibility workers and supervisors in local eligibility offices. State medicaid eligibility staff usually set up the interviews and selected local offices that were in counties where a significant amount of medicaid planning activity was taking place or that had undertaken a specific response to the problem. In Massachusetts, however, only three eligibility offices in the entire state processed applications for long-term care coverage; all three were visited.

TABLE 4-2. Selected Characteristics of Case Study States

State	Income cap state [a]	Estate recovery program before OBRA 93	Centralized estate recovery	Uses liens [b]	1994 CSRA [c] minimum (dollars)	1994 MMMNA [d] maximum (dollars)	Medicaid nursing home expenditures per elderly state resident, 1992 [e] (state rank)
California	No	Yes	Yes	No	$72,660	$1,817	$474 (35)
Florida	Yes	Yes, but minimal	No	No	72,660	1,179	$302 (49)
Massachusetts	No	Yes	Yes	Yes	14,532	1,179	$1,185 (5)
New York	No	Yes	No	Yes, at county discretion	72,660	1,817	$1,353 (2)

OBRA 93 = Omnibus Budget Reconciliation Act of 1993.

a. An income cap state does not provide nursing home coverage to medically needy medicaid applicants but does to persons whose countable incomes fall below a special income level, which under federal law cannot exceed 300 percent of the federal supplemental security income (SSI) benefit level.

b. Liens are imposed on real property (usually the home) and protect the interests of the state in recovering incurred medicaid costs from the property upon the sale of the home or upon the death of the medicaid recipient.

c. Community Spouse Resource Allowance (CSRA) is the amount of assets retained by a noninstitutionalized spouse of a medicaid applicant and is excluded in determining eligibility for the institutionalized spouse.

d. Minimum Monthly Maintenance Needs Allowance (MMMNA) is the amount of countable income (either income of the applicant or joint income) that can be retained by the noninstitutionalized spouse. All remaining countable income, excluding a personal needs allowance, must be used as the medicaid recipient's contribution to his or her nursing home care. Unlike the treatment of assets, in which a married couple's total combined assets are considered available to the medicaid applicant, medicaid eligibility rules treat a couple's income separately. Thus, if the noninstitutionalized spouse has independent income in excess of the MMMNA, he or she is not required to contribute to the cost of the institutionalized spouse's nursing home care beyond the first month of institutionalization.

e. Mean medicaid nursing home expenditures per elderly resident nationwide were $633 in 1992.

FINDINGS

We made no effort to measure the magnitude of medicaid estate planning in the case study states, other than asking eligibility workers
their opinions about the extent to which they believed applicants had
participated in medicaid estate planning activities before submitting
their medicaid applications. The statements made here about the
magnitude of medicaid estate planning were primarily based on the
subjective opinions of the individuals interviewed during the site
visits, as well as on our observations.

Although clear evidence of medicaid estate planning activity
existed in all four states, the majority of people who applied for medicaid long-term care benefits did not purposefully divest or shelter
their assets beforehand. Other than perhaps a home, a car, and some
personal property, which were exempt in determining eligibility for
medicaid, most elderly people in need of nursing home care did not
have many financial assets. This was particularly true for persons
without living spouses, who were also the least likely to know about
the opportunities that medicaid estate planning offered. People with
low levels of assets did not use financial planners, lawyers, or other
financial experts.

In general, a strong relationship was found between the level of
medicaid estate planning reported by local eligibility offices and the
level of financial wealth within a geographical area. The higher the socioeconomic status of a geographical area, the more medicaid estate
planning was reported. In addition, medicaid estate planning attorneys concentrated their practices in upper-middle-class areas. The following three things generally went together: an area with a large population of upper-middle-class elderly persons, the presence of a
number of attorneys who practiced elder law and medicaid planning
as a specialty, and a high level of medicaid estate planning activity.

In every interview with eligibility workers and their supervisors,
we asked the following question: "What percentage of applicants do
you think have done something purposively to divest or shelter their
assets before coming in and applying for medicaid?" In cases involving single applicants without spouses, responses ranged from 5 to 25
percent, with most workers estimating that 5 to 10 percent of single
applicants did some kind of medicaid estate planning in the preap-
plication period. For cases involving married applicants, workers

consistently estimated a much higher rate, ranging from 20 percent to "almost every" application in some counties. Most estimates, however, fell into the 20 to 25 percent range. Note that these responses were from states and counties where the general perception was that a higher level of medicaid estate planning activity was going on. If states and counties had been selected randomly, workers probably would have reported a lower level of medicaid estate planning activity.

The magnitude of medicaid estate planning was not uniform across the four states. More medicaid planning activity was evident in New York than the other three states. Although considerable activity and a healthy elder law industry were found in Massachusetts, recent policy initiatives taken by the Massachusetts medicaid program had made an impact on reducing the magnitude of medicaid planning there.

In California, the level of medicaid planning activity was more sporadic. Although most of the visited counties reported some amount of medicaid planning by long-term care applicants, the levels of activity were nowhere near those reported by eligibility workers in New York and Massachusetts. In only San Luis Obispo and Los Angeles counties did eligibility workers report a high level of medicaid planning among long-term care applicants.

Similarly, in Florida, the level of medicaid planning reported by local offices was less than reported in New York and Massachusetts. Because Florida was an income cap state, the medicaid estate planning industry was hindered; even if individuals depleted their countable assets, many were left with incomes that exceeded Florida's income cap.[12] However, with the enactment of the income trust provision in OBRA 93, the level of planning activity in Florida has increased.

MEDICAID PLANNING TECHNIQUES FOR MARRIED COUPLES

Several medicaid estate planning techniques used in cases involving a spouse living in the community stemmed from the spousal impoverishment provisions of MCCA. Under these provisions, financial assets held by either spouse are totaled, then divided equally between the institutionalized and noninstitutionalized spouses. The noninstitutionalized spouse is allowed to retain half, subject to both a minimum and maximum amount.[13] At their option, states can set the minimum amount (called the Community Spouse Resource Allowance, or CSRA) anywhere between the established federal minimum and maximum. Both the minimum and maximum CSRA levels are indexed to inflation.[14]

The medicaid spousal impoverishment provisions also established federal rules regarding how the income of married couples would be divided, once the institutionalized spouse became eligible for medicaid. These provisions were designed to ensure that the spouse living in the community retained an adequate level of income on which to live. The amount of income that the noninstitutionalized spouse is allowed to retain is called the Minimum Monthly Maintenance Needs Allowance (MMMNA). Like the CSRA, the MMMNA is subject to both a federal minimum and a maximum.[15] If the income of the noninstitutionalized spouse is below the MMMNA, income from the institutionalized spouse can be diverted to the other spouse, to bring the noninstitutionalized spouse's income up to the MMMNA.

The "Just Say No" Strategy

Of all the medicaid planning techniques, the "just say no" strategy was, by far, the most egregious. Under the "just say no" strategy, the institutionalized spouse first transfers all assets (and sometimes income) to the spouse living in the community, as specifically permitted under MCCA. Then the noninstitutionalized spouse simply refuses to make any resources available to support the institutionalized spouse. In addition, the institutionalized spouse executes an agreement that reassigns his or her support rights from the spouse living in the community to the state medicaid program.

Use of the "just say no" technique virtually eliminated medicaid means-testing for married couples when one spouse needed nursing home care. With this technique, the noninstitutionalized spouse retained all of the couple's assets, regardless of the total amount, while the institutionalized spouse obtained medicaid coverage for nursing home care.

This strategy emanated from a long-standing medicaid eligibility policy that allowed states to provide medicaid coverage to applicants who had been abandoned by a financially responsible relative, usually a spouse. Historically, these cases usually involved instances in which a mother and a child or children were abandoned by a husband and father. The elder law industry adopted the provision as a medicaid estate planning technique for nursing home residents with noninstitutionalized spouses.

Eligibility workers in California, Florida, and Massachusetts reported that the "just say no" strategy was rarely attempted, but in New York, workers said that it was widely used. In Monroe, Nassau, New York (Manhattan), and Suffolk counties, workers said that "virtually every application" for a married applicant involved the use of the "just say no" strategy. Operationally, the technique often required nothing more than the noninstitutionalized spouse checking a box on a form provided to him or her by an attorney or adviser indicating that he or she did not wish to make any income or resources available to the institutionalized spouse.

Elder law attorneys claimed that the New York regulations only reflected the intent of MCCA, which they said included specific language allowing for the use of the "just say no" strategy. MCCA did require states to extend eligibility to an institutionalized spouse who assigned his or her support rights from the noninstitutionalized spouse to the state: "The institutionalized spouse shall not be ineligible by reason of resources determined under paragraph (2) to be available for the cost of care where (A) the institutionalized spouse has assigned to the state any rights to support from the community spouse."[16] However, MCCA was silent on the circumstances under which an assignment of support rights was legitimate and on the right of a spouse living in the community to refuse to support his or her institutionalized spouse. In states other than New York, a simple verbal refusal by the noninstitutionalized spouse to support the institutionalized spouse was not accepted as a case of true spousal abandonment, and the medicaid application was denied for excess resources. One state—Maryland—enacted a law in 1992 that restricted the assignment of support rights provisions to situations in which the institutionalized spouse needed protection, such as when the spouse living in the community had truly abandoned the institutionalized spouse and refused to provide any financial support for his or her care. The Maryland law also provided for penalties against a noninstitutionalized spouse who refused to pay for his or her spouse's care.

Raising the CSRA through Fair Hearings

If the noninstitutionalized spouse's income was below the MMMNA, MCCA stated that that spouse could receive additional income and resources from the institutionalized spouse to bring his or her income up to the MMMNA.[17] Through a fair hearing process, the noninstitutionalized spouse could have the CSRA raised above the state's CSRA maximum to the asset level that was necessary to produce enough income to bring his or her income up to the MMMNA.

At face value, the policy was reasonable as long as the institution-alized spouse's income was looked to as the first available resource for increasing the noninstitutionalized spouse's income up to the MMMNA. However, the section of MCCA dealing with allowable de-ductions from the institutionalized spouse's income stated that the deduction for the support of the spouse living in the community could be deducted only "to the extent income of the institutionalized spouse is made available to (or for the benefit of) the community spouse." Medicaid estate planning attorneys argued that this section implied that the institutionalized spouse did not have to make his or her income available to the noninstitutionalized spouse before deter-mining the additional resources that the noninstitutionalized spouse would need to bring his or her income up to the MMMNA.

If the income of the institutionalized spouse was not tapped first to bring the income of the noninstitutionalized spouse up to the MMMNA, significant amounts of assets could be preserved by having the institutionalized spouse not make his or her income avail-able to his or her spouse. For example, assume that all of the income of an institutionalized spouse was used to pay for the cost of nursing home care, and the spouse living in the community had zero income of his or her own. If the total assets of both spouses were invested in holdings yielding 5 percent per year, the noninstitutionalized spouse could retain assets of $448,920 and still have an income below the 1995 maximum MMMNA of $1,871 per month.

Elder law attorneys argued that the policy should be to raise the CSRA of the noninstitutionalized spouse without looking first to the income from the institutionalized spouse, because the institutional-ized spouse's income could be transitory. As a result, allowing the spouse living in the community to retain enough assets to support himself or herself if the institutionalized spouse should die was important. This argument has some merit. However, income support from the institutionalized spouse may not necessarily cease at his or her death. For example, spousal benefits under social security would continue to be paid following the death of the institutionalized spouse, as would survivors benefits from private pensions (if they have been elected). Some income sources, such as life insurance benefits, could become available only upon the death of the institutionalized spouse.

The strategy of raising the CSRA level through the fair hearing process was most frequently cited by eligibility workers in Massachusetts. Medicaid applicants in the other three states generally did not use the approach, partly because other techniques were equally successful and did not require applicants to go through a fair hearing process. The three eligibility offices in Massachusetts reported five to fifteen fair hearings appeals per month to raise the CSRA in this manner. The workers also found the whole process frustrating because they were forced to initially deny eligibility to the applicant, then looked like the bad guys when the application was approved during the fair hearing process.

At the time of our site visit in December 1993, Massachusetts was not first looking to the income of the institutionalized spouse to increase the income of the noninstitutionalized spouse up to the MMMNA before increasing the CSRA. However, the state was in the process of issuing new regulations to change the methodology by applying the "income first" rule and subsequently implemented that change in June 1994.

In March 1994 the Medicaid Bureau of the Health Care Financing Administration (HCFA) issued a memorandum stating that because MCCA was not specific on the income first rule, states were free to adopt their own reasonable interpretation of MCCA on the issue: "We would now like to clarify that states have the option to use the 'income first' rule or to apply some other reasonable interpretation of the law until we have issued final regulations which specifically address this issue."[18]

The income first rule was also being contested in the courts. In a series of court cases in Ohio, the state initially won a case that determined that the state had the right to apply the income first rule, but two subsequent appeals court decisions said that MCCA was "unambiguous" on the issue and that the statute called for increasing the MMMNA through a raising of the CSRA level first, before tapping the institutionalized spouse's income.[19] In 1995 a federal class action suit was also pending in Pennsylvania contending that the state had not provided applicants with any information regarding their rights to seek an increase in the MMMNA by raising the CSRA above the federal maximum.[20]

Raising the CSRA through Court Orders

Another medicaid planning technique for raising the CSRA above the federal maximum was through a court order. MCCA stated that, if a court issued an order that required an institutionalized spouse to provide monthly income or assets to the spouse living in the community, the court order took precedence over the usual medicaid CSRA limits. As with the income first rule, however, the use of court orders to raise the CSRA above the allowed maximums was controversial and subject to various interpretations.

During our site visits, we had found evidence of court orders to raise the CSRA in California, Massachusetts, and New York. This technique was particularly common in California, and had become a routine strategy in some counties. Without further congressional clarification, the use of this medicaid planning technique could grow dramatically.

MEDICAID PLANNING TECHNIQUES FOR SINGLE PERSONS

Unlike married persons, medicaid applicants who were single could not take advantage of strategies that involved diverting assets or income to a nonapplicant spouse. Thus, other planning techniques were more frequently used by unmarried applicants.

Planned Gifting

Perhaps the largest loophole in medicaid law and regulation that allowed significant transfers of assets was, ironically, the policy on transfer of asset penalties itself. MCCA amended the medicaid statute to clarify how states should treat cases in which asset transfers took place, including the imposition of transfer of asset penalties. In general, states were required to impose periods of ineligibility when an applicant transferred a substantial amount of assets in the thirty-month period before applying for medicaid coverage. For example, if John Smith transferred $100,000 to his daughter on Monday and then applied for medicaid on Tuesday, claiming he had no assets of his own, the state was required to impose a period of ineligibility on Mr. Smith, which would render him ineligible for medicaid coverage until the penalty period ran out. The loophole was created in how Congress required states to determine the period of ineligibility. First, the length of the period of ineligibility was determined by dividing the amount of the transfer by the average monthly cost of private nursing home care. If the average private cost of nursing home care was $3,000 per month and an applicant transferred $12,000 before applying for medicaid, then a four-month period of ineligibility would be imposed. More important, however, MCCA stipulated that the period of ineligibility for asset transfers must be imposed from the *date of the transfer.* In effect, it allowed any applicant to protect at least half of his or her total assets (see box on transfer of assets penalty policy on page 77).

The transfer of asset penalty policy allowed any individual to transfer half of his or her assets at any time, to use the remaining half to pay for private nursing home care, and to always have the period of ineligibility expire by the time the remaining assets were depleted. The elder law industry commonly referred to this planning technique as the "half a loaf" method, because one could always save at least half of one's assets through this technique, and "half a loaf is better than none."

In our site visits, the "half a loaf" method was by far the most common medicaid planning technique being used by nonmarried applicants. It was simple, foolproof, and entirely in compliance with medicaid law. Eligibility workers indicated that only rarely did they identify an asset transfer in a medicaid application that resulted in a delay in approving medicaid eligibility, because in almost all cases, the period of ineligibility on an identified transfer expired by the time the application was made.

Congressional staff agreed that computing the period of ineligibility from the date of the transfer created a loophole for the medicaid estate planning industry, but they claimed that the policy was

TRANSFER OF ASSETS PENALTY POLICY

The following scenario demonstrates how the medicaid transfer of asset penalty policy allows applicants to protect at least half of their total assets:

In July 1994 Mrs. Gage, an eighty-six-year-old widow, fell in her apartment and broke her hip. After a hospitalization, she was admitted to a nursing home. Medicare covered her first twenty-one days in the nursing home in full, and Mrs. Gage's medigap coverage paid the $87.50 medicare copayment requirement for the twenty-second to the one hundredth day. However, after one hundred days in a nursing home, Mrs. Gage still could not get up or walk without assistance and therefore could not be discharged. She thus had to pay the $120 per day nursing home charge out of her own resources. She had $42,000 in savings in certificates of deposit.

At this point, Mrs. Gage's son sought the counsel of a medicaid estate planning attorney to inquire what he can do to prevent his mother from depleting all of her assets in paying for her care. The attorney counseled Mrs. Gage's son to have his mother transfer half of her assets to her children. As counseled, Mrs. Gage transferred $21,000 to her son and daughter. Almost six months later, Mrs. Gage depleted her remaining assets to $2,000, and she applied for medicaid. For having transferred the $21,000 to her children six months previously, the medicaid eligibility worker imposed a period of ineligibility on Mrs. Gage. The worker computed the period of ineligibility by dividing the amount transferred ($21,000) by the average private cost of nursing home care in the state, which was determined to be $3,600. The penalty period was thus 5.83 months. By statute, the period of ineligibility was also stipulated to begin on the date of the transfer, which was six months before the date that Mrs. Gage applied for medicaid. As a result, by the time Mrs. Gage applied for medicaid, the period of ineligibility had already expired and the eligibility worker approved Mrs. Gage's medicaid coverage effective immediately.

consistent with congressional intent. The provision was fashioned to protect the little guy from being unduly penalized for ingenuous transfers. One example would be if a grandmother made a $10,000 gift to her son and six months later needed to go to a nursing home. Congress wanted to protect such individuals from having states impose periods of ineligibility when relatively small amounts of funds were transferred or given away without any intent of depleting assets for medicaid planning purposes. The application of penalty periods in such cases could result in real hardship—for example, if applicants depleted their assets yet were also denied eligibility for medicaid.

Trusts

A major thrust of OBRA 93 was to limit the use of trusts as a medicaid planning device. In September 1994, HCFA issued state Medicaid Manual instructions implementing the OBRA 93 trust provisions, which, while not having the force of law, reflected HCFA's regulatory intent. These provisions provided important clarifications to states on how assets held in a trust, as well as income generated by the principal in a trust, were to be counted in the medicaid eligibility process.[21] Important components of the new provisions included the following:

—Assets held in a revocable trust were always counted as available to the applicant for medicaid eligibility purposes;

—Payments made from a revocable trust to any individual or third party other than the applicant were to be treated as a transfer of assets;

—Any income or principal that could be paid from an irrevocable trust to the applicant was counted as an available resource;

—If no circumstances existed under which income or principal from an irrevocable trust could be paid to the applicant, then income and principal were not considered available to the applicant. All such income and principal was considered a transfer of assets for sixty months before the medicaid application date;

—Transfers of a home into an irrevocable trust was to be counted as a transfer of assets, because a home no longer was considered an excluded asset when transferred; and

—Certain types of trusts were exempted from OBRA 93, including special needs trusts, pooled trusts, and income-only or Miller trusts.

Our site visits to the four states were conducted before the issuance of the HCFA state Medicaid Manual instructions, but the OBRA 93 provisions clearly had made an impact on reducing the number of trusts being written for medicaid planning purposes. For example, presenters at a continuing legal education seminar in Boston recommended that attorneys not write any medicaid planning trusts until HCFA implementing instructions were issued, and one elder law attorney said he stopped writing trust instruments altogether, because, as an attorney, his fiduciary obligation was not to bring his client's financial interests into jeopardy.

Although trusts were used as a medicaid planning tool in some cases, their use before implementation of the OBRA 93 provisions was not widespread. Eligibility workers reported seeing trusts relatively infrequently, maybe one or two per month in their normal caseload. Trusts were more often encountered by workers in Massachusetts and New York than in California or Florida.

Annuities

An annuity is a financial instrument that pays a fixed income stream over a defined period of time in return for an initial payment of principal. For example, an individual may buy an annuity for $50,000 that pays him a fixed income of $420 per month over his remaining lifetime. Annuities have been used as a medicaid planning tool because they are an easy and effective way to quickly convert assets to income.

However, a medicaid applicant who purchased an irrevocable annuity that paid a fixed income stream over his remaining lifetime has not sheltered any assets, because the income from the annuity must be used to partially offset the cost of his nursing home care. In this manner, purchasing an annuity only allowed a prospective medicaid applicant to pay later rather than sooner. Instead of depleting one's assets and then applying for medicaid, an individual could purchase an annuity, immediately become medicaid eligible, and pay a higher proportion of his nursing home bill because his monthly income was augmented by annuity payments.

Annuities were effective medicaid planning devices, however, if the income received from the annuity was not actuarially equivalent to the principal payment. For example, if an eighty-year-old male purchased a twenty-year annuity, with any remaining payments to be made to heirs upon the purchaser's death, then the purchaser successfully sheltered assets for heirs.

In our study, we found that annuities were most frequently used as a medicaid planning tool in California. Under existing California regulations, irrevocable annuities were not considered an available resource as long as the purchaser was receiving "periodic payments of interest and principal" from the annuity. However, the regulations were silent on whether the periodic payments had to be actuarially equivalent to the purchase price of the annuity. An obvious and relatively common technique of medicaid planners was to use an applicant's excess assets to purchase an annuity, but then have the annuity make periodic payments of interest and principal of minimal amounts, with any remaining principal and interest passing to heirs on the purchaser's death. For example, one eligibility office in California encountered an annuity worth more than $500,000, which only made payments of principal and interest of $5,000 per year (about 1 percent).

The OBRA 93 provisions required that, in regard to transfer of asset rules and the countability of resources, annuities be treated in a manner similar to trusts. In a state Medicaid Manual transmission issued in November 1994, HCFA provided clarification on how annuities were to be treated for medicaid eligibility purposes. The transmittal adopted the position that to be excluded as a countable resource the expected return on the annuity must be commensurate with a reasonable estimate of the life expectancy of the beneficiary. If not, the beneficiary was presumed not to have received fair market value for the annuity, and a transfer of assets penalty should be imposed on the difference between the fair market value and the actual rate of return. For example, if an eighty-year-old male purchased a $10,000 annuity with a payout period of ten years, but the remaining life expectancy for an eighty-year-old male was only 6.98 years, a transfer of assets penalty should be applied to the amount that would be paid to the beneficiary between 6.98 years and 10 years. In the state Medicaid Manual transmission, HCFA included life expectancy tables by age and gender that states and local eligibility offices could use to assess the actuarial equivalency of annuities.

Spending

Spending money, although not a medicaid estate planning strategy per se, was a simple way for medicaid applicants to reduce their assets to medicaid eligibility thresholds. Medicaid eligibility workers indicated that applications often were denied because of excess resources of relatively small amounts. For example, an applicant with savings of $9,000 would be $7,000 over the medicaid eligibility level of $2,000. In these cases, workers would often advise applicants to spend excess resources on purchases that were excluded in the eligibility determination process. Applicants could be advised to pay off mortgages, credit card debt, and automobile loans; to make home repairs or improvements; or to make some major purchases, such as appliances, furniture, and so forth.

There is nothing illegal about depleting one's assets through simply spending money, and unlike other medicaid planning techniques, the amount of assets involved were generally minimal. Reducing assets to medicaid eligibility levels was easy through these kinds of purchases for applicants who had relatively few assets. Though not required to do so, eligibility workers reported that they often felt an obligation to inform applicants with few assets of the things they could do to deplete their assets by spending money, instead of depleting assets on private nursing home care, particularly when workers saw other applicants sheltering significant amounts of wealth with the assistance of elder law attorneys.

Joint Accounts

Before enactment of OBRA 93, another medicaid planning technique in some states was to transfer assets through joint bank accounts. For example, in Florida, assets could be quickly transferred by adding a joint signatory to an applicant's bank account and then having the joint signatory withdraw all funds from the account. Until OBRA 93 was enacted, medicaid policy in Florida ruled that such actions could not be considered as transfers of assets, because the applicant himself had not actively transferred the funds, and the joint owner of the account had every right to withdraw the funds without the applicant's approval.

OBRA 93 clarified that transfers of jointly held assets that reduced the applicant's ownership or control of the assets was an illegal transfer subject to penalties. Joint signatories had the right to withdraw funds from a joint account, but the applicant must demonstrate that the withdrawal of those funds did not constitute a transfer of assets previously owned by the applicant. After OBRA 93 was enacted, Florida changed its policy expeditiously, and this medicaid planning technique was no longer a viable option.

Burial Trusts

Most states allowed funds in an irrevocable burial trust to be excluded in determining eligibility for medicaid, so that applicants could set aside funds to prepay their funeral expenses without having their eligibility for medicaid affected. These excluded funds were in addition to the $1,500 allowed under federal medicaid law that could be excluded for the purchase of a burial plot. Anecdotes described applicants sheltering significant amounts of assets in irrevocable burial accounts, with the implication that the trustees of such accounts (for example, a funeral home) could transfer funds not used for funeral expenses to the heirs of the medicaid recipient after the funeral was over.

Although eligibility workers in all the case study states were asked whether they ever observed funds being sheltered in irrevocable burial accounts, little evidence existed that this was happening. The most notable exception was in Suffolk County, New York, where eligibility workers reported that they occasionally saw very large prepaid burial accounts (for example, bronze caskets costing $20,000 to $30,000). In general, however, a worker could, albeit rarely, come across a burial contract for an amount that seemed excessive, but we uncovered little evidence that burial accounts were being used as a medicaid planning tool in the four states.

ESTATE RECOVERY PROGRAMS

Another component of medicaid estate planning was protecting assets still held by medicaid recipients while they were alive (primarily the medicaid recipient's home, but also other assets that were excluded in the medicaid eligibility determination process) from being recovered by states after the medicaid recipient died. The process of recouping costs incurred by medicaid recipients in nursing homes from their estates after their death is called estate recovery. Before OBRA 93, medicaid estate planning to protect these assets from state recovery was not needed in many instances, because half the states did not operate estate recovery programs. However, an important provision of OBRA was to require all states to implement estate recovery programs.

In most states that operate estate recovery programs the process works something like this:

—Medicaid recovery staff collect information from various sources on all recent decedents, all recent decedents who were enrolled in medicaid before their death, or all decedents in nursing homes;

—Names (and other identifying information) of decedents are matched against medicaid enrollment and claims files to determine the amount of medicaid payments made for medicaid-covered services used by decedents before their death;

—If a match is found, a notification letter is sent to the executor of the estate and to prospective heirs indicating the amount of the state's claim against the medicaid recipient's estate;

—The state's claim against the estate is resolved in accordance with state law regarding the relative precedence of alternative creditors against an estate. For example, the claim of medicaid estate recovery programs against the estate is usually secondary to the claims of funeral homes and estate administrators; and

—In addition, if the state imposed a lien on the home of the medicaid recipient, the lien is not released (and, therefore, the home cannot be sold) until the state's claim is settled.

Although most states that operated recovery programs used a process similar to this, the estate recovery programs of the four case study states differed widely in their characteristics and effectiveness. California and Massachusetts administrated aggressive estate recovery programs that were centralized at the state level. Both programs were run in a manner similar to the model outlined, with some differences.

Massachusetts placed a notification lien on the principal residence of single nursing home clients who were not likely to be discharged. Notification liens alerted the Medicaid Department of any change in the ownership of the home so that the state was able to seek recoveries for medicaid long-term care expenditures. Notification would be sent to the state upon the death of the institutionalized person and also when the institutionalized person was still living but had attempted to transfer title of the home to someone other than a spouse. The California recovery program was largely similar to that of Massachusetts. The most important difference was that California did not place liens on the principal residence of single medicaid nursing home clients. Another difference was that California sought recovery only from probated estates with assets of $500 or more. The state did not consider pursuing recovery from estates smaller than this cost efficient, because any assets were typically exhausted by the cost of administering the estate and funeral bills.

In New York, estate recovery was a county responsibility, which, predictably, resulted in considerable variability across counties. One county had no program, while others (for example, Nassau, New York [Manhattan], and Suffolk counties) had fairly aggressive programs. Like Massachusetts, most counties in New York placed liens on the homes of single nursing home clients. New York also allowed recovery from the estates of noninstitutionalized spouses when the community spouse died. Recovery from the community spouse's estate was problematic, however, because the New York Medicaid Department had no systematic way of identifying community spouses who had died and a recent court case had greatly restricted the ability of counties to seek recovery from the estates of community spouses.

Florida had the weakest estate recovery program of the four states. Florida's estate recovery program basically consisted of a contract with one attorney who was responsible for seeking medicaid recoveries across the state. Also, Florida's constitutional protection of the homestead from creditors severely restricted the ability of medicaid to seek recoveries from the home equity of deceased nursing home clients. Thus, opportunities for recovery were extremely limited. Nevertheless, Florida was attempting to step up its activities in the recovery area—even considering the possibility of changing the homestead exemption in the state constitution.

Seeking Recovery from the Surviving Spouse's Estate

In contrast to the estates of most single medicaid nursing home clients, the estates of community spouses may contain substantial financial and real property assets. As such, estate recovery programs could realize significant collections from the estates of community spouses when they die.

Two primary obstacles prevented successful medicaid recoveries from the estates of community spouses. The first problem arose because most states did not keep a registry of community spouses. Consequently, the state could have no way of knowing when the community spouse died. Without this knowledge, states had no possibility of seeking recoveries from the estates of former community spouses. The second problem was that the assets could be transferred to a third party (such as a child) before the community spouse died. As a result, the assets were no longer in the estate of the community spouse when the state attempted to recover the cost of long-term care for the institutionalized spouse.

Both obstacles could be overcome if medicaid law were amended to allow liens to be placed on the estates of surviving spouses. In 1993 only ten of the twenty-seven states operating estate recovery programs pursued recoveries from the estates of community spouses.

CONCLUSION

Although long-term care eligibility workers reported that a clear minority of medicaid applicants participated in medicaid estate planning activity, workers in all four case study states indicated that medicaid estate planning by some applicants remained a policy problem. The provisions of OBRA 93 that were designed to address medicaid estate planning strategies were generally viewed as necessary and effective, but many of the techniques used by the medicaid estate planning industry remained unaffected by existing medicaid law or were made possible by ambiguities that remained in existing statutes. Additional reforms would be needed to further mitigate opportunities for nonpoor elderly applicants to shelter or divest their assets before applying for medicaid coverage.

Options for Further Federal Reform

Should Congress decide to enact further reforms to tighten the medicaid eligibility system for long-term care coverage and to pursue estate recovery efforts more aggressively, many options are available that were not addressed in OBRA 93.

1. *Amend federal law to limit transfers from the community spouse to a third party "for the sole benefit of the community spouse."*

OBRA 93 precluded states from imposing transfer of asset penalties on transfers "from the individual's spouse to another for the sole benefit of the spouse." This provision created a loophole that allowed married couples the option of transferring all of their jointly held assets to the community spouse before applying for medicaid and then transferring all of the community spouse's assets to a third party for the sole benefit of the community spouse. For example, the community spouse could use all of the couple's assets to purchase an actuarially equivalent annuity that converted all of his or her assets to an income stream paid solely to the community spouse. Because income of married couples is treated separately in the medicaid eligibility process, no limit is imposed on the amount of assets that can be protected through this planning technique. A community spouse could potentially convert $1 million to an actuarially equivalent annuity, and thus shelter all of the assets in this manner. Further, because the community spouse is not required to contribute to the cost of care for the institutionalized spouse, none of the income received by the community spouse from such an annuity is required to help pay for the institutionalized spouse's care. One option is to limit transfers of this type to those that would increase the community spouse's assets to the maximum CSRA allowed. Transfers that would increase the community spouse's assets above the CSRA could be treated as transfers subject to penalty. An additional option would be to pool the income as well as the resources of both spouses in the initial determination of eligibility for the institutionalized spouse and only allow the community spouse to retain income up to the MMMNA level.

2. *Address the "half a loaf" strategy by changing the date on which the transfer of asset penalty period begins.*

The success of the "half a loaf" strategy is related to the penalty period for transfers, which begins on the date of the transfer. An alternative option that would preclude applicants from using this strategy is to begin the penalty period on the date the applicant would otherwise be eligible for medicaid. If an applicant transferred $20,000 in July 1994 and applied for medicaid in January 1995 (and was determined eligible), the penalty period could begin in January 1995, not July 1994. Should the asset transfer provision be so revised, some flexibility could be retained in the new provision so that applicants who had unwittingly transferred relatively small amounts of assets before application are not unduly penalized.

3. *Amend federal medicaid law to clarify the circumstances under which an institutionalized spouse in long-term care should be deemed eligible for medicaid when the community spouse refuses to support the institutionalized spouse.*

Applicants would be precluded from using the "just say no" strategy as was being used in New York state to preserve all of a married couple's assets for the community spouse. The amendment could clarify that evidence of true abandonment by the community spouse is necessary before an institutionalized spouse could be deemed eligible for medicaid without counting the resources of the community spouse as available to the institutionalized spouse.

4. *Clarify the rights of medicaid estate recovery programs to recover from the estates of surviving spouses of deceased medicaid recipients.*

Medicaid law prohibits states from placing liens on the homes of surviving spouses during the life of the institutionalized spouse receiving medicaid. At the same time, the medicaid spousal impoverishment provisions and various medicaid estate planning strategies increased opportunities for community spouses to retain much higher levels of assets while the institutionalized spouse received medicaid coverage for his or her nursing home care. Most states did not pursue recovery from the estates of surviving spouses. The legality of placing liens upon the homes of surviving spouses upon the death of the institutionalized spouse on medicaid is ambiguous in federal law. Congress should clarify federal law in regard to the right of states to protect their claims through the placement of liens on the property of surviving spouses after the death of the institutionalized spouse.

5. *Clarify federal law on the income first rule and the use of court orders for raising the CSRA.*

Congress could clarify whether the income of the institutionalized spouse needs to be looked to first in bringing the community spouse's income up to the MMMNA, before increasing the CSRA through a fair hearing process. Congress might also wish to clarify the circumstances under which asset levels specified in court orders for a community spouse are to be used in place of the usual CSRA limits.

6. *Stipulate that transfer of asset penalties can also be applied when transfers have been made to avoid estate recovery.*

This change would clarify that states can impose transfer of asset penalties on transfers of exempt assets, such as the home, as well as nonexempt assets. California does not currently apply transfer of asset penalties on transfers of the home.

7. *Allow or require medicaid applicants to provide copies of federal tax returns as documentation of their financial situation in the medicaid eligibility process.*

Federal income tax returns provide useful information that could be used to verify the income and assets reported on medicaid applications. For instance, unearned income from savings accounts, stocks, bonds, trusts, and so on are reported on Schedule B. Property taxes on real property (regardless of the location of the property) are reported as deductions on Schedule A. Gifts in excess of $10,000 are also reported. The confidentiality of federal tax return data was a barrier to requiring applicants to submit these data as part of the medicaid application process in some states.

The Future of Medicaid Estate Planning

The OBRA 93 medicaid eligibility and estate recovery provisions affected the ability of medicaid long-term care recipients to shelter or divest their assets, but they were not the final step. Medicaid estate planning is by no means dead, and it never will be, as long as medicaid coverage of nursing home care remains a means-tested benefit. Opportunities will always be available for elderly people to manage their financial assets to maximize the financial security of a community spouse or to preserve inheritances for heirs. The divestiture of financial assets by elderly persons is done for a large number of reasons other than for medicaid estate planning, so medicaid planning strategies will remain a component of an elderly individual's overall portfolio strategy. In addition, as long as the incentives created by existing public policy remain as they are, it is reasonable to expect that elderly individuals will act in an economically rational manner. Chastising the behavior of individuals who do medicaid estate planning is unfair, when the economic incentives for doing so are so compelling, and it is not illegal.

Eligibility workers were consistent in reporting a higher level of medicaid estate planning activity among married applicants than among unmarried applicants. First, a greater incentive existed to preserve financial assets in the case of married applicants. Second, married couples, on average, had more wealth to protect than applicants without spouses. And third, more opportunities were available in existing medicaid eligibility provisions to pursue medicaid estate planning in the case of married applicants. The majority of eligibility workers interviewed felt that current policy was inequitable in regard to the fairly liberal protections afforded married applicants, compared with the relatively restrictive requirement that single applicants are allowed to retain only $2,000 in liquid assets. Further, many felt that current policy was unfair to people, who while not married, shared financial resources in their households, such as siblings who had lived together for many years, or widows and widowers who lived together but preferred not to remarry.

One future trend is fairly predictable—that medicaid eligibility provisions and estate recovery policies will become increasingly specific. Elder law attorneys readily admitted that the medicaid estate planning business depended upon the nooks and crannies of medicaid eligibility policy and that compared with the Internal Revenue Service code, many more vagaries in medicaid law could be exploited to the benefit of their clientele. As the medicaid estate planning business continues to develop and devise new medicaid planning techniques, and medicaid policymakers continue to respond to these techniques, increasing specificity will be seen in medicaid law and regulation regarding allowable versus unallowable transfers, how transfer of asset penalties are to be applied, what is and what is not a countable asset, and what mechanisms are available to states to seek recovery of assets held in the estates of deceased medicaid recipients and their spouses after their deaths.

A relationship exists between the future course of public policy regarding medicaid estate planning and the potential growth of private long-term care insurance products. Both medicaid estate planning and private long-term care insurance (or similar risk protection products such as continuing care retirement communities) represent alternative asset protection strategies for elderly persons with substantial assets. To the extent that medicaid estate planning becomes a less viable option, the demand for alternative risk protection products may increase accordingly.

Aside from the overarching issue of how liberal or restrictive medicaid coverage of nursing home care should be, policymakers must address issues of fairness and equity. Medicaid estate planning is often rationalized on the basis that medicaid benefits are not only means tested—they are also basically mean. The more the perception persists that public coverage of nursing home care is unfair, the more willing people will be to circumvent the system through medicaid planning. If the means-testing of medicaid long-term care benefits was perceived as more fair, fewer applicants may feel justified in protecting their wealth through medicaid estate planning techniques. For example, some support is evident for raising the medicaid asset threshold above the existing $2,000 limit, so that single medicaid recipients can at least leave some modest inheritance to heirs. Others have argued for a homestead exemption to protect homes of modest value (for example, $50,000 or less) from estate recovery.

The policy refinements that need to be made to medicaid statutes to combat the use of medicaid estate planning techniques may seem highly technical and arcane, but their importance should not be underestimated if medicaid is to remain a health insurance program for people who are truly poor.

NOTES

1. This study represents the third in a series of studies on medicaid estate planning and public policy responses to medicaid estate planning. The two earlier studies were Brian Burwell, *Middle-Class Welfare: Medicaid Estate Planning for Long-Term Care Coverage* (Lexington, Mass.: SysteMetrics, September 1991); and Brian Burwell, *State Responses to Medicaid Estate Planning* (Cambridge, Mass.: SysteMetrics/MEDSTAT, May 1993).

2. The penalty period is the length of time an applicant who would otherwise be medicaid eligible is denied eligibility because he or she transferred assets before making an application.

3. These fifteen states are Alabama, Alaska, Arizona, Arkansas, Colorado, Delaware, Florida, Idaho, Iowa, Mississippi, Nevada, New Jersey, New Mexico, South Dakota, and Wyoming.

4. In contrast, median net worth for nonelderly households has declined.

5. A good example of such a newsletter is the *ElderLaw Report* published by Little, Brown and Company, Law Division, 34 Beacon St., Boston, Mass. 02108.

6. See, for example, Peter Kemper and Christopher Murtaugh, "Lifetime Use of Nursing Home Care," *New England Journal of Medicine*, vol. 342, no. 9 (1991), pp. 595–600.

7. See, for example, Steven Moses, *The Magic Bullet: How to Pay for Universal Long-Term Care: A Case Study of Illinois* (LTC Incorporated, February 1995).

8. See, for example, Joshua Wiener, Raymond Hanley, and Katherine Harris, "The Economic Status of Elderly Nursing Home Users," Brookings, January 1994. See also Frank A. Sloan and Mary W. Shayne, "Long-Term Care, Medicaid, and Impoverishment of the Elderly," *Milbank Quarterly*, vol. 71, no. 4 (1993), pp. 575–600.

9. See, for example, *Medicaid Estate Recovery under OBRA '93: Picking the Bones of the Poor?*, a report by the Commission on Legal Problems of the Elderly (Washington: American Bar Association, November 1994).

10. General Accounting Office, *Medicaid Estate Planning*, GAO/HRD-93-29R (1993).

11. An income cap state is one that has elected not to provide medically needy coverage for medicaid recipients in nursing homes, but instead to provide coverage for nursing home residents under a special income cap that by federal law cannot exceed 300 percent of the federal benefit level for the SSI program.

12. The income cap in Florida in 1994 was $1,338 per month, 300 percent of the federal SSI benefit level for a single individuals, which was $446.

13. In 1995 the minimum amount of assets that the spouse living in the community was allowed to retain (even if it equaled more than half of the couple's total assets) was $14,964. The maximum amount (even if it was less than half) was $74,850.

14. For a summary of medicaid eligibility for nursing home coverage see William Crown, Brian Burwell, and Lisa Maria B. Alecxih, *An Analysis of Asset Testing for Nursing Home Benefits* (Washington: American Association of Retired Persons, Public Policy Institute, 1994).

15. In January 1995 the minimum MMMNA was $1,230 per month (150 percent of the federal poverty level for a couple), and the maximum was $1,871 per month.

16. Sec. 1924(c)(3).

17. For a more detailed explanation of this provision, see, for example, Burwell, *Middle-Class Welfare*, pp. 22–23.

18. Memorandum from Sally K. Richardson, director of the Medicaid Bureau, Health Care Financing Administration, to all regional administrators, March 3, 1994.

19. See *Kimnach v. Ohio Department of Human Services* (Ct. of Common Pleas, Franklin County, No. 93CVF-06-4191, February 14, 1994); *Kimnach v. Ohio Department of Human Services* (Ohio Ct. App., Franklin County, No. 93APEO4-520, 1994 WL 484660, September 8, 1994); and *Gruber v. Ohio Dept. of Human Services* (Ohio Appt. Ct., No. 94CAE06015, 1994, WL 667869, October 28, 1994). These cases are also summarized in the *ElderLaw Report*, vol. 6 (July/August 1994), no. 3 (October 1994), and no. 6 (January 1995), respectively.

20. See Kenneth M. Coughlin, "Class Action Suit Challenges Pennsylvania's 'Income First' Rule," *ElderLaw Report*, vol. 6, no. 1 (July/August 1994).

21. For a more detailed discussion on the use of trusts as a medicaid planning device before enactment of the Omnibus Budget Reconciliation Act of 1993, see Burwell, *State Responses to Medicaid Estate Planning*.

PART 3
Use and Expenditures for Paid Services

Chapter 5

LISA MARIA B. ALECXIH, JOHN COREA,
AND DAVID L. KENNELL

♦

Implications of Health Care Financing, Delivery, and Benefit Design for Persons with Disabilities

Previous studies have found that persons with disabilities use health care services more than those without disabilities.[1] One study found that compared with persons with no limiting conditions, per capita medical expenditures were three times as high for persons with one limiting chronic condition and five times as high for persons with two or more limiting conditions.[2] Average program expenditures of medicare and medicaid, which finance much of the health care for persons with disabilities, are also higher for disabled beneficiaries than for those in other eligibility categories.[3] For medicaid beneficiaries, long-term care costs (particularly nursing home care) for persons with disabilities account for much of the difference. However, acute care costs are also higher for disabled medicare beneficiaries than for aged medicare beneficiaries.[4]

Expenditures for persons with disabilities make up a substantial portion of the total cost of government health programs, particularly medicaid. Payments for blind and disabled persons accounted for the largest share of medicaid expenditures in 1993, and, until recently, grew faster than any other medicaid eligibility category.[5]

Partly because of rising expenditures for persons with disabilities, medicare and medicaid are under heavy pressure to reduce spending. As a result, states, for example, are increasingly moving beneficiaries into health maintenance organizations as a way to achieve cost savings. Managing service use is particularly relevant for "dual eligibles"— persons covered by both medicare and medicaid, who typically have acute and long-term care needs. Services are often not well coordinated for this group, which may lead to even higher health care costs.[6] Pressures to reduce costs make understanding the utilization patterns of persons with disabilities particularly important, not only to suggest where the savings opportunities lie but also because faulty interventions could have serious adverse consequences for this vulnerable population.

In this study, we present findings from the household sample of the 1987 National Medical Expenditures Survey (NMES), the most recent data source available with utilization and expenditure information for a representative sample of the U.S. noninstitutionalized population. We examined the NMES data to see how utilization and expenditures of persons with disabilities differed from those of persons without disabilities.[7] Our findings have important implications for efforts to change the health care financing and delivery system, including limits on the growth of medicare and medicaid expenditures, increased use of managed care and integrated delivery systems, and changes in beneficiary copayment and deductibles.

METHODOLOGY

We analyzed data from the 1987 NMES to estimate health care use and expenditures for persons with and without disabilities.[8] The household sample was part of a government-sponsored national survey that provided data on the sociodemographic characteristics and annual health care use and expenditures of a representative sample of the noninstitutionalized civilian population. Respondents were interviewed five times over a sixteen-month period. Included in the survey were questions concerning the use, expenditures, and sources of payment for different types of care. Sources of payment included private insurance, medicaid, medicare, other third-party payers, and out-of-pocket expenditures. Information reported about visit charges from respondents was verified with the providers of the service.[9] Although costs for nursing home residents are an important source of expenditures for persons with disabilities, these individuals were not included in the sample population and therefore could not be included in this analysis.

The survey also included information about functional limitations often used to identify and measure the severity of disabilities for persons of all ages. In this study, we defined disability as limitation in at least one of five activities of daily living (ADLs) lasting three months or longer: bathing, dressing, using the bathroom, getting in and out of bed, and eating.[10] This definition allowed for a modest sample size (928 observations) while eliminating the majority of persons recovering from acute conditions.[11] Of the 928 persons with disabilities in the sample, 638 were age 65 or older. Persons with short-term impairments were excluded because we were interested in examining the use of services by persons with a chronic disability.

In examining health care utilization, this study focused on "users" of care. A user was defined as a person who had expenditures for any of the following: prescription medication, home and community-based care, durable medical equipment (DME), dental care, hospitalizations, physician office visits, outpatient department visits, and emergency room visits. The calculation of average expenditures for persons using any service included a small number of persons who used only prescription drugs or DME.[12]

Although significant changes have taken place in utilization and expenditure patterns since the data in the NMES were collected in 1987, differences between persons with disabilities and those without probably have not changed significantly. Our findings, however, must be viewed with the knowledge that, since 1987, expenditures increased for home and community-based care resulting from clarification of medicare payment policy and from medicaid changes, insurers continued to pressure providers to reduce expensive inpatient days, medical prices greatly escalated, and enrollment in managed care skyrocketed.

FINANCING, DELIVERY, AND BENEFIT DESIGN FOR PERSONS WITH DISABILITIES

The disproportionate use of health care resources by individuals with a disability has important implications for health care financing, delivery, and benefit design. Although persons with disabilities made up only 2 percent of the population in 1987, they accounted for about 13 percent of noninstitutional health expenditures. Per capita expenditures increased considerably with severity of disability, from $6,850 for those with one ADL limitation to approximately $12,600 for persons with two or more ADL limitations (table 5-1). The variety of

TABLE 5-1. *Per Capita Health Expenditures of Persons with Disabilities, by Level of Disability*

Dollars

Disability level	Nonelderly persons	Elderly persons	Total population
1 ADL	$ 5,671	$ 7,686	$ 6,850
2 ADLs	11,195	13,728	12,617
3+ ADLs	11,905	13,001	12,546
1+ ADLs	9,153	10,918	10,188

Source: Lewin-VHI analysis of 1987 National Medical Expenditure Survey data.
Note: Level of disability was based on the number of activities of daily living (ADLs) with which the person required assistance or supervision for three months or longer.

conditions causing disability, the wide range of medical and social interventions required by this population, and the heavy use of health care services by persons with disabilities presents distinct challenges to the health care system to provide appropriate and effective care in an efficient manner.

Financing Implications

The differences in total expenditures among persons with disabilities and those without disabilities have two major financing implications. First, higher health care use and expenditures for individuals with disabilities would affect any effort to make payments to providers on a capitated basis (that is, a fixed amount per enrollee). The higher costs for persons with disabilities underlines the need to compensate providers for anticipated differences in the resource use of covered populations in capitated payments systems. Second, financing reform designed to spread the cost of care for this population across broader segments of the populations (for example, community rating) would increase costs for those groups in which persons with disabilities are currently underrepresented (for example, those with private insurance).

Risk adjustment. Under either a voluntary or mandatory enrollment system, some health plans could attract disproportionately healthier or more impaired enrollees. Under a capitated payment method, a system that adjusts payments to account for differences in enrollees' health status will be important to encourage efficiencies and maintain quality of services. In their evaluation of medicare risk contracts with health maintenance organizations, Randall S. Brown and Jerold W. Hill highlighted the importance of an adequate risk adjustment system for medicare to achieve savings.[13] Using current methods, medicare overpays health maintenance organizations because it cannot adequately adjust for the tendency of healthier-than-average beneficiaries to enroll in managed care.

For persons who used services, overall 1987 expenditures for persons with disabilities were more than six times the level of those for persons without disabilities (figure 5-1). Some of the difference resulted from substantial demographic and economic variations. Most significantly, persons with disabilities were much more likely to be elderly, and utilization increased with advanced age. Persons with disabilities were also more likely to be female, less likely to be white, more likely to live alone, and more likely to have lower family incomes.

To control for population differences and to isolate the effect of disability on utilization and expenditures, we performed a series of regression analyses. We examined the independent effect of disability on (1) the likelihood of service use through a series of logistic regression models; (2) average expenditures through linear regressions on the logged expenditures among those using services; and (3) per capita expenditures by combining the models predicting use with those predicting expenditures among users. Each model controlled for the same set of independent effects: disability status, age, gender, race, family income, living arrangement, and insurance coverage.

Most of the difference in usage rates observed between persons with and without disabilities was preserved when controlling for differences in the populations (table 5-2). Persons with disabilities were 13 percent more likely to have health care expenditures than those without disabilities, and average expenditures for those users were 3.7 times as high for persons with disabilities. As a result, per capita health expenditures remained more than four times as high for persons with disabilities compared with persons without disabilities.

Although expenditures were higher for persons with disabilities, developing a risk adjustment system could be difficult because personal characteristics did not explain much of the variation in expenditures among patients. The regressions accounted for only 8.7

FIGURE 5-1. *Average Health Care Expenditures by Type of Service for Persons with Any Spending, Persons with and without Disabilities*

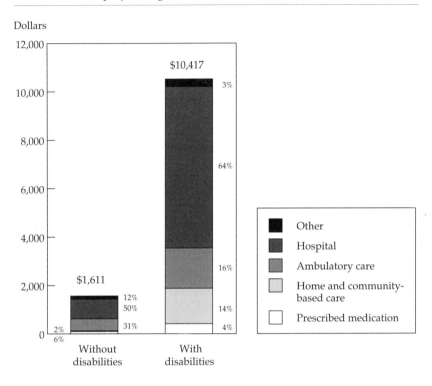

Source: Lewin-VHI analysis of 1987 National Medical Expenditure Survey data.

percent of the variation in use of services and 13.5 percent of the variation in expenditures among those using services. The limited ability to explain much of the variance in utilization or costs for individuals based on their personal characteristics has been documented by other researchers.[14] Without such a system for capitated payments, persons with disabilities could face discrimination in their attempts to join health plans and possible denial of needed services as health plans attempt to compensate for inadequate payment systems.

Community rating. Private insurers avoid much of the higher expenditures associated with disabilities because persons with disabilities often do not have private health insurance coverage. Most

TABLE 5-2. *Predicted Service Use and Expenditures*

Measure of service use	Persons without disabilities	Persons with disabilities	Ratio of persons with to those without disabilities
Probability of having expenditures[a]	0.86	0.97	1.1
Average expenditure among those with expenditures[b]	$426	$1,594	3.7
Per capita expenditures[c]	$367	$1,551	4.2

Source: Lewin-VHI analysis of 1987 National Medical Expenditure Survey data.

Note: All regressions controlled for disability status, age, gender, race, family income, living arrangement, and insurance coverage. Equations were evaluated at the mean values for the general population. See appendix for regression results.

a. Results from logistic regressions.

b. Results from linear regressions of logged expenditures. Predicted values represent median, not mean, expenditures.

c. Combined results from logistic regressions predicting use and linear regressions of logged expenditures among users.

nonelderly persons are insured through their employers, but persons with chronic disabilities are much less likely to be employed. Further, because they are less likely to be in the work force, their incomes are lower, making it difficult to purchase relatively expensive individual health insurance policies. In 1987, only 55 percent of persons with disabilities had private insurance coverage compared with 75 percent of persons without disabilities. Among nonelderly persons with disabilities, private insurance rates were even lower (43 percent versus 74 percent for those without disabilities). Elderly persons with disabilities were also substantially less likely to have private insurance to supplement medicare than those without disabilities (64 percent compared with 81 percent).

Persons with disabilities had slightly more than two-thirds (67.9 percent) of their health care expenses covered by government programs, primarily as a result of the medicare coverage for elderly persons and for some working-age individuals with disabilities (figure 5-2). Medicaid also picked up a larger share of expenditures for persons with disabilities than for those without disabilities (14 percent versus 7 percent), particularly for nonelderly individuals (26 percent versus 9 percent).[15] Expenditures for nonelderly persons with disabil-

FIGURE 5-2. *Average Expenditures by Payment Source, Persons with and without Disabilities*

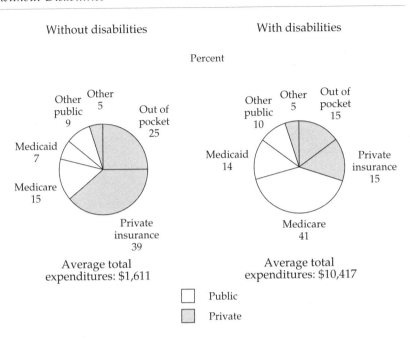

Source: Lewin-VHI analysis of 1987 National Medical Expenditure Survey data.

ities were spread more evenly among a variety of sources of payment than they were for elderly persons. Although medicare paid the majority of expenditures for elderly persons with disabilities, expenditures for nonelderly persons with disabilities came largely from medicaid and other public programs.

Public programs also disproportionately financed the difference in expenditures for persons with disabilities and those without disabilities (figure 5-3). Among elderly persons, medicare covered the majority of the difference in expenditures they faced if they had disabilities. Average health expenditures for those with disabilities were 1.9 times higher than those without disabilities ($11,164 compared with $3,853). Medicare covered 58 percent of this difference ($4,277).[16] Out-of-pocket payments covered another 18 percent ($1,287). Medicaid, private insurance, and (to a lesser extent) other sources made up the rest.

Among nonelderly persons, average health expenditures for those with disabilities were 6.2 time higher than for those persons without disabilities ($9,379 compared with $1,301). Medicaid covered the greatest portion of the large difference in expenditures between persons with and without disabilities (28 percent).[17] Medicare accounted for a slightly larger proportion (21 percent) of the difference than private insurance or other federal programs (16 percent and 15 percent, respectively). Out-of-pocket payments covered 6 percent of the difference.

During the health care reform debates of 1993 and 1994, several proposals were made to integrate younger persons with disabilities, including medicaid and medicare beneficiaries and uninsured individuals, into private insurance plans. Under these reforms, premiums for health insurance policies would be established on a community-rated basis; that is, premiums would be based on the average costs of everyone in the risk pool without regard to age, gender, preexisting condition, or disability status.

Because of the high health care expenditures of the disabled population, it was often noted that these reforms would increase health insurance premiums for nondisabled persons. However, despite these fears, including nonelderly persons with disabilities in community-rated health insurance plans would have only a limited impact on premiums because health expenditures for this population are a relatively small portion of overall health care costs. If private insurers were to absorb noninstitutional expenditures for nonelderly persons with disabilities, per capita annual spending for privately insured younger persons would have increased by only about $78 in 1987.[18] If persons with disabilities were more likely to enroll in certain health plans, the premium increase would be greater in those plans.

Delivery System Implications

Within each type of service, persons with disabilities were generally much more likely to use each type of service, and the average expenditures among users were also higher. Similar to the regressions for any use of health care services, we performed regressions for each type of service: hospital care, ambulatory care (physician, outpatient department, or emergency room visits), prescribed medication, and home and community-based care (table 5-3).

FIGURE 5-3. *Average Expenditures from Each Payment Source, by Age Group, Persons with and without Disabilities*

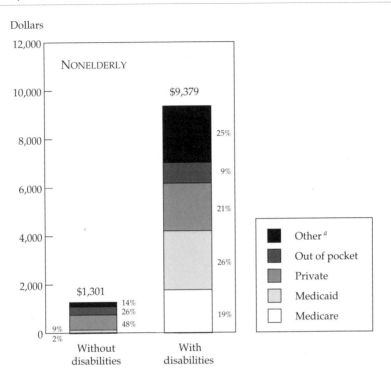

Controlling for other factors, hospital care expenditures for individuals with disabilities were nearly five times as high as for those without disabilities, as a result of both a higher probability of a hospital stay and higher expenditures for those with stays. Expenditures for prescribed medications were 3.8 times as high for persons with disabilities as those without. Finally, ambulatory care expenditures showed the least difference with a ratio of 2.3 times for persons with disabilities compared with persons without disabilities. The difference in ambulatory care expenditures stemmed primarily from the type of providers used. Among elderly persons, emergency room visits were more than twice as likely by those with disabilities (24 percent versus 11 percent), partly because the emergency room served as the entry point for many hospital stays. Among nonelderly individuals, 45 percent of persons with disabilities visited an outpa-

FIGURE 5-3. (continued)

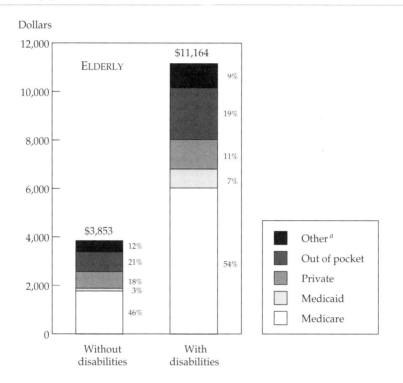

Source: Lewin-VHI analysis of 1987 National Medical Expenditure Survey data.
a.   Consisted of other federal and state programs, workers compensation, services provided free from provider, and other sources.

tient department compared with 16 percent of those without disabilities. High use of clinics by poor medicaid recipients (who had higher rates of disability) could be partly responsible for the large difference in outpatient department visits.

The most striking difference was in the use of and expenditures for home and community-based care services, which are generally targeted to people with chronic conditions that limit their activities. One-third (34 percent) of persons with disabilities used these services, while less than 2 percent of persons without disabilities used them. Nonelderly persons without disabilities either used these services after a hospital stay or received care during a short-term disability. Home and community-based care services were used more often by

TABLE 5-3. *Predicted Service Use and Expenditures by Type of Service*

Measure of service use	Persons without disabilities	Persons with disabilities	Ratio of persons with to those without disabilities
Hospitalization			
Probability of having expenditures[a]	0.07	0.18	2.7
Average expenditure among those with expenditures[b]	$4,557	$8,348	1.8
Per capita expenditures[c]	$312	$1,544	4.9
Ambulatory care			
Probability of having expenditures[a]	0.74	0.87	1.2
Average expenditure among those with expenditures[b]	$208	$405	2.0
Per capita expenditures[c]	$154	$352	2.3
Prescribed medication			
Probability of having expenditures[a]	0.58	0.86	1.5
Average expenditure among those with expenditures[b]	$61	$158	2.6
Per capita expenditures[c]	$35	$135	3.8
Home and community-based care			
Probability of having expenditures[a]	0.01	0.10	9.1
Average expenditure among those with expenditures[b]	$245	$849	3.5
Per capita expenditures[c]	$3	$83	31.7

Source: Lewin-VHI analysis of 1987 National Medical Expenditure Survey data.

Note: All regressions controlled for disability status, age, gender, race, family income, living arrangement, and insurance coverage. Equations were evaluated at the mean values for the general population. See appendix for regression results.

a. Results from logistic regressions.

b. Results from linear regressions of logged expenditures. Predicted values represent median, not mean, expenditures.

c. Combined results from logistic regressions predicting use and linear regressions of logged expenditures among users.

elderly than nonelderly persons with disabilities. The percentage of elderly persons with disabilities who used home and community-based care services was twice that for nonelderly persons with disabilities who used such services (44 percent versus 22 percent).

Persons with disabilities are an identifiable group of frequent health care users, and their high medical expenditures suggest that they could benefit from care management. In addition, although little empirical evidence exists, most researchers think that a lack of continuity in current care arrangements not only has financial consequences but could also reduce the quality of care.[19]

The existing system for financing care for persons with disabilities provides disjointed incentives. For example, nursing facility personnel could minimize the hospitalization of residents, thus providing savings to medicare. In 1987 elderly nursing facility residents used more than three times as many hospital days as noninstitutionalized elderly persons.[20] The per diem payment system used by most payers for nursing facility care provides no financial incentive for staff to reduce hospital admissions or length of stay because no payments are made to the nursing facility for these efforts. In some systems in which nursing facility and hospital care are combined under a capitated payment method, providers have been successful in reducing hospital days per 1,000 elderly persons.[21] Better coordinating services and combining payment sources could reduce some of the inefficiencies in the health care delivery system.

Benefit Design Implications

Covered benefits and associated deductibles and copayments could play a particularly important role for persons with disabilities because of their high health care expenditures. Out-of-pocket expenditures in 1987 were higher for persons with disabilities (who tended to have lower incomes) than for persons without disabilities. On average, persons with disabilities spent nearly four times as much out of pocket as persons who did not have disabilities (about 2.5 times adjusted for age), yet they were almost twice as likely (1.9 times) to have family income less than 200 percent of the poverty level (figure 5-4). Consequently, 23 percent of persons with disabilities spent more than 10 percent of family income on out-of-pocket health care expenses compared with 3 percent of persons who did not have disabilities (figure 5-5).

FIGURE 5-4. *Average Out-of-Pocket Expenditures, Persons with and without Disabilities, by Age Group*

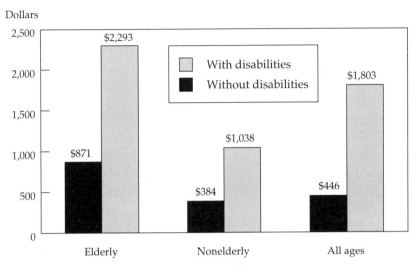

Source: Lewin-VHI analysis of 1987 National Medical Expenditure Survey data.

The largest single source of out-of-pocket expenditures for persons with disabilities was home and community-based services (figure 5-6). This is not surprising given the medical and social support needs of this population and the lack of public and private coverage for these services.

Under medicare and medicaid cost containment efforts or in the broader context of health reform, our findings suggest that the cost sharing requirements in health insurance plans could have important implications for persons with disabilities. For example, proposals have been made to institute coinsurance for the medicare home health benefit. This would likely disproportionately affect persons with disabilities because medicare beneficiaries who have high utilization of medicare home health benefits are more likely to have chronic conditions.[22] The NMES data indicated that medicare beneficiaries with disabilities already had high out-of-pocket payments, and increases in medicare home health copayments would likely increase either their direct out-of-pocket payments or the premiums they must pay for medicare supplemental insurance.

FIGURE 5-5. *Persons with Out-of-Pocket Expenditures in Excess of 10 Percent of Family Income, Persons with and without Disabilities, by Age Group*

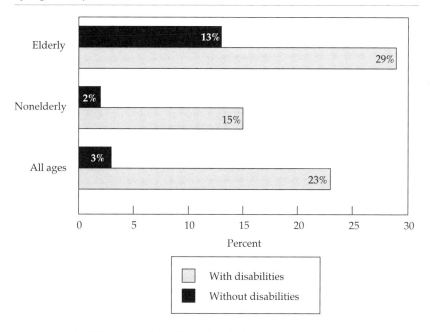

Source: Lewin-VHI analysis of 1987 National Medical Expenditure Survey data.

SUMMARY

The characteristics of health care use and expenditures of persons with disabilities have important implications for health care financing policy. The significantly higher health expenditures for persons with disabilities, relative to those without disabilities, suggest that any system with capitated payments for this population would need to adjust for the higher risk of utilization. These adjustments would be necessary to ensure adequate compensation to providers as well as access to services, choice of plans and providers, and quality care for enrollees with disabilities. If a private insurance system were developed for the nonelderly population, the added cost per policy of including payments for persons with disabilities in the pool of persons with private insurance would have been only $78 annually in 1987.

FIGURE 5-6. *Average Out-of-Pocket Expenditures by Type of Service, Persons with and without Disabilities*

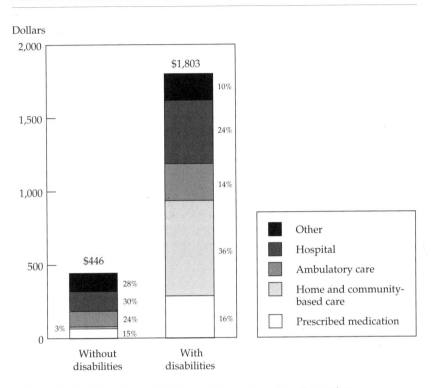

Source: Lewin-VHI analysis of 1987 National Medical Expenditure Survey data.

The propensity to use significantly more care, particularly hospital care, among persons with disabilities indicates that better care coordination and the proper financial incentives across providers might reduce costs for this population while improving the care received. Finally, the substantial health care expenditures among persons with disabilities, coupled with limited personal resources, suggests that this population could be particularly vulnerable under certain health benefit package designs.

The higher health care use and expenditures among persons with disabilities presents a challenge to policymakers, insurers, and providers. Special attention needs to be paid to this population in any plan to reform the health care financing or delivery systems, either through public or private efforts.

NOTES

1. Dorothy P. Rice and Mitchell P. Laplante, "Medical Expenditures for Disability and Disabling Comorbidity," *American Journal of Public Health,* vol. 82 (May 1992), pp. 739–41; James Lubitz and Penelope Pine, "Health Care Use by Medicare's Disabled Enrollees," *Health Care Financing Review,* vol. 7 (Summer 1986), pp. 19–30; Aaron Krute and Mary Ellen Burdette, "Prevalence of Chronic Disease, Injury, and Work Disability," in Social Security Administration, Office of Research and Statistics, *Disability Survey 72: Disabled and Nondisabled Adults, A Monograph,* Research Report No. 56, SSA Pub. No. 13-11812 (Government Printing Office, April 1981); Sandra Duchnok, "Health Insurance Coverage and Medical Care Utilization, 1972," in Social Security Administration, Office of Research and Statistics, *Disability Survey 72: Disabled and Nondisabled Adults, A Monograph,* Research Report No. 56, SSA Pub. No. 13-11812 (GPO, April 1981); Donald T. Ferron, "Medical Care Charges for the Disabled and Nondisabled, 1972," in Social Security Administration, Office of Research and Statistics, *Disability Survey 72: Disabled and Nondisabled Adults, A Monograph,* Research Report No. 56, SSA Pub. No. 13-11812 (GPO, April 1981); Henry P. Brehm and Robert H. Cormier, "Medical Care Costs for the Disabled," in Social Security Administration, Office of Research and Statistics, *Social Security Survey of the Disabled: 1966,* Report No. 8, DHEW Pub. No. (SSA) 73-11713 (GPO, January 1970); Gary L. Stanley and Idella Gwatkin Swisher, "Medicare Care Utilization by the Disabled," in Social Security Administration, Office of Research and Statistics, *Social Security Survey of the Disabled: 1966,* Report No. 5, SSA Pub. No. 77-11713 (GPO, January 1969); and Advisory Council on Social Security, *The Status of the Social Security Program and Recommendations for Its Improvement* (GPO, 1965).

2. Rice and Laplante, "Medical Expenditures for Disability and Disabling Comorbidity." This does not include nursing home expenditures.

3. Lubitz and Pine, "Health Care Use by Medicare's Disabled Enrollees"; Herbert A. Silverman, "Medicaid Recipients, Services, Utilization, and Program Payments," *Health Care Financing Review,* annual supplement (1992), pp. 311–36; and Penelope Pine, Steven Clauser, and David K. Baugh, "Trends in Medicaid Payments and Users of Covered Services," *Health Care Financing Review,* annual supplement (1992), pp. 235–69.

4. Lubitz and Pine, "Health Care Use by Medicare's Disabled Enrollees."

5. Pine and others, "Trends in Medicaid Payments and Users of Covered Services." In 1988 payments to children began increasing at a faster rate than payments to disabled persons, as a result of legislation expanding medicaid coverage to include new groups of low-income children.

6. Lewin-VHI, Inc., "The Potential of Coordinated Care Targeted to Medicare Beneficiaries with Medicaid Coverage," prepared for the Health Care Financing Administration (Fairfax, Va., July 1992); Joshua Wiener and Jason Skaggs, *The Integration of Acute and Long-Term Care Financing and Services: A Policy Synthesis* (Washington: American Association of Retired Persons, forthcoming); Susan Doerr, *Developing a Comprehensive System of Services for GHC's Chronically Ill Enrollees: Issues and Alternatives* (Seattle, Wash.: Klein/Doerr, Consultants, January 1995); Paul Saucier and Trishia Riley, *Managing Care for Older Beneficiaries of Medicaid and Medicare: Prospects and Pitfalls* (Portland, Maine: National Academy for State Health Policy, September 1994); Walter N. Leutz, Merwyn R. Greenlick, and John A. Capitman, "Integrating Acute and Long-Term Care," *Health Affairs*, vol. 13, no. 4 (1994), pp. 59–74; fact sheet issued by National Chronic Care Consortium, 1991; and Alice Rivlin and Joshua Wiener, with Raymond Hanley and Denise Spence, *Caring for the Disabled Elderly: Who Will Pay?* (Brookings, 1988).

7. In this study, we did not address the extent to which higher expenditures among persons with disabilities resulted from diseases that were unrelated to their disability (for example, cancer diagnosed for a person with Alzheimer's disease). Including expenditures related to such diseases or conditions could overstate the expenditures that resulted from disability if persons with disabilities were disproportionately affected by these conditions.

A more complete presentation of the results from the NMES data is available in our full report for the Health Care Financing Administration. See Lisa Maria B. Alecxih, John Corea, and David Kennell, *Health Care Use and Expenditures of Persons with and without Disabilities*, prepared for the Health Care Financing Administration (Fairfax, Va.: Lewin-VHI, Inc., 1995).

8. Data were analyzed using Statistical Analysis System (SAS) software. Standard errors were adjusted for the complex sample design with Survey Data Analysis (SUDAAN) software, which uses the Taylor series linearization method. All regressions were also performed using SUDAAN. See Babubhai V. Sha and others, *Statistical Methods and Mathematical Algorithms Used in SUDAAN* (Research Triangle, N.C.: Research Triangle Institute, 1993).

9. Attempts were made to verify all expenditures for medicaid beneficiaries and a sample of the nonmedicaid population.

10. An activity of daily living (ADL) was considered limited if a person reported difficulty with the activity and also required supervision or help with the activity in either Round 1 or Round 4 of the survey (the two points at which questions about functional status were asked). A sixth ADL, walking, was not incorporated into our definition of disability.

11. The distribution of persons with disabilities by level of disability in the 1987 National Medical Expenditure Survey:

	Nonelderly persons			Elderly persons		
Disability level	Percent	Records	Weighted	Percent	Records	Weighted
1 ADL	41	118	787,000	42	261	1,110,000
2 ADLs	24	71	461,000	22	142	590,000
3+ ADLs	35	101	654,000	36	235	933,200
Total	100	290	1,902,000	100	638	2,633,200

12. Average expenditures among this population would be slightly lower than average expenditures among only users of services, because drug and durable medical equipment (DME) expenditures were typically lower than other service expenditures. The difference for any service, however, was likely to be small; average total health care expenditures were less than 3 percent higher per user when drugs and DME were excluded.

13. Randall S. Brown and Jerold W. Hill, "The Effects of Medicare Risk HMOs on Medicare Costs and Service Utilization," in Harold Luft, ed., *HMOs and the Elderly* (Ann Arbor, Mich.: Health Administration Press, 1994).

14. J. William Thomas and Richard Lichtenstein, "Including Health Status in Medicare's Adjusted Average per Capita Cost Capitation Formula," *Medical Care*, vol. 26, no. 3 (March 1986), pp. 259–75; and Christina Witsberger, "Comparison of Health Services Utilization by Type of Insurance Plan," paper prepared for the 1993 annual meeting of the National Association of Health Data Organizations.

15. The percentage of total expenditures covered by medicaid for persons with disabilities was underestimated because nursing home expenditures were excluded.

16. That is, medicare payments averaged $6,066 per elderly user with a disability, and $1,789 per elderly user without a disability—a difference of $4,277. This accounts for 58 percent of the difference in total expenditures between the two groups ($7,311).

17. ($2,413 – $122)/($9,379 – $1,301) × 100 = 28 percent.

18. Aggregate expenditures from private insurance for all persons under age 65 totaled $112.7 billion in 1987. Private insurance covered 155 million individuals with per capita expenditures of $726. By adding this to total public expenditures for nonelderly persons with disabilities, and dividing by all noninstitutionalized persons (including the 1 million with disabilities not covered by private insurance), per capita expenditures would become $788, an increase of $62 per capita. After adjusting for the percentage of persons with disabilities who were uninsured, the increase becomes $78 per capita.

19. Wiener and Skaggs, *The Integration of Acute and Long-Term Care Financing and Services;* Doerr, *Developing a Comprehensive System of Services for GHC's Chronically Ill Enrollees;* Saucier and Riley, *Managing Care for Older Beneficiaries of Medicaid and Medicare;* Leutz and others, "Integrating Acute and Long-Term Care"; and fact sheet issued by National Chronic Care Consortium.

20. Vicki Frieman and Christopher Murtaugh, *Interactions between Hospital and Nursing Home Use* (Rockville, Md.: Agency for Health Care Policy and Research, 1994).

21. United HealthCare Corporation, *Managing Medical Care for Nursing Home Residents: A Demonstration Proposal* (Minneapolis, Minn.: United HealthCare Corporation, 1992); and Wiener and Skaggs, *The Integration of Acute and Long-Term Care Financing and Services.*

22. Jennifer Schore, *Patient, Agency, and Area Characteristics Associated with Regional Variation on the Use of Medicare Home Health Services* (Princeton, N.J.: Mathematica Policy Research, 1994).

TABLE 5A. *Results of Logistic Regressions Predicting Use of Service*

Variable	Any care		Hospitalization		Ambulatory care		Prescribed medication		Home and community-based care	
	Beta	P for B = 0	Beta	P for B = 0	Beta	P for B = 0	Beta	P for B = 0	Beta	P for B = 0
Intercept	2.7593	0	-1.8582	0	1.5461	0	1.3403	0	-2.7811	0
Disabled	1.7494	0	1.1261	0	0.8389	0	1.4685	0	2.3052	0
Under age 18	-1.0655	0	-1.9294	0	-0.7043	0	-1.5623	0	-2.408	0
Age 18–34	-1.1406	0	-0.5334	0	-0.7467	0	-1.4041	0	-2.1442	0
Age 35–54	-0.9771	0.001	-0.7694	0	-0.5903	0	-1.1506	0	-1.9578	0
Age 55–64	-0.6446	0.029	-0.4604	0.003	-0.2085	0.202	-0.6078	0.001	-1.4335	0
Age 65–74	-0.2977	0.300	-0.1337	0.382	0.1041	0.509	-0.2829	0.092	-0.7394	0
Age 75–84	-0.0489	0.871	0.1159	0.452	0.4067	0.017	0.1078	0.553	-0.2464	0.216
White	0.7841	0	0.1638	0.010	0.5708	0	0.5262	0	0.3348	0.018
Male	-0.7166	0	-0.4524	0	-0.6182	0	-0.6561	0	-0.469	0
Earned less than $15,000	-0.4772	0	0.4995	0	-0.1471	0.019	0.0138	0.791	0.1389	0.361
Earned $15,000–$30,000	-0.3696	0	0.2935	0	-0.1437	0.006	0.0346	0.397	-0.1493	0.333
Earned $30,000–$50,000	-0.1419	0.034	0.152	0.016	-0.0713	0.145	0.0081	0.848	-0.1406	0.414
Lived alone	0.3765	0	-0.3646	0	0.2507	0	0.2272	0	0.7313	0
Received medicaid	0.2689	0.004	0.5455	0	0.3631	0	0.3705	0	1.0667	0
Uninsured	-0.8935	0	-0.5213	0	-0.7052	0	-0.623	0	-0.4157	0.084

Source: Lewin-VHI analysis of 1987 National Medical Expenditure Survey data.

Note: For any care, the dependent variable R-squared = 0.087 and –log likelihood = 12457.91; hospitalization, R-squared = 0.045, –log likelihood = 8488.98; ambulatory care, R-squared = 0.074, –log likelihood = 17158.33; prescribed medication, R-squared = 0.108, –log likelihood = 19596.58; and home and community-based care, R-squared = 0.129, –log likelihood = 2558.22.

TABLE 5B. *Results of Linear Regressions Predicting Expenditures among Users*

Variable	Any care		Hospitalization		Ambulatory care		Prescribed medication		Home and community-based care	
	Beta	P for B = 0	Beta	P for B = 0	Beta	P for B = 0	Beta	P for B = 0	Beta	P for B = 0
Intercept	6.7082	0	8.7702	0	5.492	0	4.5556	0	5.861	0
Disabled	1.3204	0	0.6053	0	0.666	0	0.9479	0	1.2428	0
Under age 18	-1.2085	0	-0.5917	0	-0.6883	0	-1.4635	0	-0.9325	0.015
Age 18-34	-0.7617	0	-0.4317	0	-0.1814	0.043	-1.0264	0	-1.0698	0
Age 35-54	-0.5693	0	-0.1598	0.177	-0.07	0.455	-0.5478	0	-0.4703	0.065
Age 55-64	-0.1168	0.229	0.1035	0.408	0.1782	0.067	0.1596	0.072	-0.3764	0.142
Age 65-74	0.134	0.170	0.2314	0.061	0.3969	0	0.3269	0	-0.1747	0.423
Age 75-84	0.269	0.006	0.1522	0.204	0.4114	0	0.3584	0	-0.2388	0.257
White	0.2052	0	-0.1648	0.001	0.1098	0	0.1677	0	0.0257	0.867
Male	-0.2763	0	0.0754	0.076	-0.1604	0	-0.1645	0	-0.0683	0.655
Earned less than $15,000	-0.1682	0	-0.1278	0.044	-0.1494	0.001	0.0808	0.018	-0.2485	0.343
Earned $15,000-$30,000	-0.1542	0	-0.1509	0.013	-0.0892	0.014	0.0554	0.077	-0.452	0.069
Earned $30,000-$50,000	-0.0853	0.002	-0.1076	0.080	-0.0403	0.207	0.0519	0.093	-0.3725	0.214
Lived alone	0.1889	0	0.1016	0.092	0.2044	0	0.085	0.021	0.2947	0.040
Received medicaid	0.2858	0	0.0355	0.467	0.2416	0	0.2972	0	0.9172	0
Uninsured	-0.4507	0	-0.0994	0.211	-0.2927	0	-0.1778	0	-0.6676	0.028

Source: Lewin-VHI analysis of 1987 National Medical Expenditure Survey data.
Note: For total expenditures, the dependent variable R-squared = 0.135182; hospitalization, R-squared = 0.134873; ambulatory care, R-squared = 0.086146; prescribed medication, R-squared = 0.245817; and home and community-based care, R-squared = 0.225269.

Chapter 6

KENNETH G. MANTON AND ERIC STALLARD

Program Payment and Utilization Trends for Medicare Beneficiaries with Disabilities

The use of medicare part A and B services by elderly persons (age 65 and over) with chronic disabilities changed markedly since 1980.[1] The medicare-reimbursed use of home health agencies (HHAs), skilled nursing facilities (SNFs), hospital outpatient services, and physician services increased. At the same time, the use of inpatient hospital services, in terms of the number of admissions and the average length of stay (LOS), declined during the 1980s—though subsequent inpatient hospital use stabilized or increased modestly.

The service use changes were the result of a number of factors. Significant alterations in the medicare program were made, particularly the introduction of the Prospective Payment System (PPS) in 1983, which led to immediate declines in hospitalization rates and average hospital LOS. While the use of HHAs and SNFs was expected to increase as a result of PPS, General Accounting Office (GAO) and Health Care Financing Administration (HCFA) studies found that more intensive reviews of HHA claims leading to higher denial rates during the first several years of implementation of the new payment system depressed potential increases in use. While HHA and SNF use did not increase initially as expected in response to PPS, the use of outpatient and physician services by medicare beneficiaries during the phase-in of PPS increased dramatically. This growth led to further programmatic changes—for example, the implementation of the Resource Based Relative Value Scale (RBRVS), which replaced the old "customary, prevailing, and reasonable" charge system of physician reimbursement in 1991. The number of HHA visits reimbursed by medicare began to increase rapidly after promulgation of new regulations regarding HHA use by HCFA in mid-1989. The Medicare Catastrophic Care Act (MCCA) of 1988, although repealed in 1989, produced a sharp increase in the use of

SNFs by medicare-eligible persons and permanent increases (more than 75,000) in the national supply of SNF beds. Furthermore, the Omnibus Budget Reconciliation Act (OBRA) of 1987, by requiring medicaid nursing facilities to meet medicare standards, led to further de facto increases in the number of SNF beds.

Changes in medical technology and service delivery amplified changes induced by the implementation of PPS and other medicare program changes. Increases in managed care and capitated payment helped stimulate the growth of service delivery in non-inpatient settings. New methods of treatment emphasizing outpatient hospital care, such as day surgery, and home care also accelerated movement toward delivering care in non-inpatient settings.

Finally, changes in the health and functional status of elderly persons with disabilities affected their use of different medicare part A and B services. The prevalence of both chronic disability and selected chronic conditions for elderly persons with chronic disabilities declined between 1982 and 1989, before many medicare programmatic changes and advances in medical technology had taken full effect.[2] Among persons with chronic disabilities, the use of special equipment and housing increased between 1982 and 1989.[3] In addition, the educational attainment and economic status of elderly persons with disabilities were improving—and should continue to improve to 2015 and beyond.[4] Greater educational attainment and improved economic status reduced the likelihood of disability for the individual and should make elderly persons with disabilities increasingly sophisticated consumers of health care services.[5]

Changes in the medicare system, medical technology and service delivery, the health and functional status of elderly persons, and the educational attainment and economic resources of elderly persons affected the level and mix of services used by medicare beneficiaries during the 1980s and will continue to do so through the 1990s and beyond. To analyze these changes, a longitudinal survey was needed that tracked the health and functional status and medical service use of elderly medicare beneficiaries, and a multivariate statistical procedure that controlled for factors influencing the use of medicare services over time. For these reasons, we used the National Long-Term Care Survey (NLTCS), which assessed the health and functional status of elderly persons with disabilities and their medicare service use in 1982, 1984, and 1989. For each wave of the NLTCS, we used health and functional status measures to define groups with specific health and functional profiles. These profiles were defined identically for each survey, allowing changes in each individual's health and functional status to be noted over time. We then used medicare part A and B utilization data linked to NLTCS records to compare service use for a twelve-month period following each survey.

DATA

The NLTCS is a nationally representative survey of elderly medicare-eligible persons. The NLTCS, first conducted in 1982, was initially designed to identify the population of medicare-eligible persons over age 65 with chronic (more than ninety days) impairment in activities of daily living (ADLs) or instrumental activities of daily living (IADLs). For community residents classified as chronically disabled, a detailed survey determined the exact nature of the disabilities, the types of formal and informal care used to cope with the disabilities, and the social and economic characteristics of the disabled person and his or her family. Four purposes of the 1982 NLTCS were to (1) determine the prevalence of chronic disability in the U.S. elderly population in 1982, (2) describe in detail the characteristics of those persons, (3) link detailed survey data to medicare payment records to expand the information on the chronic health and functional status of medicare-eligible persons beyond that available in medicare records, and (4) provide a basis upon which the results of long-term care demonstrations could be generalized to the U.S. elderly population. To accomplish the fourth goal, a wide range of questions was asked about disability and service use so that the NLTCS asked most of the questions used in different long-term care demonstrations. For example, in the NLTCS community interview, multiple questions were asked about limitations in each of nine ADLs and ten IADLs and in the performance of eight physical tasks.[6] Disability was defined as the inability to perform any ADL or IADL for more than ninety days because of problems with health or aging. In addition, the presence of twenty-nine medical conditions and behavior and sensory problems was assessed.

The 1984 and 1989 NLTCS, explicitly designed as longitudinal surveys, had to perform several additional functions. First, an institutional interview form was developed in 1984. Though persons in institutions were identified by the screening instrument for the 1982 NLTCS, they were not given a detailed interview. In 1984 and 1989 institutionalized persons were given the institutional interview to better describe their characteristics. Second, the 1984 and 1989 NLTCS were designed to follow changes (improvements and losses) in an individual's function over time. To do this, all persons who had been identified as either chronically disabled or institutionalized in an earlier NLTCS were automatically interviewed—either in the community or in an institution—to determine details of their functional changes. Rescreening also was required of a portion of NLTCS samples who had been previously found not to be chronically disabled to identify newly emergent cases of disability. Third, the 1984 and 1989 NLTCS were designed to follow changes in the national prevalence of chronic disability and institutionalization over time. To do this, samples of roughly 5,000 persons who had passed age 65 and enrolled in medicare between the two NLTCSs were drawn so that disability in the entire U.S. population over age 65 would be represented in both 1984 and 1989.

The NLTCS was based on a list sample, not an area probability sample. That is, sampling was done from medicare enrollment files, which provided the list of names from which a probability sample of individuals was drawn. List samples have several advantages. First, all persons sampled, being drawn from medicare records, were medicare eligible. Second, sampling from medicare administrative files meant that nearly 100 percent of the sample could be tracked between surveys through the computer files. Third, because persons were sampled from medicare files, persons in all types of residences were captured in the sample. The field procedures facilitated this in both 1984 and 1989; the interviewer established residence type when he or she went to conduct a detailed interview, so the type of residence, community, or institution was directly verified in the in-person visit. In area probability samples, the households in specific residences formed the sampling unit, not specific individuals. For example, in the National Health Interview Surveys, only noninstitutional households are sampled and the respondent is not a specific individual but a respondent selected for the household. A separate survey has to be conducted for nursing homes, where the sample of institutions is drawn from a list of certified institutions. In the NLTCS list sample, given that individuals were selected, all types of residences were sampled—whether certified facilities or not. The list samples of the NLTCS also provided mortality and medicare use data for all persons sampled, including nonrespondents. Thus the nature of nonresponse bias vis-à-vis medicare service use and mortality could be determined. In area probability samples, medicare linkage is possible only for respondents.

The sample size and structure of the NLTCS were designed to have adequate power both to distinguish differences in disability prevalence estimates by age and gender and to estimate changes in disability and residential status over time. In 1982, 55,000 names were initially drawn from medicare enrollment records because the chronic disability prevalence rate was unknown. Of these, roughly 35,000 persons were screened—the number necessary to produce about 6,000 community interviews of chronically disabled persons (6,088 persons responded of 6,393 identified as disabled during the screening).

In 1984 the sample was designed with longitudinal features. About 12,100 of the 26,623 persons who were not chronically disabled in 1982 were selected for screening in 1984. Thus, with the supplementary sample of 5,000 "age-in" persons (those who passed age 65 between the two survey dates), roughly 17,000 persons were screened. From the screening and from persons who had been disabled or institutionalized in 1982, 5,934 community and 1,773 institutional interviews were produced. In 1989 a total of about 18,000 persons were screened, automatically eligible, or in an age-in sample. This produced 4,463 community and 1,354 institutional interviews.

Because some persons were tracked longitudinally and interviewed more than once, and with the subsampling of nondisabled persons, the 1982, 1984, and 1989 NLTCS-integrated longitudinal file contained information on 30,308 individuals. From linked medicare files 1982 to 1991, about 10,000 deaths (and dates of deaths) were identified. In all three years, a total of 16,485 community interviews were done (some persons were reinterviewed) along with 3,127 institutional interviews conducted in 1984 and 1989. Screening response rates varied from 96 to 97 percent and detailed interview rates from 95 to 96 percent. Thus response rates were high. The oldest-old population (persons over age 85) was well represented in the samples in each year.

We analyzed the 16,485 community responses in the three NLTCSs that yielded the most detailed morbidity and disability data. The 1984 and 1989 institutional surveys only assessed ADL and cognitive impairments, so those data were not directly used in multivariate analyses. The institutional sample had an average of 4.8 out of 6 possible ADL impairments. Thus the institutional group was designated as a separate, frail population. Survey persons in institutions were included in analyses by forming a discrete category for them.

Persons received a detailed community interview in 1982 because they reported chronic disability during the screening. The community interview was more detailed than the screening, so that some persons identified as disabled during the screening may not have been so identified on the community interview. In 1982, of the 6,088 community interviews completed, 550 persons did not qualify as chronically impaired. These persons had false positive disability responses during the screening. As a result, they might be treated as not chronically disabled. Though not chronically disabled, they still received the entire detailed community interview. In 1984 and 1989, in addition to screen-false-positives, persons who were either disabled or institutionalized on an earlier survey automatically received the detailed interview in subsequent NLTCSs, regardless of their current disability status. From the two sources, 550 persons reported no disability during the community interview in 1982, 989 in 1984 (296 from 1982, 227 screen-in, 466 previously disabled), and 945 in 1989 (371 from 1984, 288 screen-in, 286 previously disabled). Over the three years, 1,817 persons received a total of 2,484 detailed interviews but reported no chronic disability.

We evaluated the medicare service use of these persons and found that it was not significantly higher than for the 20,244 persons who had been screened out as nondisabled (in 35,686 screen interviews).[7] Thus, for some analyses, we could use the 2,484 detailed interviews to make estimates of medicare service use for nondisabled persons if their responses were reweighted to represent the total nondisabled U.S. population in each year. This approach to evaluating the nondisabled had the advantage that the detailed interview contained information not available during the screening (for example, the presence or absence of each of twenty-nine medical conditions). Hence, we could make U.S. medicare service use estimates from the multivariate analyses by applying adjusted weights to nondisabled respondents.

Another way to estimate medicare service use for the U.S. nondisabled population was to apply basic sample weights directly to persons who screened out or who reported no chronic disability on the community survey. Using medicare service data for all persons screened out as nondisabled, we could estimate their service use with basic sample weights. We used the second method to make U.S. medicare service estimates for nondisabled persons in this analysis because it afforded more efficient use of the medicare service data.

To tabulate service use, we needed to select a time period over which medicare payments and service units would be collected; we chose the twelve months after the final interview in each survey year. The 1982 NLTCS records were linked to medicare service use records for October 1, 1982, to September 30, 1983; 1984 survey records, for October 1, 1984, to September 30, 1985; and 1989 survey data, for October 1, 1989, to September 30, 1990. The service use data were collected over a common time frame after interviewing was complete to avoid variability resulting from effects peculiar to specified time periods over which service use was monitored. In 1982 and 1984, the start of service data collection coincided with the end of interviewing. Because the exact ages of death for persons were available from medicare records, we could adjust the sample weights for survivors for the mortality that occurred during the interview period. In 1989, interviewing ended two months earlier than in 1982 and 1984. This required that an additional mortality adjustment be made to the 1989 sample weights. All services and payments occurring in a twelve-month period after the end of interviewing were collected for each person. The procedure did not overlap the interview period, involve services used before the survey, or become confounded with medicare program changes.

METHODS

From the NLTCS, fifty-six measures of health and functional status were selected for each individual, including ADL and IADL impairments, difficulty with normal activities (such as climbing stairs, bending over, and lifting objects), and a series of medical conditions or illnesses. Using these characteristics, a number of groups were defined whose members had similar health and functional statuses.

A number of problems arose. First, data collected from self- and proxy reports of health and functional status were categorical and subject to error.[8] Second, because many health and functional measures were needed to describe elderly persons, there was potentially serious collinearity. Third, representing disability by discrete, homogeneous categories could be misleading at late ages because many elderly persons with a few functional limitations remained capable of independent living.[9] Given these limitations, we needed to use a continuous scoring system to reflect each individual's degree of disability along several dimensions.[10]

Many standard grouping algorithms did not deal with the measurement characteristics of these data, so forming groups using the NLTCS measures was inappropriate. For example, if categorical data were reported without error, procedures for analyzing contingency tables could have been used to identify groups and subgroups for analysis.[11] If variables were reported with error, a more general procedure—latent class analysis (LCA)—would be needed.[12] In LCA, two types of parameters are estimated: cell probabilities as in contingency tables; and scores of zero or 1 indicating membership in one of the K groups identified by the analysis from the original measures. A third way to identify groups was auto-group, a clustering procedure in which a single criterion variable (for example, service costs) was partitioned using trial subdivisions defined from explanatory variables introduced one at a time. This provided the best explanation of a single criterion variable using a measure of fit based on making the sum of squared deviations from the model as small as possible.

Instead, we used the grade of membership (GOM) model to form seven groups from the fifty-six health and functional status measures. GOM extended LCA by allowing the membership scores to vary continuously from zero to 1, subject to the restriction that the K scores for each individual sum to 1. GOM provided two types of parameters:

1. GOM scores indicating each individual's membership in each of the K groups. For some purposes, GOM scores could be viewed as probabilities.

2. Group-specific marginal probabilities for each category of each variable in the analysis.

In GOM, the overall marginal probabilities were weighted averages of the group-specific marginal probabilities, with weights equal to the average GOM score for each group.

Although the groups were based on the fifty-six health and functional status measures, GOM also could provide estimates of group-specific marginal probabilities for nonhealth variables measuring utilization and payments for medicare-covered services. These were used to estimate average utilization and program payments on a per enrollee and per beneficiary basis.

RESULTS

A series of analyses were performed. First, we conducted the GOM analysis of the health and functional variables to identify K multivariate health profiles. Second, we examined how program payments and utilization changed over time for the K profiles.

Multivariate Estimates of Health and Functional Status Profiles

Analyses of health differences in service use were based on groups identified from fifty-six health and functional status items in the 1982, 1984, and 1989 NLTCS. We pooled the surveys to define seven health and functional groups describing health variation over time. The joint analysis of disability and health measures was conducted using the GOM model, a multivariate procedure. The overall and group-specific marginal probabilities for the fifty-six variables were tallied (table 6-1).

The overall marginal probability was the unweighted population frequency for each characteristic among 16,485 respondents to the detailed NLTCS community survey. It was also the weighted average of the seven group-specific marginal probabilities. The characteristics of the seven groups could be identified by examining relative values of their marginal probabilities:

1. The active and healthy group had no ADL or IADL problems, little physical impairment, and few health problems.

2. The circulatory problem group had no ADLs, one IADL, and few physical impairments. The most serious problems included cardiovascular disease, stroke, and diabetes.

3. The acutely ill group had trouble with one ADL (bathing) and three IADLs and were physically impaired. The group members had multiple health problems, for example, cancer (21.6 percent), heart attack (33.1 percent), and other heart trouble (100 percent).

TABLE 6-1. Overall and Group-Specific Marginal Probabilities of Fifty-Six Health and Functioning Variables from the 1982, 1984, and 1989 National Long-Term Care Surveys

Characteristic	Unweighted population frequency	Group						
		1	2	3	4	5	6	7
		Active and healthy	Circulatory problems	Acutely ill	IADL, vision impaired, and demented[a]	IADL impaired with physical problems[a]	ADL mobility impaired[b]	ADL frail[b]
Person is confined to								
1. Bed	0.8	0.0	0.0	0.0	0.0	0.0	0.0	6.1
2. Chair or bed	1.5	0.0	0.0	0.0	0.0	0.0	0.0	11.2
3. Wheelchair	7.0	0.0	0.0	0.0	0.0	0.0	23.0	26.4
Person needs help with								
4. Eating	7.0	0.0	0.0	0.0	0.0	0.0	0.0	63.0
5. Getting in and out of bed	26.2	0.0	0.0	0.0	0.0	0.0	100.0	100.0
6. Walking around inside	39.9	0.0	0.0	0.0	0.0	0.0	100.0	100.0
7. Dressing	19.4	0.0	0.0	0.0	0.0	0.0	0.0	100.0
8. Bathing	43.1	0.0	0.0	60.1	0.0	0.0	100.0	100.0
9. Toileting	21.7	0.0	0.0	0.0	0.0	0.0	62.8	100.0
10. Heavy work	71.9	0.0	100.0	100.0	100.0	100.0	100.0	100.0
11. Light work	22.6	0.0	0.0	0.0	0.0	0.0	0.0	100.0
12. Laundry	22.6	0.0	0.0	0.0	0.0	0.0	0.0	100.0
13. Cooking	29.8	0.0	0.0	100.0	100.0	0.0	0.0	100.0
14. Grocery shopping	56.9	0.0	0.0	100.0	100.0	100.0	100.0	100.0
15. Getting around outside	59.1	0.0	0.0	0.0	69.8	100.0	100.0	100.0

16. Traveling	52.9	0.0	100.0	100.0	100.0	100.0	78.8
17. Managing money	26.8	0.0	0.0	100.0	0.0	0.0	100.0
18. Taking medicine	23.5	0.0	0.0	0.0	0.0	0.0	100.0
19. Using telephone	16.0	0.0	0.0	100.0	0.0	0.0	100.0
Degree of difficulty with							
20. Climbing stairs							
None	18.6	61.9	0.0	0.0	0.0	0.0	0.0
Some	29.1	38.1	86.1	0.0	0.0	0.0	0.0
Very	31.4	0.0	13.9	0.0	100.0	55.3	0.0
Cannot	21.0	0.0	0.0	0.0	0.0	44.7	100.0
21. Bending over							
None	43.5	100.0	0.0	0.0	100.0	34.3	0.0
Some	27.9	0.0	100.0	0.0	0.0	0.0	0.0
Very	18.0	0.0	0.0	100.0	0.0	65.7	14.3
Cannot	10.6	0.0	0.0	0.0	0.0	0.0	85.7
22. Holding a ten-pound package							
None	29.6	100.0	0.0	0.0	0.0	0.0	0.0
Some	18.1	0.0	100.0	0.0	0.0	0.0	0.0
Very	15.9	0.0	0.0	100.0	0.0	0.0	0.0
Cannot	36.4	0.0	0.0	100.0	100.0	100.0	100.0
23. Reaching overhead							
None	56.1	100.0	0.0	0.0	0.0	100.0	0.0
Some	21.2	0.0	100.0	0.0	84.0	0.0	0.0
Very	13.9	0.0	0.0	72.7	16.0	0.0	35.0
Cannot	8.8	0.0	0.0	27.3	0.0	0.0	65.0

TABLE 6-1. (continued)

24. Combing hair								
None	71.6	100.0	100.0	0.0	100.0	0.0	100.0	0.0
Some	16.0	0.0	0.0	0.0	0.0	100.0	0.0	13.4
Very	7.0	0.0	0.0	100.0	0.0	0.0	0.0	28.3
Cannot	5.4	0.0	0.0	0.0	0.0	0.0	0.0	58.3
25. Washing hair								
None	55.8	100.0	100.0	0.0	100.0	0.0	100.0	0.0
Some	14.8	0.0	0.0	0.0	0.0	58.9	0.0	0.0
Very	9.4	0.0	0.0	100.0	0.0	14.1	0.0	0.0
Cannot	20.0	0.0	0.0	0.0	0.0	0.0	0.0	100.0
26. Grasping small objects								
None	66.0	100.0	100.0	0.0	100.0	0.0	100.0	14.4
Some	20.3	0.0	0.0	0.0	0.0	100.0	0.0	18.3
Very	10.1	0.0	0.0	100.0	0.0	0.0	0.0	31.6
Cannot	3.6	0.0	0.0	0.0	0.0	0.0	0.0	35.7
27. See well enough to read newspaper	74.3	100.0	100.0	100.0	0.0	100.0	100.0	41.6
Person has								
28. Rheumatism or arthritis	72.8	53.6	100.0	100.0	0.8	100.0	100.0	66.6
29. Paralysis	8.5	0.0	2.3	0.0	0.0	0.0	12.5	45.3
30. Permanent stiffness	23.4	0.0	76.0	95.3	0.0	0.0	13.1	38.0
31. Multiple sclerosis	0.6	0.0	0.0	2.8	0.0	0.0	1.8	1.1
32. Cerebral palsy	0.4	0.0	0.0	3.4	0.0	0.0	0.0	0.9
33. Epilepsy	0.8	0.0	0.0	8.1	0.0	0.0	0.0	1.9
34. Parkinson's disease	2.8	0.0	7.7	0.0	0.0	0.0	0.0	12.3
35. Glaucoma	9.2	0.0	0.0	0.0	67.2	0.0	0.0	0.0
36. Diabetes	16.3	0.0	83.3	0.0	0.0	0.0	0.0	33.1

	Col1	Col2	Col3	Col4	Col5	Col6	Col7	Col8
37. Cancer	6.0	4.2	8.1	21.6	4.5	0.0	0.0	12.2
38. Constipation	30.8	0.0	100.0	100.0	0.0	0.0	0.0	52.6
39. Insomnia	39.3	0.0	100.0	100.0	0.0	0.0	0.0	44.1
40. Headache	16.6	0.0	0.0	100.0	0.0	0.0	0.0	0.0
41. Obesity	23.6	9.8	100.0	18.9	0.0	0.0	22.0	12.8
42. Arteriosclerosis	27.8	0.0	100.0	60.5	33.9	0.0	0.0	59.4
43. Mental retardation	1.4	0.0	0.0	0.0	6.9	0.0	0.0	5.3
44. Dementia	7.8	0.0	0.0	0.0	37.0	0.0	0.0	38.3
45. Heart attack	5.8	0.0	19.9	33.1	0.0	0.0	0.0	7.2
46. Other heart problems	29.3	0.0	100.0	100.0	0.0	0.0	0.0	37.4
47. Hypertension	45.6	20.2	100.0	98.8	0.0	18.4	37.1	47.1
48. Stroke	6.6	0.0	14.6	0.0	0.0	0.0	0.0	33.3
49. Circulation trouble	50.2	0.0	100.0	100.0	0.0	44.9	11.3	79.0
50. Pneumonia	5.8	0.0	0.0	89.2	0.0	0.0	0.0	0.0
51. Bronchitis	13.6	0.0	0.0	100.0	0.0	0.0	0.0	0.0
52. Influenza	17.8	0.0	0.0	100.0	0.0	0.0	0.0	0.0
53. Emphysema	9.7	0.0	0.0	100.0	0.0	0.0	0.0	0.0
54. Asthma	7.3	0.0	0.0	100.0	0.0	0.0	0.0	0.0
55. Broken hip	2.1	0.0	0.0	0.0	0.0	0.0	11.3	3.1
56. Other broken bones	5.2	2.6	0.0	25.3	0.0	2.8	12.1	5.2

Sources: Duke University, Center for Demographic Studies, analysis of the 1982, 1984, and 1989 National Long-Term Care Survey; and derived from Kenneth G. Manton, Eric Stallard, and Max A. Woodbury, "Home Health and Skilled Nursing Facility Use: 1983–90," *Health Care Financing Review*, vol. 16, no. 1 (1994), pp. 155–86, tables 8 and 9.

a. IADL = instrumental activities of daily living.

b. ADL = activities of daily living.

4. The IADL, vision impaired, and demented group had IADL impairments, poor vision, glaucoma, and dementia.

5. The IADL impaired with physical problem group had mobility problems, moderate difficulty with physical performance, and arthritis and circulatory problems.

6. The ADL mobility impaired group had ADL and IADL impairments related to mobility, physical performance limitations related to lower limb problems, arthritis, some paralysis, and the highest likelihood of hip fractures.

7. The ADL frail group was impaired on most ADLs and IADLs and in most physical functions. Members had multiple health problems, including the most stroke and dementia.

Groups 2 through 7 could be examined in pairs. Groups 2 and 3 were distinguished by illnesses; Groups 4 and 5 by IADL impairments; and Groups 6 and 7 by ADL impairments. In each pair, severity was greater in the second group.

The overall and group-specific marginal probabilities of seven variables used to assess the predictive validity of the seven groups also were derived (table 6-2). In this elderly (over age 65) sample, the mean ages of the groups varied by fifteen years. The acutely ill were the youngest (mean age 71.8 years); the IADL, vision impaired, and demented were the oldest (mean age 86.5 years). The ADL frail were the second oldest (mean age 81.6 years), with the ADL mobility impaired the third oldest (mean age 81.4 years). The active and healthy group had a mean age of 76.2 years. The two IADL groups and the ADL mobility impaired were least likely to be married. The ADL frail had a significant proportion of married persons. Females predominated in the acutely ill, the circulatory problem, the ADL mobility impaired, and the IADL impaired with physical problem groups. The best educated were the active and healthy group. The least educated were the acutely ill and the IADL, vision impaired, and demented groups. The seven groups had distinctive sociodemographic profiles.

The subjective health and nursing home variables supported the multidimensional characterization of the groups, with 91 percent of the circulatory problem and 100 percent of the acutely ill groups reporting fair or poor health, but little use of nursing homes. Eighty-eight percent of the active and healthy, 67 percent of the IADL, vision impaired, and demented, and 60 percent of the ADL mobility impaired groups reported good or excellent health; 90 percent of the

ADL frail and 75 percent of the IADL impaired with physical problem groups reported fair or poor health. The only significant nursing home use was for the ADL mobility impaired and ADL frail groups. In each pair of groups (2 and 3, 4 and 5, and 6 and 7), the subjective health for the second group was significantly poorer. The seven groups were distinguished by the two health measures.

In addition to the analysis of 16,485 detailed community interviews, 35,686 screen interviews were conducted with persons who screened out for disability and 4,945 screening or detailed institutional interviews with persons who were institutionalized at one or more of the interview dates in 1982, 1984, and 1989. Screen-out persons were assigned to the active and healthy group. Institutionalized persons defined an eighth group. With these adjustments, GOM scores were defined for the entire NLTCS sample, and with the sampling weights, GOM scores were estimated for the national medicare-enrolled aged (over age 65) population. Although GOM allowed individuals to belong to more than one group, the average GOM score could be interpreted as the percent of the population in a group. For the averages for 1982, 1984, and 1989, see table 6-3.

About 80 percent of these elderly persons were active and healthy. The 1.3 percent improvement from 1982 to 1989 was similar to the 1.1 percent non-age-standardized improvement in the nondisabled population when using summary counts of disabilities. About 3 percent had circulatory problems; about 1.3 percent were acutely ill; about 3.5 percent had IADL problems, with both IADL groups decreasing in prevalence from 1982 to 1989; about 6.2 percent had ADL problems, with one ADL group decreasing and the other increasing in prevalence from 1982 to 1989; and 5.5 percent were institutionalized in 1989, a small decline from 1982.

Program Payment and Utilization Trends

Data also were collected describing changes in use of, and payment for, specific medicare services from 1982–83 to 1989–90. Presentation of the information was based on the eight groups defined in table 6-3. Three issues were considered:

1. Changes from 1982–83 to 1989–90 for short stay hospital, SNF, HHA, hospital outpatient, physician, durable medical equipment

TABLE 6-2. *Overall and Group-Specific Marginal Probabilities of Seven Variables Used to Assess the Predictive Validity of Seven Groups Generated from Fifty-Six Health and Functioning Variables from the 1982 and 1989 National Long-Term Care Surveys*

		Group						
		1	2	3	4	5	6	7
Characteristic	Unweighted population frequency	Active and healthy	Circulatory problems	Acutely ill	IADL, vision impaired, and demented[a]	IADL impaired with physical problems[a]	ADL mobility impaired[b]	ADL frail[b]
1. Sex								
Male	34.5	52.6	24.9	30.1	49.1	6.3	12.6	43.6
Female	65.5	47.4	75.1	69.9	50.9	93.7	87.4	56.4
2. Age								
65–66	4.5	4.9	6.5	13.6	0.0	4.3	2.6	2.1
67–69	11.1	14.3	17.6	24.6	0.0	7.0	5.7	7.3
70–74	21.7	27.3	34.1	38.5	0.2	20.9	12.6	15.1
75–79	22.6	26.3	32.4	23.3	11.5	18.4	19.2	19.6
80–84	19.6	18.3	9.3	0.0	30.9	25.3	28.2	22.0
85–89	13.3	7.8	0.0	0.0	33.9	19.5	21.4	16.8
90+	7.3	1.2	0.0	0.0	23.5	4.5	10.4	17.0
Mean (in years)	78.5	76.2	73.9	71.8	86.5	79.3	81.4	81.6
3. Marital status								
Married	42.7	56.9	56.4	56.5	22.1	18.5	19.6	52.1
Not married	57.3	43.1	43.6	43.5	77.9	81.5	80.4	48.0

4.	Education								
	None	3.2	2.1	0.1	1.6	9.2	2.7	2.3	7.0
	Grade school	21.6	13.8	20.3	50.8	46.0	23.5	8.6	21.6
	Junior high school	32.6	29.6	38.3	39.8	23.7	38.0	33.6	31.0
	High school	29.4	37.1	32.0	7.6	13.6	26.1	35.6	27.7
	College	11.0	13.8	8.2	0.0	6.5	9.1	16.8	11.5
	Graduate school	2.1	3.7	1.1	0.2	1.1	0.6	3.1	1.3
5.	Income								
	$0–4,999	16.9	9.8	15.2	40.0	13.9	30.9	20.5	9.7
	$5,000–6,999	14.2	11.7	20.7	24.8	11.6	15.0	15.2	7.9
	$7,000–9,999	15.9	15.2	20.1	18.9	11.7	13.7	14.8	17.4
	$10,000–14,999	16.0	20.4	20.5	9.7	9.2	6.9	13.6	19.9
	$15,000–29,000	12.9	16.5	13.8	3.8	14.3	7.8	6.7	18.9
	$30,000+	5.0	6.3	1.9	0.0	9.2	1.0	4.7	7.8
	Refused to answer	6.9	9.7	1.4	0.0	7.9	8.3	8.5	6.1
	Don't know	12.3	10.5	6.4	2.7	22.2	16.4	16.0	12.3
6.	Subjective health								
	Excellent	13.3	32.3	0.0	0.0	17.5	1.7	13.8	1.6
	Good	23.2	56.1	9.1	0.0	49.4	23.9	46.2	8.1
	Fair	33.4	11.6	75.7	33.4	29.5	54.7	34.2	20.2
	Poor	21.1	0.0	15.2	66.6	3.5	19.7	5.8	70.0
7.	Have you ever been a patient in a nursing home?								
	Yes	17.1	2.1	1.7	3.4	7.3	3.3	53.0	44.3
	No	82.9	97.9	98.3	96.6	92.7	96.7	47.0	55.7

Source: Duke University, Center for Demographic Studies, analysis of the 1982, 1984, and 1989 National Long-Term Care Survey; and derived from Kenneth G. Manton, Eric Stallard, and Max A. Woodbury, "Home Health and Skilled Nursing Facility Use: 1983–90," *Health Care Financing Review*, vol. 16, no. 1 (1994), pp. 155–86, tables 8 and 9.

a. IADL = instrumental activities of daily living.

b. ADL = activities of daily living.

TABLE 6-3. *Total and Group-Specific Grade of Membership Scores Generated from Fifty-Six Health and Functioning Variables from the 1982, 1984, and 1989 National Long-Term Care Surveys*

						Group		
Year	Total	1 Active and healthy	2 Circulatory problems	3 Acutely ill	4 IADL, vision impaired, and demented[a]	5 IADL impaired with physical problems[a]	6 ADL mobility impaired[b]	7 ADL frail[b]	8 Institutional
1982	100.0	79.3	2.8	1.4	2.2	2.2	3.1	3.3	5.7
1984	100.0	79.5	3.2	1.3	2.3	2.2	3.2	2.7	5.5
1989	100.0	80.6	2.9	1.3	1.6	1.9	3.3	2.9	5.5

Source: Duke University, Center for Demographic Studies, analysis of the 1982, 1984, and 1989 National Long-Term Care Survey; and derived from Kenneth G. Manton, Eric Stallard, and Max A. Woodbury, "Home Health and Skilled Nursing Facility Use: 1983–90," *Health Care Financing Review*, vol. 16, no. 1 (1994), pp. 155–86, tables 8 and 9.

a. IADL = instrumental activities of daily living.

b. ADL = activities of daily living.

(DME), and other (primarily renal and therapy) services: Medicare services could be grouped several ways. Dividing part A services into short stay hospital, SNF, and HHA services was standard. How to categorize part B services was less obvious. Often ancillary services were included with physician services defining a heterogeneous set of services. We divided part B services into four types: hospital outpatient, physician, DME, and other—primarily renal and therapy—services. These service categories were strongly differentiated by the eight health and functioning groups.

2. Changes in the percentage of enrollees using services, the use per enrollee, the use per beneficiary, and total volume of specific medicare services used by each group in the two time periods: For part A services, changes were examined in both the units of each service consumed and the medicare program payments for those services. Because defining service units for part B was difficult, only medicare program payments for those services were examined. The percentage of enrollees using services was the ratio of the number of beneficiaries for that service to the number of enrollees, multiplied by 100. The payment (use) per enrollee was the payment (use) per beneficiary times the percent using services. The total payment was the payment per enrollee times the number of aged persons enrolled in medicare. The group specific total payment was the group's payment per enrollee times the number in the group enrolled in medicare. The number in the group enrolled in medicare was the number of aged persons enrolled in medicare times the average GOM score for the group (table 6-3).

3. Relation of changes from 1982 to 1990 in service use and program payments to population health dynamics and medicare program changes: Changes in medicare affected the type and kind of services used over the period. The NLTCS measured population health changes and was linked to medicare files so both cross-sectional and longitudinal estimates of service use by health groups could be made. We evaluated the impact of changes in the regulatory environment on service use; changes in the levels of services used and program payments across service types in the presence of population growth and aging; health and functional groups that experienced similar or coordinated changes in levels of use and payments over time; and correlations in payments for each of the seven services.

Program payments for 1982–83 and 1989–90 included the dollar amounts paid by medicare on behalf of aged beneficiaries for the indicated services but did not include the costs of deductibles, copayments, balance billing, out-of-pocket expenses for noncovered services, noncovered days, or medicare part A or B premiums. Dollar values for 1982–83 were inflated 29.3 percent to be comparable with dollar values for 1989–90. This factor was the increase from 1983 to 1990 of the consumer price index for urban wage earners and clerical workers, which was the basis of cost-of-living increases for social security beneficiaries.[13]

Short Stay Hospital Use

Short stay hospital use and medicare program payment varied across groups and over time (table 6-4).

Service changes from 1982–83 to 1989–90 overlapped the phase in of PPS from 1983 to 1987. A 22 percent decline was evident in total hospital days used, and a 32 percent decline in hospital days per enrollee. These figures were derived from the ratios .78 and .68 in the total population column of table 6-4. (The original data for the ratios in tables 6-4–6-8 are in appendix tables 6A-1 through 6A-5.) The 32 percent decline in hospital days per enrollee reflected an 18 percent decline in percentage of enrollees using hospital days combined with a 17 percent decline in the number of hospital days per beneficiary.

Changes across groups in hospital days per beneficiary were similar for the first six groups; that is, from –18 percent for the active and healthy to –24 percent for the two IADL groups. The ADL frail group had a smaller decline (–11 percent) in days per beneficiary. The largest declines in total days used were for the acutely ill (–34 percent), the IADL, vision impaired, and demented (–50 percent), and the IADL impaired with physical problem (–36 percent) groups. The institutional group had a 19 percent increase in total days used with only –1 percent change in hospital days per beneficiary.

While use declined, overall and for most groups (by differing amounts), the average payment per beneficiary (+11 percent; in constant dollars) and total payments (+4 percent) increased modestly. Increases were not uniform. The three groups with the largest reductions in total days used also had reductions in total payments. Increases occurred for the active and healthy, those with circulatory problems,

TABLE 6-4. *Ratios of Short Stay Hospital Days and Payments, 1989–90 to 1982–83, for Health and Functioning Groups Defined from the 1982, 1984, and 1989 National Long-Term Care Surveys*

					Group				
		1	2	3	4	5	6	7	8
Item in ratio	Total population	Active and healthy	Circulatory problems	Acutely ill	IADL, vision impaired, and demented[a]	IADL impaired with physical problems[a]	ADL mobility impaired[b]	ADL frail[b]	Institutional
Days spent in hospital									
Percentage using services	0.82	0.81	0.87	0.79	0.81	0.85	0.83	0.78	1.09
Average days per beneficiary	0.83	0.82	0.78	0.79	0.76	0.76	0.79	0.89	0.99
Average days per enrollee	0.68	0.66	0.68	0.63	0.61	0.64	0.66	0.70	1.08
Total days used (millions)	0.78	0.76	0.81	0.66	0.50	0.64	0.82	0.76	1.19
Total days used (percent)	1.00	0.98	1.04	0.86	0.64	0.82	1.05	0.97	1.53
Hospital payments (1990 dollars)									
Percentage using services	0.82	0.80	0.87	0.78	0.81	0.84	0.82	0.78	1.09
Average payment per beneficiary	1.11	1.16	1.08	1.00	0.89	0.99	0.98	0.98	1.16
Average payment per enrollee	0.91	0.94	0.93	0.78	0.72	0.83	0.80	0.76	1.27
Total payment (millions)	1.04	1.08	1.11	0.83	0.58	0.83	1.00	0.83	1.39
Total payment (percent)	1.00	1.04	1.06	0.79	0.56	0.80	0.96	0.79	1.34

Source: Duke University, Center for Demographic Studies, analysis of the 1982, 1984, and 1989 National Long-Term Care Survey; original data are in appendix table 6A-1.

a. IADL = instrumental activities of daily living.

b. ADL = activities of daily living.

and the institutional groups. Thus the reduction in use produced decreases in total payments for more chronically impaired groups. Other types of service use were expected to increase in these groups.

As PPS was implemented, beginning October 1, 1983, and extending to 1987, initial reductions in hospital use were large, then declined over time. This could indicate changes in the behavior of short stay hospitals as they learned how the system functioned; for example, the higher reimbursement Diagnosis Related Groups (DRGs) tended to increase over time. Volume of use decreased from 100.4 million days in 1982-83 to 77.9 million days by 1989–90 (see appendix table 6A-1), but program payments increased 4 percent. The active and healthy, those with circulatory problems, and the institutional groups contributed to the increase in total payments, with the active and healthy dominating in each period using 62.2 percent of hospital days in 1989–90, a slight decline from 1982–83 (63.2 percent of days).

PPS was phased in according to a schedule of uniform reporting periods in effect at individual facilities. Periodic adjustments (at least annually) of PPS have taken place since 1986 (for example, as mandated by the 1987 Omnibus Budget Reconciliation Act, P.L. 100-203); DRG weights and other adjustments (for example, teaching hospital, facilities' cost of capital) were evaluated. Additional DRGs were added to reflect emerging medical technologies since PPS's introduction. PPS could be interpreted as modestly reducing variance in payment per enrollee, by discouraging use by the less sick, resulting in slower payment increases after initial reductions.

Skilled Nursing Facility Use

Use and payment of SNFs showed more variation over time and group than did hospital use. SNFs responded to different legislative and regulatory changes (table 6-5).

First, SNFs showed a large increase across groups in total days used from 1982–83 to 1989–90—most strongly for the ADL mobility impaired and the institutional groups. All groups had large increases in the percentage using SNF services. Only the acutely ill and the IADL impaired with physical problem groups used fewer SNF days per beneficiary.

Increases in total payment reflected tremendous volume increases in SNF use from 1982–83 to 1989–90 (350 percent increase in constant

TABLE 6-5. *Ratios of Skilled Nursing Facility Service Days and Payments, 1989–90 to 1982–83, for Health and Functioning Groups Defined from the 1982 and 1989 National Long-Term Care Surveys*

		Group							
		1	2	3	4	5	6	7	8
Item in ratio	Total population	Active and healthy	Circulatory problems	Acutely ill	IADL, vision impaired, and demented[a]	IADL impaired with physical problems[a]	ADL mobility impaired[b]	ADL frail[b]	Institutional
Days spent in a skilled nursing facility									
Percentage using services	2.16	2.04	2.10	2.23	1.92	2.04	2.57	1.79	2.86
Average days per beneficiary	1.29	1.08	1.01	0.89	1.26	0.98	1.15	1.16	1.77
Average days per enrollee	2.80	2.13	2.12	1.97	2.41	1.98	2.97	2.08	5.03
Total days used (millions)	3.17	2.57	2.50	2.09	1.96	1.98	3.65	2.26	5.52
Total days used (percent)	1.00	0.81	0.79	0.66	0.62	0.62	1.15	0.71	1.74
Skilled nursing facility payments (1990 dollars)									
Percentage using services	2.14	2.04	2.06	2.22	1.83	2.00	2.46	1.76	2.87
Average payment per beneficiary	1.84	1.63	1.48	1.35	1.97	1.56	1.66	1.96	2.53
Average payment per enrollee	3.93	3.31	3.04	3.00	3.61	3.11	4.09	3.45	7.25
Total payment (millions)	4.50	3.84	3.61	3.19	2.91	3.12	5.08	3.74	7.95
Total payment (percent)	1.00	0.85	0.80	0.71	0.65	0.69	1.13	0.83	1.77

Source: Duke University, Center for Demographic Studies, analysis of the 1982, 1984, and 1989 National Long-Term Care Survey; original data are in appendix table 6A-2.

a. IADL = instrumental activities of daily living.

b. ADL = activities of daily living.

dollars). Increases occurred for all groups, with the ADL mobility impaired and the institutional groups having larger total payment increases.

The increase from 3.5 to 10.0 percent of the institutional group using SNF services in the year following the NLTCS interview could represent reclassification of already institutionalized patients, in combination with greater illness and disability (see appendix table 6A-2). The institutional group using short stay hospitals increased by 9 percent, whereas the general population had an 18 percent decrease for the same period (table 6-4). This suggested that the institutional group in 1989 had poorer health and functioning than in 1982—consistent with the earlier discharge of patients from short stay hospitals in 1989–90. Much of the change could be attributed to MCCA, which liberalized the SNF benefit and stimulated the certification of institutions as SNFs. In response to the liberalized SNF benefits in MCCA, 1,624 nursing homes, with 75,000 beds, became SNF certified and were concentrated in previously underserved areas.[14] Even though MCCA was repealed in 1989 (effective January 1, 1990), the investments in staff and capital plant necessary to receive the higher SNF payment rate had been incurred, allowing a rapid increase in SNF use. In sum, increases in SNF use were contemporaneous with SNF rule changes and the short-term stimulus of MCCA legislation.

Home Health Agency Use

During 1982–89, HHA use grew rapidly, but unevenly, in the eight groups (table 6-6). HHA likely shifted from being posthospital subacute care, less expensive than SNF, to a service provided to chronically disabled persons that could help them cope with constraints on institutional growth in the period examined. Only the institutional group showed a decline in percentage using HHA services. The other groups had varying increases. From 1982 to 1990, the average number of visits per beneficiary increased for all groups, by variable amounts. The acutely ill increase was the smallest, followed by the ADL mobility impaired and the active and healthy groups. The acutely ill group also had the smallest increase in total HHA visits. The greatest increases in total visits were for the active and healthy and the circulatory problem groups.

TABLE 6-6. *Ratios of Home Health Agency Service Visits and Payments, 1989–90 to 1982–83, for Health and Functioning Groups Defined from the 1982 and 1989 National Long-Term Care Surveys*

		Group							
		1	2	3	4	5	6	7	8
Item in ratio	Total population	Active and healthy	Circulatory problems	Acutely ill	IADL, vision impaired, and demented[a]	IADL impaired with physical problems[a]	ADL mobility impaired[b]	ADL frail[b]	Institutional
Home health agency visits									
Percentage using services	1.24	1.36	1.51	1.12	1.19	1.32	1.20	1.05	0.77
Average visits per beneficiary	1.40	1.42	1.61	1.24	1.58	1.50	1.39	1.48	1.73
Average visits per enrollee	1.75	1.93	2.42	1.38	1.88	1.98	1.66	1.56	1.33
Total visits used (millions)	2.00	2.24	2.86	1.47	1.52	1.99	2.07	1.69	1.47
Total visits used (percent)	1.00	1.12	1.43	0.74	0.76	0.99	1.03	0.85	0.73
Home health agency payments (1990 dollars)									
Percentage using services	1.24	1.35	1.51	1.12	1.19	1.32	1.21	1.05	0.77
Average payment per beneficiary	1.49	1.51	1.73	1.27	1.71	1.67	1.48	1.50	2.06
Average payment per enrollee	1.85	2.05	2.60	1.42	2.04	2.20	1.79	1.58	1.59
Total payment (millions)	2.12	2.38	3.08	1.50	1.64	2.20	2.22	1.71	1.74
Total payment (percent)	1.00	1.12	1.45	0.71	0.78	1.04	1.05	0.81	0.82

Source: Duke University, Center for Demographic Studies, analysis of the 1982, 1984, and 1989 National Long-Term Care Survey; original data are in appendix table 6A-3.

a. IADL = instrumental activities of daily living.

b. ADL = activities of daily living.

HHA payments provided a complementary picture of change over time by groups. Average payments per enrollee and per beneficiary increased for all groups, as did total payment. HHA use did not rise as rapidly as SNF use during the 1982–90 period, nor did the pattern of change favor the chronically disabled group over the active and healthy or the circulatory problem groups. The largest increases were for the active and healthy and the circulatory problem groups. The increases reflected the liberalization of HHA benefits in the Omnibus Reconciliation Act of 1980, effective July 1, 1981 (for example, removal of restrictions on the annual number of HHA visits and the elimination of the three-day prior hospitalization requirement), and the regulatory attempt to control costs in 1983–87 via claims denial.

Medicare Part B Services

Ratios describing changes in medicare part B payments by year and disability group are presented in table 6-7.

For hospital outpatient, physician, DME, and other services, service units were not easily identifiable from medicare files. The percentage using hospital outpatient services showed large increases overall (124 percent) and across all groups over time (from 60 to 142 percent). The variation across groups declined markedly over time (from a 2 to 1 ratio in 1982–83 to a 1.3 to 1 ratio in 1989–90; see appendix table 6A-4). The largest increases in total payments were for the active and healthy and those with circulatory problems. The active and healthy group accounted for $4.6 billion of a total $6.4 billion spent in 1989–90 (71.6 percent versus 65.5 percent in 1982–83). By groups, from 1982–83 to 1989–90, the acutely ill, the IADL, vision impaired, and demented, and the ADL mobility impaired had the smallest increases in total payment and payment per beneficiary.

The legislative and regulatory environment for hospital outpatient services was partly driven by PPS. The 1986 OBRA mandated a change in the reasonable cost methodology for outpatient surgery, which had increased substantially in use after PPS. A prospective payment system—ambulatory care groups for surgery and other services based on *Current Procedural Terminology, Fourth Edition* categories—was being assessed at the end of the study period. The incentive to substitute hospital outpatient for inpatient services, particularly surgery, drove the reimbursement changes. While use increased 124 percent, from 1982 to 1990, program payments increased 262 percent in constant dollars. Cost shifting from hospital inpatient use to outpatient services (especially surgery) as a result of PPS was evident.

Each major legislative initiative since the mid-1980s, mainly continued increases in the average annual payments for such services, has had an impact on the amounts paid to physicians to provide covered services. To that end, a freeze in customary, usual, and reasonable charges was implemented for fifteen months in the 1984–86 period and a system to moderate cost increases by encouraging assignment was in place during the latter part of the 1982–89 period. The national relative value scale approach to physician payment was not in place by 1990.

Each group's average physician payment per beneficiary had a similar increase from 1982–83 to 1989–90. Increases were smallest for the IADL, vision impaired, and demented and the ADL frail groups. The uniformity of the increase in the percentage using services from 59.1 to 77.3 percent was notable (see appendix table 6A-4). The use of physician services was becoming nearly universal with the active and healthy, the IADL, vision impaired, and demented, and the institutional groups having smaller payments per beneficiary.

DME included such diverse items as wheelchairs, braces, oxygen tubing, and walkers. A low-volume service, it showed a decline (–53 percent) in payment per beneficiary (from $380 in 1982–83 to $178 in 1989–90). Despite that drop, total costs increased 533 percent, as a result of a fifteenfold increase in the percentage of persons using DME. DME use was concentrated in both the acutely ill and the circulatory problem groups as well as in the four IADL and ADL groups. Payment per beneficiary was highest for the acutely ill group ($433 each in 1989–90).

Other services was a residual medicare category (primarily renal services and therapy), given the definition of the previous six service types. The average payment per beneficiary and total payment increases were large (1,177 percent and 984 percent, respectively). Increases were smallest for the institutional and the IADL, vision impaired, and demented groups. Total payment grew from $116 million in 1982–83 to $1.3 billion in 1989–90, with very high payments per beneficiary ($4,709 overall). Most of the growth in this category stemmed from increased renal care payment because of a rapid increase in the

TABLE 6-7. *Ratios of Hospital Outpatient, Physician, Durable Medical Equipment, and Other (Renal and Therapy) Service Payments, 1989–90 to 1982–83, for Health and Functioning Groups Defined from the 1982 and 1989 National Long-Term Care Surveys*

		Group							
Item in ratio	Total population	1 Active and healthy	2 Circulatory problems	3 Acutely ill	4 IADL, vision impaired, and demented[a]	5 IADL impaired with physical problems[a]	6 ADL mobility impaired[b]	7 ADL frail[b]	8 Institutional
Hospital outpatient payments (1990 dollars)									
Percentage using services	2.24	2.42	2.08	1.94	1.99	2.00	2.04	1.78	1.60
Average payment per beneficiary	1.41	1.41	1.80	1.31	1.02	1.77	1.09	1.57	1.72
Average payment per enrollee	3.17	3.42	3.75	2.54	2.03	3.56	2.23	2.79	2.76
Total payment (millions)	3.62	3.96	4.44	2.70	1.64	3.56	2.77	3.02	3.03
Total payment (percent)	1.00	1.09	1.23	0.75	0.45	0.98	0.77	0.83	0.84
Physician payments (1990 dollars)									
Percentage using services	1.31	1.36	1.19	1.12	1.22	1.22	1.18	1.07	1.12
Average payment per beneficiary	2.26	2.27	2.48	2.30	1.96	2.35	2.37	2.16	2.58
Average payment per enrollee	2.95	3.09	2.95	2.57	2.39	2.87	2.81	2.31	2.88
Total payment (millions)	3.38	3.58	3.49	2.73	1.93	2.88	3.49	2.50	3.16
Total payment (percent)	1.00	1.06	1.03	0.81	0.57	0.85	1.03	0.74	0.94

Durable medical equipment payments (1990 dollars)

Percentage using services	15.00	0.0	8.00	9.13	3.00	9.00	4.54	6.50	0.0
Average payment per beneficiary	0.47	0.0	0.97	1.94	1.35	0.91	0.31	0.47	0.0
Average payment per enrollee	5.22	0.0	6.85	17.51	3.80	8.26	1.39	2.93	0.0
Total payment (millions)	6.33	0.0	8.35	18.87	3.22	8.30	1.76	3.19	0.0
Total payment (percent)	1.00	0.0	1.32	2.98	0.51	1.31	0.28	0.50	0.0

Other payments (1990 dollars)

Percentage using services	0.74	0.62	1.07	0.92	0.60	1.37	1.20	2.13	1.20
Average payment per beneficiary	12.77	17.17	7.27	12.76	5.41	17.18	27.47	10.70	1.44
Average payment per enrollee	9.47	10.53	7.71	11.69	3.28	23.59	33.02	22.85	1.71
Total payment (millions)	10.84	12.19	9.12	12.38	2.65	23.63	41.06	24.69	1.88
Total payment (percent)	1.00	1.12	0.84	1.14	0.24	2.18	3.79	2.28	0.17

Source: Duke University, Center for Demographic Studies, analysis of the 1982, 1984, and 1989 National Long-Term Care Survey; original data are in appendix table 6A-4.

a. IADL = instrumental activities of daily living.

b. ADL = activities of daily living.

TABLE 6-8. Ratios of Total Payments and Percentages of Total Payments, 1989–90 to 1982–83, and Percentages of Total Change in Total Payments (in Constant Dollars), for Seven Medicare Service Types, for Health and Functioning Groups Defined from the 1982 and 1989 National Long-Term Care Surveys

| | | Group | | | | | | | |
| | | 1 | 2 | 3 | 4 | 5 | 6 | 7 | 8 |
Service	Total population	Active and healthy	Circulatory problems	Acutely ill	IADL, vision impaired, and demented[a]	IADL impaired with physical problems[a]	ADL mobility impaired[b]	ADL frail[b]	Institutional
					Ratio of total payments (millions)				
Short stay hospital	1.04	1.08	1.11	0.83	0.58	0.83	1.00	0.83	1.39
Skilled nursing facility	4.50	3.84	3.61	3.19	2.91	3.12	5.08	3.74	7.95
Home health agency	2.12	2.38	3.08	1.50	1.64	2.20	2.22	1.71	1.74
Hospital outpatient	3.62	3.96	4.44	2.70	1.64	3.56	2.77	3.02	3.03
Physician	3.38	3.58	3.49	2.73	1.93	2.88	3.49	2.50	3.16
Durable medical equipment	6.33	0.0	8.35	18.87	3.22	8.30	1.76	3.19	0.0
Other (renal and therapy)	10.84	12.19	9.12	12.38	2.65	23.63	41.06	24.69	1.88
Total (all services)	1.58	1.66	1.66	1.20	0.88	1.28	1.53	1.24	1.95

Ratio of total payments (percent)

Short stay hospital	1.00	1.04	1.06	0.79	0.56	0.80	0.96	0.79	1.34
Skilled nursing facility	1.00	0.85	0.80	0.71	0.65	0.69	1.13	0.83	1.77
Home health agency	1.00	1.12	1.45	0.71	0.78	1.04	1.05	0.81	0.82
Hospital outpatient	1.00	1.09	1.23	0.75	0.45	0.98	0.77	0.83	0.84
Physician	1.00	1.06	1.03	0.81	0.57	0.85	1.03	0.74	0.94
Durable medical equipment	1.00	0.0	1.32	2.98	0.51	1.31	0.28	0.50	0.0
Other (renal and therapy)	1.00	1.12	0.84	1.14	0.24	2.18	3.79	2.28	0.17
Total (all services)	1.00	1.05	1.05	0.76	0.56	0.81	0.97	0.79	1.23

Percentage of total change in total payments

Short stay hospital	100.0	129.2	11.7	-12.1	-40.5	-17.0	-0.5	-29.6	58.9
Skilled nursing facility	100.0	33.6	4.6	1.8	3.3	4.2	8.3	9.4	34.9
Home health agency	100.0	50.4	9.9	2.5	3.3	6.1	10.8	15.4	1.6
Hospital outpatient	100.0	73.9	4.8	1.6	1.1	3.2	3.8	4.7	6.9
Physician	100.0	74.5	4.3	1.8	1.3	2.7	4.8	3.7	6.8
Durable medical equipment	100.0	39.9	6.9	16.8	2.5	15.0	5.6	13.5	0.0
Other (renal and therapy)	100.0	69.4	5.2	2.0	1.1	4.3	10.3	6.3	1.6
Total (all services)	100.0	73.4	5.2	1.0	-0.8	2.0	5.2	3.2	10.8

Source: Duke University, Center for Demographic Studies, analysis of the 1982, 1984, and 1989 National Long-Term Care Survey; original data are in appendix table 6A-5.
a. IADL = instrumental activities of daily living.
b. ADL = activities of daily living.

over-age-65 renal care population. The payments were distributed over all groups, suggesting renal dysfunction was not necessarily a chronic disabling (in terms of ADL and IADL functions) condition.

System Shifts

Ratios of total payments from 1989–90 to 1982–83 for each of the seven medicare services and for the aggregate of all services provided an overview of system changes (table 6-8).

The average increase in payment for all services was 58 percent. At the extremes, the IADL, vision impaired, and demented group had a 12 percent decrease in payments, and the institutional group had a 95 percent increase. The only other groups above the average increase were the active and healthy group and the circulatory problem group. In contrast, three groups reporting primarily fair or poor health—the acutely ill, the IADL impaired with physical problems, and the ADL frail groups—all had increases in a narrow range (20 to 28 percent).

In comparing group ratios with total population ratios for specific services, distinctive patterns emerged. The active and healthy group had higher than average ratios for short stay hospital, HHA, hospital outpatient, physician, and other services. The circulatory problem group had higher ratios for short stay hospital, HHA, hospital outpatient, physician, and DME services. The acutely ill group had higher ratios only for DME and other services. The IADL, vision impaired, and demented group had no ratios higher than average. The IADL impaired with physical problems group had higher ratios for HHA, DME, and other services. The ADL mobility impaired group had higher ratios for SNF, HHA, physician, and other services. The ADL frail group had higher ratios only for other services. The institutional group had higher ratios for short stay hospital and SNF services. Thus a correlation existed in the relation (to total trends) of different services with the health characteristics of the groups.

Although the largest overall contribution to the total increase in medicare program payments (73.4 percent) was by the active and healthy group, that was less than its 80.6 percent share of the population (table 6-3). The institutional group (with 5.5 percent share) accounted for 10.8 percent of the overall increase, 58.9 percent of the short stay hospital increase, and 34.9 percent of the SNF increase. The two ADL groups (with 6.2 percent share) accounted for 8.4 percent of the overall increase, 26.2 percent of the HHA increase, and 17.7 percent of the SNF increase. The two IADL groups (with 3.5 percent share) accounted for 1.2 percent of the overall increase, 9.4 percent of the HHA increase, and 7.5 percent of the SNF increase. The acutely ill group (with 1.3 percent share) accounted for 1.0 percent of the overall increase and 16.8 percent of the DME increase.

SUMMARY

Changes in medicare part A and B service use for 1982 to 1990 were examined using health and functional groups defined from NLTCS data. In making comparisons we stratified the service data on health defined by eight groups identified from fifty-six health and functional measures and by institutionalization. We tabulated medicare service use records for the twelve months after each survey. By forming such external variables, we generated health and functional status specific estimates for seven types of service use, in 1982–83 and 1989–90, for eight health and functioning groups. By using sample weights, we estimated the amount of services in each category used by the U.S. elderly population. Differences existed between groups as a result of changes in both the likelihood of using a service and the volume of service used per beneficiary. Thus disability predicted variation in the use of medicare services by community residents—a predictability persisting from 1982 to 1990. The addition of health measures explicated more of the internal variation of use in the community population and clarified the use patterns of an acutely ill group.

In terms of changes in the health and functional status of the population, the proportion in the most active group increased. Services in the lowest service use groups tended to increase, but those effects were dominated by the changes in the services used per enrollee of functionally impaired groups. Increases were evident (but at lower levels) in the nondisabled and active subgroups. The size of those populations caused large, absolute increases in service use. For the institutional group, total SNF and HHA use increased, while the percentage of such persons using HHA services declined. The HHA use per enrollee in this group increased. The ADL frail group had a large increase in HHA use per enrollee. Overall, the increase for the two ADL groups was a considerable portion of the total increase in HHA payments—that is, 26.2 percent, compared with 50.4 percent of the increase coming from the active and healthy group, which was twenty-eight times larger.

Analysis of the use of the seven medicare services over time for the eight disability groups identified relations between hospital, SNF, and HHA changes to the regulatory environment suggesting that legislative changes redistributed service use over groups. Specific targeting for specific services could achieve a stronger result. Nonetheless, we observed a tendency for the more disabled groups to increase their use of certain services more than in less disabled groups, while the volume of SNF and HHA payments was often shifted from the healthiest group. We also presented physician, hospital outpatient, DME, and other service payments. Physician and hospital outpatient data revealed increases in payments across groups, consistent with aged population growth and medical inflation. DME and other services experienced growth and uneven patterns of increase and decline, which were much more difficult to correlate with specific legislative or demographic explanations.

NOTES

1. We acknowledge the helpful comments and suggestions of Judy Sangl and Nancy Miller of the Office of Research and Demonstrations, Health Care Financing Administration. This research was supported by HCFA grant no. 500-89-0047 and NIA grant nos. AG01159 and AG07025.

2. Kenneth G. Manton, Larry S. Corder, and Eric Stallard, "Estimates of Change in Chronic Disability and Institutional Incidence and Prevalence Rates in the U.S. Elderly Population from the 1982, 1984, and 1989 National Long Term Care Survey," *Journal of Gerontology:Social Sciences*, vol. 47, no. 4 (1993), pp. S153–S166; and Kenneth G. Manton, Eric Stallard, and Larry S. Corder, "Changes in Morbidity and Chronic Disability in the U.S. Elderly Population: Evidence from the 1982, 1984, and 1989 National Long Term Care Surveys," *Journal of Gerontology:Social Sciences*, vol. 50, no. 4 (1995), pp. S194–S204.

3. Kenneth G. Manton, Larry S. Corder, and Eric Stallard, "Changes in the Use of Personal Assistance and Special Equipment 1982 to 1989: Results from the 1982 and 1989 NLTCS," *Gerontologist*, vol. 33, no. 2 (1993), pp. 168–76.

4. Samuel H. Preston, "Demographic Change in the United States, 1970–2050," in Kenneth G. Manton, Burton H. Singer, and Richard Suzman, eds., *Forecasting the Health of Elderly Populations* (New York: Springer-Verlag, 1992), pp. 51–78.

5. Kenneth G. Manton and Eric Stallard, "Medical Demography: Interaction of Disability Dynamics and Mortality," in L. Martin, ed., *The Demography of Aging* (Washington: National Research Council Committee on Population, 1994), pp. 217–77.

6. Sidney Katz and Camachi Akpom, "A Measure of Primary Socio-biological Functions," *International Journal of Health Services*, vol. 6, no. 3 (1976), pp. 493–508; and M. Powell Lawton and Elaine M. Brody, "Assessment of Older People: Self-Maintaining and Instrumental Activities of Daily Living," *Gerontologist*, vol. 9, no. 2 (1969), pp. 179–86.

7. Manton, Stallard, and Corder, "Changes in Morbidity and Chronic Disability in the U.S. Elderly Population."

8. M. I. Dorevitch and others, "The Accuracy of Self and Informant Ratings of Physical Functional Capacity in the Elderly," *Journal of Clinical Epidemiology*, vol. 45, no. 7 (1992), pp. 791–98. See also David B. Reuben, Albert L. Siu, and Sokkun Kimpau, "The Predictive Validity of Self-Support and Performance-Based Measures of Function and Health," *Journal of Gerontology:Medical Sciences*, vol. 47, no. 4 (1992), pp. M106–M110.

9. Kenneth G. Manton and others, "Time Varying Covariates of Human Mortality and Aging: Multidimensional Generalization of the Gompertz," *Journal of Gerontology:Biological Sciences*, vol. 49, no. 4 (1994), pp. B169–B190; and Manton and Stallard, "Medical Demography."

10. Kenneth G. Manton, Max A. Woodbury, and Eric Stallard, "Statistical and Measurement Issues in Assessing the Welfare Status of Aged Individuals and Populations," *Journal of Econometrics*, vol. 50 (1991), pp. 151–81; and Kenneth G. Manton, Max A. Woodbury, and H. Dennis Tolley, *Statistical Applications Using Fuzzy Sets* (New York: Wiley-Interscience Publication, 1994).

11. Yvonne Bishop, Stephen Fienberg, and Paul Holland, *Discrete Multivariate Analysis: Theory and Practice* (MIT Press, 1975).

12. Paul Lazarsfeld and Neil Henry, *Latent Structure Analysis* (Boston: Houghton Mifflin, 1968).

13. Steven F. McKay, *Short-Range Actuarial Projections of the Old-Age, Survivors, and Disability Insurance Program, 1991: Actuarial Study No. 104*, SSA Pub. No. 11-11550 (Baltimore, Md.: Social Security Administration, October 1990).

14. *Long Term Care: Emerging Trends*, special issue of *Health Care Financing Review*, vol. 14, no. 4 (Summer 1993).

TABLE 6A-1. *Short Stay Hospital Use, for Health and Functioning Groups Defined from the 1982, 1984, and 1989 National Long-Term Care Surveys*

		Group							
		1	2	3	4	5	6	7	8
Item	*Total population*	*Active and healthy*	*Circulatory problems*	*Acutely ill*	*IADL, vision impaired, and demented[a]*	*IADL impaired with physical problems[a]*	*ADL mobility impaired[b]*	*ADL frail[b]*	*Institutional*
Days spent in hospital in 1982–83									
Percentage using services	24.7	21.3	38.3	43.8	40.6	40.7	39.9	47.9	27.1
Average days per beneficiary	15.6	14.3	17.2	19.6	18.2	18.8	19.0	19.7	16.5
Average days per enrollee	3.8	3.1	6.6	8.6	7.4	7.7	7.6	9.4	4.5
Total days used (millions)	100.4	63.5	4.9	3.1	4.3	4.4	6.0	7.5	6.7
Total days used (percent)	100.0	63.2	4.9	3.1	4.3	4.4	6.0	7.4	6.6
Days spent in hospital in 1989–90									
Percentage using services	20.3	17.2	33.4	34.6	32.8	34.5	33.1	37.3	29.5
Average days per beneficiary	12.9	11.7	13.5	15.6	13.8	14.2	15.0	17.6	16.4
Average days per enrollee	2.6	2.0	4.5	5.4	4.5	4.9	5.0	6.6	4.8
Total days used (millions)	77.9	48.4	4.0	2.1	2.1	2.8	4.9	5.6	7.9
Total days used (percent)	100.0	62.2	5.1	2.7	2.7	3.6	6.3	7.2	10.1

Hospital payments in 1982–83 (1990 dollars)

Percentage using services	24.4	21.1	38.0	43.5	40.3	40.5	39.5	47.5	26.9
Average payment per beneficiary	6,237.2	5,898.4	6,557.1	7,493.7	6,906.8	7,237.7	7,175.4	7,562.7	6,267.4
Average payment per enrollee	1,524.6	1,244.9	2,491.6	3,258.8	2,786.2	2,932.5	2,833.6	3,594.1	1,683.3
Total payment (millions)	39,815.5	25,864.5	1,849.8	1,185.8	1,626.7	1,692.5	2,253.4	2,841.4	2,501.5
Total payment (percent)	100.0	65.0	4.6	3.0	4.1	4.3	5.7	7.1	6.3

Hospital payments in 1989–90 (1990 dollars)

Percentage using services	20.0	17.0	33.0	34.1	32.6	34.0	32.4	36.9	29.4
Average payment per beneficiary	6,945.8	6,858.4	7,056.3	7,459.7	6,170.3	7,144.7	7,024.0	7,407.3	7,294.1
Average payment per enrollee	1,389.2	1,164.2	2,326.1	2,543.7	2,010.1	2,431.9	2,273.8	2,734.8	2,140.6
Total payment (millions)	41,493.5	28,033.3	2,045.8	982.0	947.6	1,406.5	2,244.7	2,344.6	3,489.1
Total payment (percent)	100.0	67.6	4.9	2.4	2.3	3.4	5.4	5.7	8.4

Source: Duke University, Center for Demographic Studies, analysis of the 1982, 1984, and 1989 National Long-Term Care Survey.

a. IADL = instrumental activities of daily living.

b. ADL = activities of daily living.

TABLE 6A-2. Skilled Nursing Facility Service Use, for Health and Functioning Groups Defined from the 1982 and 1989 National Long-Term Care Surveys

| | | | | | Group | | | | |
| | | 1 | 2 | 3 | 4 | 5 | 6 | 7 | 8 |
Item	Total population	Active and healthy	Circulatory problems	Acutely ill	IADL, vision impaired, and demented[a]	IADL impaired with physical problems[a]	ADL mobility impaired[b]	ADL frail[b]	Institutional
Days spent in a skilled nursing facility in 1982–83									
Percentage using services	1.0	0.5	1.6	1.9	2.7	2.5	2.1	4.2	3.5
Average days per beneficiary	32.0	30.9	32.3	32.8	28.9	35.7	28.7	33.1	34.1
Average days per enrollee	0.3	0.2	0.5	0.6	0.8	0.9	0.6	1.4	1.2
Total days used (millions)	7.9	3.0	0.4	0.2	0.5	0.5	0.5	1.1	1.8
Total days used (percent)	100.0	38.1	4.8	2.8	5.7	6.4	6.2	13.7	22.4
Days spent in a skilled nursing facility in 1989–90									
Percentage using services	2.1	1.0	3.3	4.1	5.2	5.0	5.5	7.5	10.0
Average days per beneficiary	41.1	33.4	32.5	29.1	36.3	34.9	33.1	38.4	60.1
Average days per enrollee	0.8	0.3	1.1	1.2	1.9	1.7	1.8	2.9	6.0
Total days used (millions)	25.1	7.8	1.0	0.5	0.9	1.0	1.8	2.5	9.8
Total days used (percent)	100.0	30.8	3.8	1.8	3.5	4.0	7.1	9.8	39.1

Skilled nursing facility payments in 1982–83 (1990 dollars)

Percentage using services	0.9	0.5	1.6	1.9	2.7	2.5	2.1	4.2	3.5
Average payment per beneficiary	1,924.2	2,047.2	2,465.8	1,976.4	1,810.4	2,340.7	1,993.4	1,726.9	1,592.2
Average payment per enrollee	18.2	9.5	39.2	36.6	48.6	57.4	42.4	72.0	55.9
Total payment (millions)	474.3	196.6	29.1	13.3	28.4	33.1	33.7	56.9	83.2
Total payment (percent)	100.0	41.5	6.1	2.8	6.0	7.0	7.1	12.0	17.5

Skilled nursing facility payments in 1989–90 (1990 dollars)

Percentage using services	2.0	0.9	3.3	4.1	4.9	4.9	5.2	7.3	10.1
Average payment per beneficiary	3,547.3	3,333.8	3,652.1	2,670.7	3,575.0	3,646.7	3,312.3	3,382.7	4,023.5
Average payment per enrollee	71.4	31.3	119.3	109.9	175.5	178.5	173.7	248.1	405.6
Total payment (millions)	2,132.6	754.0	104.9	42.4	82.7	103.2	171.4	212.7	661.2
Total payment (percent)	100.0	35.4	4.9	2.0	3.9	4.8	8.0	10.0	31.0

Source: Duke University, Center for Demographic Studies, analysis of the 1982, 1984, and 1989 National Long-Term Care Survey.

a. IADL = instrumental activities of daily living.

b. ADL = activities of daily living.

TABLE 6A-3. *Home Health Agency Service Use, for Health and Functioning Groups Defined from the 1982 and 1989 National Long-Term Care Surveys*

| | | Group | | | | | | | |
| | | 1 | 2 | 3 | 4 | 5 | 6 | 7 | 8 |
Item	Total population	Active and healthy	Circulatory problems	Acutely ill	IADL, vision impaired, and demented[a]	IADL impaired with physical problems[a]	ADL mobility impaired[b]	ADL frail[b]	Institutional
Home health agency visits in 1982–83									
Percentage using services	5.0	3.1	10.3	14.7	13.7	13.3	15.5	26.6	2.4
Average days per beneficiary	27.6	21.9	25.4	38.4	26.6	28.2	29.9	42.8	25.8
Average days per enrollee	1.4	0.7	2.6	5.6	3.7	3.7	4.6	11.4	0.6
Total days used (millions)	36.1	14.3	2.0	2.1	2.1	2.2	3.7	9.0	0.9
Total days used (percent)	100.0	39.5	5.4	5.7	5.9	6.0	10.2	24.9	2.5
Home health agency visits in 1989–90									
Percentage using services	6.2	4.3	15.6	16.4	16.3	17.5	18.6	27.9	1.8
Average days per beneficiary	38.8	31.0	40.7	47.5	42.1	42.3	41.4	63.2	44.6
Average days per enrollee	2.4	1.3	6.3	7.8	6.9	7.4	7.7	17.7	0.8
Total days used (millions)	72.1	32.0	5.6	3.0	3.2	4.3	7.6	15.2	1.3
Total days used (percent)	100.0	44.3	7.7	4.2	4.5	5.9	10.5	21.0	1.8

Home health agency payments in 1982–83 (1990 dollars)

Percentage using services	5.0	3.1	10.3	14.7	13.7	13.3	15.4	26.5	2.4
Average payment per beneficiary	1,335.2	1,098.1	1,211.5	1,849.6	1,250.5	1,297.4	1,401.8	2,011.7	1,224.2
Average payment per enrollee	66.7	34.4	125.1	271.3	170.9	171.9	215.9	533.6	28.9
Total payment (millions)	1,742.8	715.8	92.9	98.7	99.8	99.2	171.7	421.9	42.9
Total payment (percent)	100.0	41.1	5.3	5.7	5.7	5.7	9.9	24.2	2.5

Home health agency payments in 1989–90 (1990 dollars)

Percentage using services	6.2	4.3	15.6	16.4	16.3	17.5	18.6	27.9	1.8
Average payment per beneficiary	1,994.8	1,663.4	2,093.0	2,347.2	2,134.0	2,161.2	2,080.6	3,015.0	2,521.7
Average payment per enrollee	123.8	70.6	325.5	384.1	347.9	377.4	386.7	842.4	45.8
Total payment (millions)	3,696.4	1,701.0	286.3	148.3	164.0	218.3	381.8	722.2	74.6
Total payment (percent)	100.0	46.0	7.7	4.0	4.4	5.9	10.3	19.5	2.0

Source: Duke University, Center for Demographic Studies, analysis of the 1982, 1984, and 1989 National Long-Term Care Survey.
a. IADL = instrumental activities of daily living.
b. ADL = activities of daily living.

TABLE 6A-4. Hospital Outpatient, Physician, Durable Medical Equipment, and Other (Renal and Therapy) Service Use, for Health and Functioning Groups Defined from the 1982 and 1989 National Long-Term Care Surveys

		Group							
Item	Total population	1 Active and healthy	2 Circulatory problems	3 Acutely ill	4 IADL, vision impaired, and demented[a]	5 IADL impaired with physical problems[a]	6 ADL mobility impaired[b]	7 ADL frail[b]	8 Institutional
Hospital outpatient payments in 1982–83 (1990 dollars)									
Percentage using services	19.8	17.5	26.8	28.4	24.9	27.1	25.8	28.7	34.7
Average payment per beneficiary	343.5	321.2	326.5	424.3	545.6	374.6	488.0	480.4	306.2
Average payment per enrollee	68.1	56.1	87.5	120.6	135.7	101.4	125.9	138.0	106.2
Total payment (millions)	1,778.2	1,164.5	65.0	43.9	79.2	58.5	100.1	109.1	157.8
Total payment (percent)	100.0	65.5	3.7	2.5	4.5	3.3	5.6	6.1	8.9
Hospital outpatient payments in 1989–90 (1990 dollars)									
Percentage using services	44.4	42.2	55.8	55.2	49.5	54.3	52.7	51.0	55.6
Average payment per beneficiary	485.7	454.4	588.2	556.6	554.8	664.6	534.3	753.8	528.1
Average payment per enrollee	215.7	191.5	328.4	307.0	274.9	360.6	281.4	384.5	293.7
Total payment (millions)	6,443.3	4,611.8	288.8	118.5	129.6	208.6	277.8	329.6	478.7
Total payment (percent)	100.0	71.6	4.5	1.8	2.0	3.2	4.3	5.1	7.4

Physician payments in 1982–83 (1990 dollars)

Percentage using services	59.1	55.5	72.5	72.8	67.3	69.6	69.8	73.8	78.4
Average payment per beneficiary	511.4	469.7	602.3	740.6	669.7	673.5	657.8	793.3	509.9
Average payment per enrollee	302.2	260.7	436.6	539.4	450.5	469.0	459.4	585.1	399.6
Total payment (millions)	7,892.7	5,417.0	324.1	196.3	263.0	270.7	365.3	462.6	593.8
Total payment (percent)	100.0	68.6	4.1	2.5	3.3	3.4	4.6	5.9	7.5

Physician payments in 1989–90 (1990 dollars)

Percentage using services	77.3	75.6	86.1	81.5	82.1	85.2	82.7	78.9	87.4
Average payment per beneficiary	1,154.9	1,064.8	1,496.4	1,703.5	1,312.9	1,582.1	1,560.6	1,710.5	1,316.9
Average payment per enrollee	892.4	805.3	1,287.6	1,388.8	1,077.6	1,347.4	1,291.0	1,348.9	1,150.7
Total payment (millions)	26,654.2	19,391.8	1,132.4	536.2	508.0	779.3	1,274.5	1,156.4	1,875.6
Total payment (percent)	100.0	72.8	4.2	2.0	1.9	2.9	4.8	4.3	7.0

Durable medical equipment payments in 1982–83 (1990 dollars)

Percentage using services	0.0	0.0	0.0	0.1	0.1	0.1	0.1	0.1	0.0
Average payment per beneficiary	380.4	0.0	271.6	223.3	165.7	277.5	490.9	518.9	0.0
Average payment per enrollee	0.1	0.0	0.1	0.2	0.1	0.2	0.6	0.5	0.0
Total payment (millions)	1.3	0.0	0.1	0.1	0.1	0.1	0.5	0.4	0.0
Total payment (percent)	100.0	0.0	5.0	5.0	6.0	11.0	39.0	33.0	0.0

Durable medical equipment payments in 1989–90 (1990 dollars)

Percentage using services	0.2	0.1	0.2	0.7	0.2	0.8	0.6	0.7	0.0
Average payment per beneficiary	178.1	114.7	262.8	433.0	223.5	252.2	152.3	245.6	0.0
Average payment per enrollee	0.3	0.1	0.6	3.2	0.5	2.0	0.9	1.6	0.0
Total payment (millions)	8.2	2.8	0.5	1.2	0.3	1.2	0.9	1.4	0.0
Total payment (percent)	100.0	33.6	6.6	14.9	3.1	14.4	10.9	16.6	0.0

TABLE 6A-4. (continued)

Other payments in 1982–83 (1990 dollars)

Percentage using services	1.2	1.2	1.5	1.8	2.0	1.6	1.3	1.3	0.9
Average payment per beneficiary	368.9	292.2	640.0	294.5	663.7	236.8	287.7	295.8	1,519.1
Average payment per enrollee	4.5	3.4	9.8	5.4	13.0	3.8	3.7	3.8	13.7
Total payment (millions)	116.4	71.1	7.3	2.0	7.6	2.2	2.9	3.0	20.4
Total payment (percent)	100.0	61.0	6.3	1.7	6.5	1.9	2.5	2.6	17.5

Other payments in 1989–90 (1990 dollars)

Percentage using services	0.9	0.7	1.6	1.7	1.2	2.2	1.5	2.8	1.1
Average payment per beneficiary	4,708.7	5,017.4	4,651.1	3,756.9	3,588.8	4,067.3	7,904.6	3,165.0	2,188.4
Average payment per enrollee	42.3	36.0	75.7	63.0	42.8	88.8	122.1	87.1	23.5
Total payment (millions)	1,262.0	866.0	66.5	24.3	20.2	51.3	120.5	74.7	38.4
Total payment (percent)	100.0	68.6	5.3	1.9	1.6	4.1	9.5	5.9	3.0

Source: Duke University, Center for Demographic Studies, analysis of the 1982, 1984, and 1989 National Long-Term Care Survey.

a. IADL = instrumental activities of daily living.

b. ADL = activities of daily living.

TABLE 6A-5. Total Payments, Percentages of Total Payments, and Change in Total Payments (in Constant Dollars) for Seven Medicare Service Types, for Health and Functioning Groups Defined from the 1982 and 1989 National Long-Term Care Surveys

					Group				
Item	Total population	1 Active and healthy	2 Circulatory problems	3 Acutely ill	4 IADL, vision impaired, and demented[a]	5 IADL impaired with physical problems[a]	6 ADL mobility impaired[b]	7 ADL frail[b]	8 Institutional
					Total payments 1982–83 (millions)				
Short stay hospital	39,815.5	25,864.5	1,849.8	1,185.8	1,626.7	1,692.5	2,253.4	2,841.4	2,501.5
Skilled nursing facility	474.3	196.6	29.1	13.3	28.4	33.1	33.7	56.9	83.2
Home health agency	1,742.8	715.8	92.9	98.7	99.8	99.2	171.7	421.9	42.9
Hospital outpatient	1,778.2	1,164.5	65.0	43.9	79.2	58.5	100.1	109.1	157.8
Physician	7,892.7	5,417.0	324.1	196.3	263.0	270.7	365.3	462.6	593.8
Durable medical equipment	1.3	0.0	0.1	0.1	0.1	0.1	0.5	0.4	0.0
Other (renal and therapy)	116.4	71.1	7.3	2.0	7.6	2.2	2.9	3.0	20.4
Total (all services)	51,821.3	33,429.3	2,368.2	1,540.0	2,104.8	2,156.4	2,927.7	3,895.3	3,399.6

Total payments 1989–90 (in millions)

Short stay hospital	41,493.5	28,033.3	2,045.8	982.0	947.6	1,406.5	2,244.7	2,344.6	3,489.1
Skilled nursing facility	2,132.6	754.0	104.9	42.4	82.7	103.2	171.4	212.7	661.2
Home health agency	3,696.4	1,701.0	286.3	148.3	164.0	218.3	381.8	722.2	74.6
Hospital outpatient	6,443.3	4,611.8	288.8	118.5	129.6	208.6	277.8	329.6	478.7
Physician	26,654.2	19,391.8	1,132.4	536.2	508.0	779.3	1,274.5	1,156.4	1,875.6
Durable medical equipment	8.2	2.8	0.5	1.2	0.3	1.2	0.9	1.4	0.0
Other (renal and therapy)	1,262.0	866.0	66.5	24.3	20.2	51.3	120.5	74.7	38.4
Total (all services)	81,690.2	55,360.6	3,925.3	1,852.9	1,852.4	2,768.3	4,471.5	4,841.7	6,617.6

Total payments 1982–83 (percent)

Short stay hospital	100.0	6.5	4.6	3.0	4.1	4.3	5.7	7.1	6.3
Skilled nursing facility	100.0	41.5	6.1	2.8	6.0	7.0	7.1	12.0	17.5
Home health agency	100.0	41.1	5.3	5.7	5.7	5.7	9.9	24.2	2.5
Hospital outpatient	100.0	65.5	3.7	2.5	4.5	3.3	5.6	6.1	8.9
Physician	100.0	68.6	4.1	2.5	3.3	3.4	4.6	5.9	7.5
Durable medical equipment	100.0	0.0	5.0	5.0	6.0	11.0	39.0	33.0	0.0
Other (renal and therapy)	100.0	61.0	6.3	1.7	6.5	1.9	2.5	2.6	17.5
Total (all services)	100.0	64.5	4.6	3.0	4.1	4.2	5.6	7.5	6.6

Total payments 1989–90 (percent)

Short stay hospital	100.0	67.6	4.9	2.4	2.3	3.4	5.4	5.7	8.4
Skilled nursing facility	100.0	35.4	4.9	2.0	3.9	4.8	8.0	10.0	31.0
Home health agency	100.0	46.0	7.7	4.0	4.4	5.9	10.3	19.5	2.0
Hospital outpatient	100.0	71.6	4.5	1.8	2.0	3.2	4.3	5.1	7.4
Physician	100.0	72.8	4.2	2.0	1.9	2.9	4.8	4.3	7.0
Durable medical equipment	100.0	33.6	6.6	14.9	3.1	14.4	10.9	16.6	0.0
Other (renal and therapy)	100.0	68.6	5.3	1.9	1.6	4.1	9.5	5.9	3.0
Total (all services)	100.0	67.8	4.8	2.3	2.3	3.4	5.5	5.9	8.1

				Change in total payments (millions)				
Short stay hospital	1,678.0	2,168.8	196.0	−203.8	−679.1	−286.1	−8.7	−496.8	987.6
Skilled nursing facility	1,658.3	557.4	75.8	29.1	54.3	70.1	137.7	155.8	578.0
Home health agency	1,953.6	985.2	193.4	49.5	64.3	119.1	210.1	300.4	31.7
Hospital outpatient	4,665.1	3,447.3	223.8	74.6	50.4	150.1	177.7	220.5	320.8
Physician	18,761.4	13,974.9	808.3	339.9	245.0	508.5	909.1	693.9	1,281.8
Durable medical equipment	6.9	2.8	0.5	1.2	0.2	1.0	0.4	0.9	0.0
Other (renal and therapy)	1,145.6	794.9	59.2	22.4	12.6	49.2	117.6	71.7	18.0
Total (all services)	29,868.9	21,931.3	1,557.1	312.9	−252.4	611.9	1,543.8	946.3	3,217.9

Source: Duke University, Center for Demographic Studies, analysis of the 1982, 1984, and 1989 National Long-Term Care Survey.

a. IADL = instrumental activities of daily living.

b. ADL = activities of daily living.

Chapter 7

JUDITH D. KASPER

Cognitive Impairment in Older People and Use of Physician Services and Inpatient Care

Cognitive impairment, which is often caused by dementia, results in substantial need for assistance in many different areas of functioning over long periods of time. The difficult management issues surrounding progressive dementia and the need for continuous care over a period of years has received considerable attention and has rightfully taken priority as the focus of research and policy concerns.[1] In this chapter I address a topic that is important in the overall care of older cognitively impaired people, but about which much less is known—access to physician care and use of hospital services, or so-called "acute care providers."

Ideally, access to physician care should be a function of a person's health status and need for such care.[2] Inadequate financing and service availability are among the barriers to access, particularly for younger people; but cognitive impairment is a potential barrier to appropriate physician and hospital care for elderly people. Seeking and obtaining care may be complicated in several ways by the presence of cognitive impairment or dementia. Cognitive impairment can interfere with an elderly individual's ability to recognize and talk about health problems, as well as with a caregiver's ability to attribute symptoms to such problems. The process of getting to a provider may be complicated by physical disability, but also by patient resistance or disorientation. Finally, for some of the same reasons, a physician may find it difficult to diagnose and treat these individuals, and some doctors may be reluctant to take them on as patients.

Because elderly people with dementia are concentrated in the oldest age groups,[3] comorbidity (the presence of more than one disease or health condition) is common. Cognitive impairment and dementia may not be subject to medical intervention, but comorbidities and many of the noncognitive symptoms that accompany dementia are. Comorbidity has been shown to be an important contributor to disability among older people.[4] The presence of other illnesses, both physical and psychological, may exacerbate the effects of dementia—increasing functional impairment and contributing to a poorer quality of life for patients and caregivers.[5] In addition to improvement of patient and family circumstances, appropriate and timely access to community-based physician care is also generally believed to reduce the need for more costly care in inpatient settings or emergency rooms (ERs).[6]

Few studies have analyzed access to physician care or use of other acute care services by older people with cognitive impairment. Of a small number of elderly people tracked in the Epidemiologic Catchment Area Study, those with cognitive impairment were less likely than others to see a health professional (controlling for age, sex, and marital status).[7] A more recent study of persons with probable or possible Alzheimer's disease found differences in service use by living arrangement. Persons who lived alone were more likely to use community-based social services but less likely to use physician, hospital, or adult day care compared with persons living with others.[8] However, this analysis did not address differences in service use between persons with and without dementia.

Regarding inpatient care, there is some evidence that, once admitted to a facility, elderly patients with dementia may have longer stays than others. In a study of frail elderly people admitted to an acute care unit for treatment, patients with dementia had a mean total length of stay twice that of patients without dementia.[9] A study of British Columbia's hospital system found that over a 15-year period, increases in hospital days for elderly patients were largely accounted for by patients with very long stays. A handful of conditions, including senility and senile dementia, was responsible.[10] There is no evidence concerning whether admissions could be avoided among elderly people with cognitive impairment, but these studies indicate that once admitted, these individuals are more likely to be high-cost patients.

Inappropriate ER use also is viewed, in part, as a consequence of failure to gain access to community-based primary care. In general, elderly people are less likely to use emergency room services than younger people.[11] Studies based on the experience of individual emergency rooms have suggested that their use among elderly people is partly in response to failed community supports, self-care problems, and psychiatric illness.[12] A larger study of one regional trauma facility found that compared with younger people, elderly ER patients were more likely to have a serious medical illness and to be admitted to the hospital.[13]

Meeting the long-term care needs of people with cognitive impairment puts extreme demands on their family and friends. Much of the ongoing assistance that needs to be provided falls outside of the acute care paradigm, and the role of physicians (and acute care services generally) is often ill defined. For patients with dementia such as Alzheimer's disease, the picture is further complicated by the lack of medical treatments that substantially alter the disease process itself. Efforts to better integrate acute and long-term care generally acknowledge the need for physicians to play a greater role in long-term care.[14] Experience in models of integrated care is growing. However, much can still be learned about the interface of acute and long-term care, particularly for subgroups of elderly people in long-term care, such as those with cognitive impairment.

DATA AND METHODS

The data for this analysis are taken from the 1989 National Long-Term Care Survey (NLTCS). Like the previous waves of this survey, the objective is to provide detailed information on functioning, as well as assistance to persons over age 65 who have activity of daily living (ADL) or instrumental activity of daily living (IADL) limitations. The original sample (1982) was drawn from medicare enrollment files. The population interviewed in 1989 consisted of persons from previous waves of the survey (1982 and 1984) as well as individuals newly screened (a sample of previously nondisabled persons and one of new medicare enrollees). The screening interview was used to determine eligibility for interview in the community resident population. Eligible persons were those who indicated a problem in performing an ADL without help, or the need for help with IADLs lasting or expected to last three months or longer. This complex design yields a nationally representative sample of elderly people with ADL and IADL limitations. (Both the design and demographic characteristics of the sampled population are described more fully elsewhere.[15])

Separate interviews were conducted to obtain information on persons living in nursing homes.

Nursing home residents in the 1989 NLTCS were excluded from this analysis. Other studies indicate a sizeable proportion of the nursing home population is cognitively impaired.[16] Evidence suggests that cognitive status may affect some aspects of nursing home care. For example, researchers have observed that residents with dementia were less likely than others to be evaluated for infections based on diagnostic criteria established by an expert panel.[17] Little is known, in general, about the influence of cognitive impairment on aspects of care and service use by nursing home residents. Limitations in the NLTCS data for nursing home residents, however, preclude an examination of the effects of cognitive impairment on physician or inpatient use. For about 40 percent of the nursing home sample, no information is available on cognitive status. Neither is any information available from the survey on physician use or other ambulatory care for this population. Future waves of the NLTCS may be able to use resident assessment information from the Minimum Data Set (now in place in most U.S. nursing homes) to better characterize cognitive status and functioning. Detailed information on physician, hospital, and other medicare-covered services should be available as well, as a result of improvements in the Medicare Statistical System.

The sample for this study consists of 3,972 persons with functional limitations in the 1989 community sample; 462 interviewees with no ADL or IADL impairment and 21 persons with missing information on key variables were excluded. Of these, 2,820 were designated as cognitively intact, 525 as mildly cognitively impaired, and 627 as moderately to severely cognitively impaired. These categorizations were based on administration of the Short Portable Mental Status Questionnaire (SPMSQ) during the interview, or an indication of senility reported by the proxy respondent if the SPMSQ was not administered. This approach has been used in numerous analyses of data from the NLTCS.[18] Slightly more than one-quarter of the disabled elderly population could be considered mild, moderately, or severely cognitively impaired (table 7-1). There is considerable variability among studies in prevalence estimates of cognitive impairment, particularly when mild impairment is included.[19] The estimates of cognitive impairment in this study sample (within a population subgroup in which cognitive impairment is no doubt overrepresented) is within

TABLE 7-1. *Disability and Chronic Conditions by Cognitive Status among Functionally Impaired Elderly People in the Community*[a]

| | | Cognitive status | | |
| | | | Mild | Moderate to |
Characteristic	Total	Intact	impairment	severe impairment
Total percent	100.0	71.5	12.9	15.6
N	3,972	2,820	525	627
Disability level[b]				
Mobility only	1.2	1.3	1.4	1.0
IADL only	42.7	45.3	41.5	32.0
1–2 ADLs	34.3	35.2	39.4	26.1
3–5 ADLs	21.7	18.3	17.8	40.8
Chronic conditions[c]				
0	9.5	8.5	8.7	14.5
1 condition	27.6	27.1	26.8	31.0
2 conditions	30.4	31.9	28.9	25.2
3+ conditions	32.4	32.5	35.7	29.4

Source: 1989 National Long-Term Care Survey.

a. Estimates are based on weighted data. Persons who were interviewed but not disabled in ADL, IADL, or mobility are excluded.

b. These are mutually exclusive categories. Persons with "mobility only" have no other IADL (instrumental activity of daily living) or ADL (activity of daily living) limitations. Persons with "IADL only" have no ADL difficulties, but may have mobility limitations in addition. Persons with ADL limitations may have in addition mobility or IADL difficulties. ADLs include bathing, dressing, eating, getting in and out of bed, and using the toilet. IADLs include heavy housework, light housework, shopping, meal preparation, telephone use, doing laundry, taking medicine, and money management.

c. The seven conditions included are diabetes, rheumatism or arthritis, and occurrence in the past twelve months of the following: heart attack or heart problems; high blood pressure or hypertension; stroke; emphysema, asthma, or bronchitis; and broken hip or other bones.

the range of estimates from other studies as well as other estimates derived from the 1982 and 1984 NLTCS waves.[20]

The measure of disability level used in this analysis classifies persons into four mutually exclusive categories:

—Persons with mobility limitations only (that is, those who use equipment or need help from others in getting around inside or getting around outside);

—Those with at least one IADL limitation (in doing heavy or light housework, shopping, preparing meals, using the telephone, doing laundry, taking medicine, and managing money) but no ADL limitations;

—Those with one or two of five ADL limitations (bathing, dressing, eating, getting in and out of bed, and using the toilet); and
—Those with three to five ADL limitations.

There is face validity to a hierarchy of severity among these levels, and some research that suggests IADLs and ADLs are hierarchical.[21] In the logistic regression analysis, a dichotomous variable is used; the most disabled individuals (that is, persons with three to five ADL limitations) are contrasted with all others.

Utilization data are taken from two sources. Use of inpatient care uses medicare claims data linked to the surveyed population. Hospital stays with admission dates within one year of the interview date were used to estimate probability of a hospital stay in this period, as well as the number of admissions per 1,000 people and the average length of stay (ALOS) per admission. Measures of ambulatory care—whether a physician was seen in the past month, whether a regular source of care was reported, and whether the person had visited the ER without an admission in the last month—are taken from the community resident interview. Recall on physician use and ER visits in the NLTCS interview was restricted to one month before the interview. Medicare claims reflecting ambulatory use are certainly preferable to patient reports. Claims data provide both greater accuracy and a picture of use of services over longer periods, such as six months or one year. However, data on individual ambulatory visits are not available from medicare files before 1991.

RESULTS

Among older people with some functional limitation, a very small percentage have only mobility problems, and two out of five have IADL but no ADL limitations (table 7-1). The prevalence of severe disability, defined as limitations in three to five ADLs, is highest among persons with moderate to severe cognitive impairment (41 percent), twice that of people with no or only mild impairment.

Ninety percent of elderly people with functional limitations had at least one of seven major chronic conditions (diabetes, rheumatism or arthritis, or the occurence in the past year of heart attack or coronary problems, high blood pressure, stroke, chronic respiratory illness, or a broken hip or other broken bones). These chronic illnesses account for

TABLE 7-2. *Prevalence of Specific Chronic Conditions Among Cognitively Intact and Moderate to Severely Cognitively Impaired Older People*

Percent (unless otherwise indicated)

	Cognitive status	
Chronic condition	Intact	Moderate to severe impairment
Total N	2,820	627
Arthritis	75	64
Diabetes	16	16
Last 12 months		
Heart attack or heart problem	34	28
Hypertension	45	39
Stroke	6	13
Chronic respiratory	23	20
Broken hip or other fractures	7	8

Source: 1989 National Long-Term Care Survey.

considerable morbidity and disability among older people. Not surprisingly, the prevalence of chronic illness is considerably higher in this functionally limited subset of elderly people than from a cross-section of people age 65 or older.[22] Comorbidity is high as well. About 60 percent had two or more conditions. The presence of two or more of these seven conditions is slightly higher among those who are not seriously cognitively impaired. Comorbidity of cognitive impairment with at least one of these seven conditions, however, occurs in 90 percent of persons with mild impairment and 85 percent of those who are moderately to severely impaired.

Compared with those with moderate to severe impairment, persons with no cognitive impairment are reported to have a somewhat higher prevalence of arthritis, a heart attack, or a heart problem in the past year, or hypertension in the past year (table 7-2). However, the prevalence of stroke among people who are moderately to severely cognitively impaired is twice that of persons with no impairment. Although dementia accounts for the largest proportion of cognitive impairment in older people, such impairment is also among

TABLE 7-3. *Inpatient Care In a One-Year Period for Elderly People in the Community by Disability Level, Chronic Conditions, and Cognitive Status*

Characteristic	Percent with admission[a]	Admissions per 1,000 persons[a]	Average length of stay[a] (days)
Total	33.3	537	9.4
Disability level			
Mobility only	26.5	426	9.1
IADL only	26.4	417	8.4
1–2 ADLs	35.6	581	8.8
3–5 ADLs	41.5	674	11.3
Chronic conditions[b]			
0	25.2	384	8.8
1 condition	29.0	453	9.5
2 conditions	32.2	507	9.8
3+ conditions	39.8	671	9.2
Cognitive status			
Intact	32.4	524	9.3
Mild	33.1	552	8.2
Moderate to severe	37.5	581	10.9

Source: 1989 National Long-Term Care Survey.
a. Based on medicare inpatient claims for one year after interview date.
b. The seven conditions included are diabetes, rheumatism or arthritis, and occurrence in the past 12 months of the following: heart attack or heart problem; high blood pressure or hypertension; stroke; emphysema, asthma, or bronchitis; and broken hip or other bones.

the neurologic effects of stroke. As with dementia, the prevalence of stroke rises with age.[23]

In addition to contributing significantly to disability, these same diseases account for a substantial portion of health care expenditures for older people. For example, heart failure, angina pectoris, and cerebrovascular disorders have been among the top five diagnostic groups accounting for hospital stays among medicare patients in recent years.[24]

Tables 7-3 and 7-4 provide descriptive data on inpatient and ambulatory service use by disability level, number of chronic conditions, and cognitive status. Table 7-3 shows indicators of inpatient care in a one-year period following the 1989 interview date, based on medicare claims. In the overall NLTCS community sample of older people with functional limitations, about one-third had a hospital admission in the past year, with 537 admissions per 1,000 people. This is considerably

TABLE 7-4. *Ambulatory Care by Disability, Chronic Conditions, and Cognitive Status[a]*

Percent

Characteristic	Physician visit in past month	Regular source of care	ER visit without admission in past month
Total percent	45.1	91.6	7.0
Disability level			
Mobility only	32.2	86.7	9.6
IADL only	41.6	89.7	6.6
1–2 ADLs	47.0	92.5	6.0
3–5 ADLs	49.9	94.1	9.0
Chronic conditions[b]			
0	28.9	86.5	3.2
1 condition	36.4	88.3	5.6
2 conditions	47.8	93.5	7.3
3+ conditions	56.1	95.4	9.0
Cognitive status			
Intact	46.2	92.4	7.2
Mild	46.3	91.3	6.4
Moderate to severe[c]	39.5	88.3	6.7
Self-report	40.2	84.7	4.8
Proxy report	38.7	92.4	8.8

Source: 1989 National Long-Term Care Survey.

a. Persons who were interviewed but not disabled in ADL, IADL, or mobility are excluded.

b. The seven conditions included are diabetes, rheumatism or arthritis, and occurrence in the past twelve months of the following: heart attack or heart problem; high blood pressure or hypertension; stroke; emphysema, asthma, or bronchitis; and broken hip or other bones.

c. Forty-seven percent of respondents were from proxies. Differences in self- and proxy reports were significant at the .05 level for regular source of care and ER visits but not for physician visit in the past month.

higher than for the medicare population as a whole (in calendar year 1990, 313 discharges per 1,000 enrollees of all ages). The percentage of persons with a hospital admission in a one-year period rises with severity of disability and number of chronic conditions, with about 40 percent of those with three to five ADL limitations and those with three or more chronic conditions being hospitalized in the previous year. The likelihood of a hospital stay among persons with moderate to severe cognitive impairment also appears greater compared to others.

The ALOS per admission in the NLTCS population is 9.4 days,

slightly higher than the ALOS of 9.0 in 1990 for all medicare enrollees.[25] Average length of stay was highest for persons with three to five ADL limitations (11.3 days) and persons with moderate to severe cognitive impairment (10.9 days).

Three indicators of ambulatory care use are shown in table 7-4, a physician visit in the past month, a regular source of care, and an ER visit without a hospital admission in the past month. About 45 percent of disabled elderly people in the NLTCS had seen a physician in the past month. The percentage of persons seeing a physician increased with severity of disability and number of chronic conditions. However, persons with moderate to severe cognitive impairment were less likely than others to have seen a physician in the past month (40 percent versus 46 percent, respectively).

Overall, a very high percentage of those surveyed (92 percent) reported a regular source of care. The percentage with a regular source of care increased with disability and number of conditions. However, the percentage among persons with moderate to severe cognitive impairment who had a regular source of care was somewhat lower (88 percent). This same pattern was observed for likelihood of a visit to a physician.

Persons with three or more conditions, and those with both the greatest (three to five ADLs) and least amount of disability (mobility only) were most likely to have had an ER visit in the past month that did not result in a hospital admission. No trend by cognitive status was observed. Data on patterns of use of emergency rooms are scarce. The 1980 National Medical Care Utilization and Expenditure Survey, though dated, indicated that 3.5 percent to 4 percent of persons over age 65 had an ER visit within a year.[26] Using this benchmark, the incidence of ER visits among disabled elderly people in a one-month period seems quite high. ER visits that do not result in a hospital admission are presumed to be less medically serious than those that do, but it cannot be assumed that such visits are unneccessary or inappropriate.

As has been noted, information on ambulatory care use is taken from community interviews with disabled individuals or their proxy respondents. Although the recall period is short—that is, service use in the past month—there is reason to be concerned about the accuracy of the information reported, especially for persons with cognitive impairment. Among those who were moderately to severely impaired, the use of proxy respondents was quite high (close to half). Among those with moderate to severe cognitive impairment (table 7-4), the percentage reporting a visit to a physician in the past month did not differ by whether the information was self-reported or given by proxy (40 percent of self-respondents and 39 percent of proxy respondents reported a visit). However, type of respondent was related to reporting a regular source of care and an ER visit in the past month. In both instances, the percentage differences are small; but in the case of an ER visit, the proxy report is double the percentage for self-respondents (4.8 percent versus 8.8 percent, respectively). Use of proxy respondents in the NLTCS is associated with increases in level of disability.[27] In the 1989 community resident interview, among persons with three to five ADLs, 70 percent had proxy respondents compared with about 25 percent of those with IADLs only.

From the information available it is impossible to evaluate the accuracy of reports of ambulatory service use by either self- or proxy respondents, in instances where individuals are moderately to severely cognitively impaired. Given the relationship between use of a proxy respondent and level of the older person's disability, greater ER use reported by proxy respondents may reflect a true difference related to severity of the sample person's disease or disability. On the other hand, the availability of a proxy respondent may indicate more oversight of the sample person's condition and a greater related propensity to seek care. The fact that those persons with proxy respondents were more likely to be reported as having a regular source of care could be seen as supporting this interpretation. Still another possibility is inaccurate reporting of use—for example, underreporting by self-respondents. This might apply to physician contacts (where no differences by type of respondent were observed) as well as to ER visits and availability of a regular source of care.

The analyses that follow combine self-report and proxy information on service use. There were no significant differences in reporting physician contact in the past month between self- and proxy respondents, and relatively small differences for the other ambulatory care indicators. However, the preceding discussion illustrates the importance of a linkage to medicare data as an accurate and continuous record of health care service use. This is particularly true for analyses of access and use in subpopulations of elderly persons who, because of severe disability or cognitive impairment, may provide information that is subject to response bias.

TABLE 7-5. *Correlations of Disability Level, Comorbidity, and Cognitive Status with Service Use*[a]

Characteristic	Physician visit in past month	Regular source of care	ER visit without admission in past month	Inpatient stay in past year
Disability level (1 = mobility only, 4 = 3–5 activities of daily living [ADLs])	.06**	.06**	.05*	.13**
Number of chronic conditions (0–7)	.18**	.11**	.08**	.12**
Cognitive status (1 = intact, 3 = moderate to severe impairment)	−.03*	−.05**	−.01	.04*

Source: 1989 National Long-Term Care Survey.
a. Persons who were interviewed but not disabled in ADLs, instrumental activities of daily living (IADLs), or mobility are excluded.
* Significant at the .05 level.
** Significant at the .01 level.

Table 7-5 shows correlations of disability level, chronic conditions, and cognitive status with measures of service use and access to care. Increases in disability level and number of chronic conditions were both positively correlated with use of physician, ER, and inpatient care, as well as with probability of having a regular source of care. Moderate to severe cognitive impairment, however, was negatively correlated with a physician visit in the past month and a regular source of care, and positively correlated with an inpatient stay in the past year. Table 7-6 examines whether the relationships between cognitive status and service use hold up after controlling for other factors.

Odds ratios based on logistic regression models for each type of service use are shown in table 7-6. A logistic model was used because of the dichotomous nature of the dependent variable. Logistic coefficients represent the logarithm of the odds ratio for a given independent variable.[28] Raising e to the power of the coefficient provides an estimate of the increased probability of having used physician services (for example, for persons with the characteristic in question relative to those without). For the two ordinal variables (number of chronic conditions and number of caregivers), the odds ratio represents the increased risk of seeing a physician for someone with n medical condi-

TABLE 7-6. *Odds of Service Use among Functionally Impaired Elderly People in the Community by Selected Characteristics (Logistic Regression Results)[a]*

Characteristic	Physician visit in past month	Regular source of care	ER visit without admission in past month	Inpatient stay in past year
3–5 activities of daily living (ADLs)	1.15	1.45*	1.48**	1.38**
	(0.98, 1.35)	(1.05, 2.02)	(1.11, 1.97)	(1.17, 1.62)
Number of chronic conditions (0–7)	1.34**	1.40**	1.25**	1.21**
	(1.27, 1.41)	(1.26, 1.56)	(1.13, 1.38)	(1.14, 1.28)
Lives alone	0.97	0.96	1.03	1.09
	(0.85, 1.11)	(0.74, 1.23)	(0.79, 1.35)	(0.99, 1.25)
Medicaid coverage[b]	1.50**	1.53*	0.78	1.21*
	(1.25, 1.81)	(1.10, 2.13)	(0.53, 1.13)	(1.00, 1.47)
Private insurance[b]	1.34**	3.06**	1.19	1.29**
	(1.15, 1.55)	(2.37, 2.95)	(0.89, 1.60)	(1.10, 1.52)
Number of caregivers (0–6)	1.01	1.12*	1.16**	1.12**
	(0.96, 1.07)	(1.00, 1.24)	(1.06, 1.27)	(1.06, 1.18)
Moderate to severe cognitive impairment	0.82*	0.79	0.89	1.20*
	(0.68, 0.98)	(0.58, 1.07)	(0.62, 1.27)	(1.00, 1.45)

Source: 1989 National Long-Term Care Survey.
a. Odds ratios and confidence intervals are shown.
b. Reference group is people with medicare only.
* Significant at the .05 level.
** Significant at the .01 level.

tions or helpers relative to someone with $n - 1$ conditions. The variables included in the models are severe disability versus lesser levels, number of chronic conditions, moderate to severe cognitive impairment versus mild or no impairment, insurance coverage (private supplemental and medicaid, with medicare only as the reference group) and two variables reflecting informal care—living arrangement (alone versus with others) and number of caregivers. The literature on predictors of use of acute care services by elderly persons (including hospital, physician, and ER) indicate that neither predisposing variables (for example, race, sex, or age) nor enabling characteristics (for example, income) account for much variation in service use.[29] One enabling characteristic—insurance coverage, which has been shown to influence physician use—is included.

Both severe disability (in contrast to lesser disability levels) and greater numbers of chronic conditions increase the risk of service use after controlling for other factors. (The only exception is for disability level and a physician visit in the past month.) Both medicaid coverage and private insurance, relative to medicare coverage only, also raise the odds of a physician visit, an inpatient stay, and a regular source of care. Private supplemental insurance coverage in addition to medicare results in a threefold increase in the likelihood of having a regular source of care after controlling for other factors.

Of the two indicators of informal care, only number of caregivers is associated with service use. Living alone versus living with others does not alter the odds of service use once other factors are introduced. However, with each increase in the number of caregivers there is an increased risk of an ER visit, an inpatient stay, and a regular source of care, but the number of caregivers is not related to a physician visit in the past month. Controlling for other variables in the model, moderate to severe cognitive impairment both reduces the likelihood of a physician visit in the past month and increases the likelihood of an inpatient stay.

DISCUSSION

The role acute medical care plays in the health and well-being of older persons with cognitive impairment is not well understood. Integration of acute and long-term care services for persons with chronic illness and continuing care needs is only beginning to be addressed. Persons with cognitive impairment are a subset of the long-term care population for whom issues of appropriate access to acute care may prove even more complicated.

This analysis indicates that among people with functional limitations, prevalence of chronic conditions such as heart disease and arthritis is high. This applies to those with severe cognitive impairment as well as those who are cognitively intact. A few studies have indicated that there may be less comorbidity among persons with dementia than others, as well as variation by type of dementia.[30] Using a selected set of chronic conditions, this study also indicates a lower prevalence of some conditions (for example, heart attack or coronary problem, and hypertension). It is important to keep in mind, however, that these are self-reported (or proxy-reported) data. Much is still to be learned about the relationship between comorbidity and cognitive impairment or dementia. This is illustrated by a recent study of the Framingham population indicating that for some types of tasks, comorbidity accounted for much of the disability among persons with cognitive impairment.[31]

Basic questions have yet to be addressed, including whether physician access is adequate and timely, and whether obstacles to access lead to inappropriate or unnecessary use of other services, such as inpatient or emergency care. Preliminary evidence shows that severe cognitive impairment represents a barrier to physician access. After controlling for disability and the presence of other chronic conditions, moderate to severe cognitive impairment reduced the likelihood of an older disabled person visiting a physician. At the same time, such impairment appears to be a risk factor for hospitalization and for a longer ALOS. These findings illustrate the need for further investigation of these relationships using data (for ambulatory service use in particular) that provide a longitudinal perspective and that are of better quality.

NOTES

1. Nancy Mace and Peter Rabins, *The 36-Hour Day*, revised, 2d ed. (Johns Hopkins University Press, 1991); and U.S. Congress, Office of Technology Assessment, *Losing a Million Minds: Confronting the Tragedy of Alzheimer's Disease and Other Dementias*, OTA-BA-323 (Government Printing Office, April 1987).

2. LuAnn Aday, Ronald Andersen, and Gretchen V. Fleming, *Health Care in the U.S.: Equitable for Whom?* (Beverly Hills, Calif.: Sage Publishers, 1980).

3. George W. Rebok and Marshal F. Folstein, "Dementia," *Journal of Neuropsychiatry and Clinical Neurosciences*, vol. 5, no. 3 (1993), pp. 265–76.

4. Jack M. Guralnik and others, *Aging in the Eighties: The Prevalence of Comorbidity and Its Association with Disability* (advance data), series 16, no. 170 (Hyattsville, Md.: National Center for Health Statistics, 1989); and Lois M. Verbrugge, James M. Lepkowski, and Yuichi Imanaka, "Comorbidity and Its Impact on Disability," *Milbank Quarterly*, vol. 67, nos. 3–4 (1989), pp. 450–84.

5. Burton V. Reiffler and others, "Double-Blind Trial of Imipramine in Alzheimer's Disease Patients with and without Depression," *American Journal of Psychiatry*, vol. 146, no. 1 (1989), pp. 45–49.

6. Barbara Starfield, *Primary Care: Concepts, Evaluation, and Policy* (Oxford University Press, 1992).

7. Richard G. Frank and others, "Use of Services by Cognitively Impaired Elderly Persons Residing in the Community," *Hospital and Community Psychiatry*, vol. 39, no. 5 (1988), pp. 555–57.

8. Pamela A. Webber, Patrick Fox, and Denise Burnette, "Living Alone with Alzheimer's Disease: Effects on Health and Social Service Utilization Patterns," *Gerontologist*, vol. 34, no. 1 (1994), pp. 8–14.

9. Lucia Torian and others, "The Effect of Dementia on Acute Care in a Geriatric Medical Unit," *International Psychogeriatrics*, vol. 4, no. 2 (1992), pp. 231–39.

10. C. Hertzman and others, "Flat on Your Back or Back to Your Flat? Sources of Increased Hospital Services Utilization Among the Elderly in British Columbia," *Social Science and Medicine*, vol. 30, no. 7 (1990), pp. 819–28.

11. Judith D. Kasper, *Perspectives on Health Care: United States, 1980 National Medical Care Utilization and Expenditure Survey*, Series B, Descriptive Report No. 14 (Office of Research and Demonstrations, Health Care Financing Administration, September 1986).

12. Steven R. Lowenstein and others, "Care of the Elderly in the Emergency Department," *Annals of Emergency Medicine*, vol. 15, no. 5 (1986), pp. 528–35; and Ellen L. Bassuk, Sara Minden and Robert Apsler, "Geriatric Emergencies: Psychiatric or Medical?", *American Journal of Psychiatry*, vol. 140, no. 5 (1983), pp. 539–42.

13. Walter H. Ettinger and others, "Patterns of Use of the Emergency Department by Elderly Patients," *Journal of Gerontology*, vol. 42, no. 6 (1987), pp. 638–42.

14. Bruce Vladeck, "Overview: The Case for Integration," in *Conference Proceedings Integrating Acute and Long-Term Care: Advancing the Health Care Reform Agenda* (Washington: American Association of Retired Persons, August 1994), pp. 3–4.

15. Kenneth G. Manton, Larry S. Corder, and Eric Stallard, "Estimates of Change in Chronic Disability and Institutional Incidence and Prevalence Rates in the U.S. Elderly Population from the 1982, 1984, and 1989 National Long Term Care Survey," *Journal of Gerontology:Social Sciences*, vol. 48, no. 4 (1993), pp. S153–66.

16. Joan F. van Nostrand, Baila Miller, and Sylvia E. Furner, "Selected Issues in Long-Term Care: Profile of Cognitive Disability of Nursing Home Residents and the Use of Informal and Formal Care by Elderly in the Community," *Health Data on Older Americans: United States, 1992*, series 3, no. 27 (Hyattsville, Md.: National Center for Health Statistics, January 1993), pp. 143–85.

17. Jay Magaziner and others, "Prevalence and Characteristics of Nursing Home-Aquired Infections in the Aged," *Journal of the American Geriatrics Society*, vol. 39, no. 11 (1991), pp. 1071–78.

18. Judith D. Kasper, "Cognitive Impairment among Functionally Limited Elderly People in the Community: Future Considerations for Long-Term Care Policy," *Milbank Quarterly*, vol. 68, no. 1 (1990), pp. 81–109; William D. Spector, "Cognitive Impairment and Disruptive Behaviors Among Community-Based Elderly Persons: Implications for Targeting Long-Term Care," *Gerontologist*, vol. 31, no. 1 (1991), pp. 51–59; and Teresa A. Coughlin and Korbin Liu, "Health Care Costs of Older Persons with Cognitive Impairments," *Gerontologist*, vol. 29, no. 2 (1989), pp. 173–82.

19. Guralnik and others, *Aging in the Eighties;* and Verbrugge and others, "Comorbidity and its Impact on Disability."

20. Kasper, "Cognitive Impairment among Functionally Limited Elderly People"; Spector, "Cognitive Impairment and Disruptive Behaviors."

21. William D. Spector and others, "The Hierarchical Relationship Between Activities of Daily Living and Instrumental Activities of Daily Living," *Journal of Chronic Disease*, vol. 40, no. 6 (1987), pp. 481–89.

22. Reiffler and others, "Double-Blind Trial of Imipramine"; Robin Mermelstein and others, "Measures of Health," *Health Data on Older Americans: United States, 1992*, series 3, no. 27 (Hyattsville, Md.: National Center for Health Statistics, January 1993), pp. 9–21; and Joan Coroni-Huntley and others, *Established Populations for Epidemiologic Studies of the Elderly*, NIH Pub. No. 86-2443 (Bethesda, Md.: National Institutes of Health, 1986).

23. Patricia F. Adams and Veronica Benson, "Current Estimates from the National Health Interview Survey," *Vital Health Statistics*, series 10, no. 184 (Hyattsville, Md.: National Center for Health Statistics, 1991), pp. 1–232.

24. Bureau of Data Management Strategy, *1994 Data Compendium* (Health Care Financing Administration, March 1994).

25. Ibid.

26. Kasper, *Perspectives on Health Care.*

27. Kenneth G. Manton and Korbin Liu, "The 1982 and 1984 National Long-Term Care Surveys: Their Structure and Analytic Uses," paper presented for the National Conference on Long Term Care Data Bases, Washington, May 21–22, 1987.

28. David Hosner and Stanley Lemeshow, *Applied Logistic Regression* (John Wiley & Sons, 1989).

29. Laurence Branch and others, "Toward Understanding Elders' Health Service Utilization," *Journal of Community Health*, vol. 7, no. 2 (1981), pp. 80–92; and Frederic D. Wolinsky and others, "Health Services Utilization

among the Noninstitutionalized Elderly," *Journal of Health and Social Behavior,* vol. 24, no. 4 (1983), pp. 325–37.

30. Josiane Holstein and others, "Prevalence of Associated Diseases in Different Types of Dementia Among Elderly Institutionalized Patients: Analysis of 3447 Records," *Journal of the American Geriatrics Society,* vol. 42, no. 9 (1994), pp. 972–77; and Gisele P. Wolf-Klein and others, "Are Alzheimer Patients Healthier?", *Journal of the American Geriatrics Society,* vol. 36, no. 3 (1988), pp. 219–24.

31. Andres A. Guccione and others, "The Effects of Specific Medical Conditions on the Functional Limitations of Elderly in the Framingham Study," *American Journal of Public Health,* vol. 84, no. 3 (1994), pp. 351–58.

Chapter 8

JOSHUA M. WIENER, CATHERINE M. SULLIVAN,
AND LISA MARIA B. ALECXIH

Catastrophic Costs of Long-Term Care for Elderly Americans

Concern about the financial hardship that high out-of-pocket health care costs impose on elderly persons has been a long-standing health policy issue. Indeed, it was the driving force behind the creation of the medicare program. Without doubt, the financial burden on elderly Americans would be much greater absent medicare; nevertheless, elderly persons in this country still endure considerable financial hardship because of rising out-of-pocket costs for health care and uncovered services.[1] Out-of-pocket spending for long-term care, primarily nursing home stays, is a major contributor to the current problem of catastrophic health care costs for elderly persons.

Total long-term care expenditures for nursing home and home health care for elderly Americans were estimated at $75.4 billion in 1993.[2] Of that amount, less than 1 percent was financed through private long-term care insurance. Slightly more than half of long-term care expenditures were covered by either medicare or medicaid. Medicare mainly covers postacute care—primarily short-term stays in skilled nursing facilities and limited home health care. By law, medicaid is available only to those who meet means-tested eligibility rules, generally those who are poor or who incur high medical expenses relative to their incomes.[3] Given these restrictions, medicare covered just 18 percent, and medicaid 34 percent, of long-term care expenditures for elderly persons in 1993. The principal source of funding for elderly long-term care in 1993 was individual out-of-pocket spending (44 percent).[4]

Although home health care expenditures have grown rapidly in recent years, nursing home costs continue to dominate public and private long-term care spending by elderly persons. Their total expenditures for nursing home and home care in 1993 were estimated at $54.7 billion and $20.7 billion, respectively. Of these totals, about one-half of nursing home care expenses ($28.0 billion) and about one-quarter of home health care expenses ($5.5 billion) were paid out of pocket by elderly Americans.[5] With average costs of a nursing home stay estimated at $37,000 per year in 1993,[6] a stay of even moderate length can have financially devastating consequences for elderly individuals and their families.

The chances that an elderly person will use nursing home care are substantial. Although only about 5 percent of elderly people are residents of nursing homes at any one time, Kemper and Murtaugh estimate that about four out of ten elderly people will require nursing home care at least once in their lives.[7] Given the high cost of nursing home care and the lack of public or private insurance, it is not surprising that 61 percent of all nursing home residents in 1987 depended on medicaid to help pay for their care.[8] Impoverishment resulting from extended nursing home stays has, in effect, become a normal risk of aging.

This chapter focuses on the financial burden that out-of-pocket long-term care costs will have on elderly Americans over the next twenty-five years, absent any change in public or private financing. Using the Brookings–ICF Long-Term Care Financing Model, out-of-pocket spending by elderly people was projected for the period 1993 to 2018. We analyze results of these long-term care spending projections for both nursing home and community-based care. Catastrophic nursing home spending patterns for selected elderly groups (divided by age, gender, income and financial assets, marital status, length of stay, and discharge status) are also discussed.

LITERATURE REVIEW

Researchers have chosen a number of different strategies to define and measure catastrophic out-of-pocket spending by elderly persons. Wyszewianski provides a framework for evaluating studies of catastrophic spending that focuses on two basic issues: (1) what service expenditures (for example, acute care, long-term care, or both) are included in the calculations of out-of-pocket spending, and (2) what measures (such as absolute dollars or dollars relative to some measure of ability to pay) are used to determine whether spending is considered catastrophic.[9]

Scope of Expenditures

Until recently, most of the analytic work on out-of-pocket medical care spending by elderly persons has focused on acute care costs. Using measures of absolute out-of-pocket expenses,[10] expenses as a share of income,[11] and, in some cases, both measures,[12] these studies provide evidence that, despite medicare's extensive coverage of physician and hospital services, out-of-pocket spending on acute care services can be quite burdensome for elderly patients. As a group, the propensity of older people to use more acute care services (particularly prescription drugs) than younger people and to have lower average incomes compared with younger people make them susceptible to high out-of-pocket health care costs.

In their analysis of data from the 1980 National Medical Care Utilization and Expenditure Survey (adjusted to approximate the conditions in 1986), Feder, Moon, and Scanlon estimated that 24 percent of elderly individuals had acute care medical bills that exceeded 15 percent of their per capita income, a relative measure of catastrophic spending.[13] Feder and colleagues found the major components of acute care out-of-pocket spending were medicare cost sharing (that is, copayments and part B premiums), prescription drugs, and supplemental insurance premiums.

A limited number of studies have investigated out-of-pocket expenses paid by elderly people for long-term care.[14] As is true of catastrophic spending for acute care, both absolute and relative measures of out-of-pocket spending for long-term care have been adopted by investigators. For example, using an absolute measure derived from combined data sources from 1976 to 1980, Rice and Gabel found that nursing home costs were the single greatest expense in out-of-pocket spending for elderly persons who paid more than $2,000 a year on out-of-pocket acute and long-term care services.[15] Rice reported similar results based on an analysis of the 1985 National Nursing Home Survey. He found that nursing home charges were responsible for more than 80 percent of the out-of-pocket health care liabilities for the 1 million elderly persons whose out-of-pocket expenses totaled $3,000 or more in 1985.[16]

Using a relative measure of catastrophic costs, Coughlin, Liu, and McBride found that prescription drug costs and nursing home expenses accounted for the largest share of expenses among severely disabled elderly persons who spent 20 percent or more of family income on out-of-pocket acute and long-term care.[17] Although the sample population was highly impaired and therefore not representative of the elderly population, the analysis of data from the 1981–1982 Channeling Demonstration project shows the dramatic impact that both acute and long-term care out-of-pocket expenses have on this vulnerable subgroup. Prescription drugs accounted for 57 percent of total out-of-pocket spending, followed by 22 percent for nursing home care. The remaining 21 percent of out-of-pocket spending was divided among hospital care, physician and ancillary services, and insurance expenses. (Home care expenses were excluded from the analysis because the Channeling intervention subsidized care for some recipients.) Although out-of-pocket health care expenses as a share of income were high for the Channeling population as a whole (accounting for about 42 percent of total family income), severely disabled persons who used nursing homes spent almost 90 percent of their incomes on out-of-pocket medical expenses. The authors conclude that prescription drugs place a disproportionate burden on low-income disabled elderly persons, but nursing home costs tend to have more financially ruinous effects for all disabled elderly individuals regardless of income.

In one of the few studies of catastrophic spending to analyze out-of-pocket costs for home care as well as nursing home services, Liu, Perozek, and Manton found that 20 percent of chronically disabled elderly people with out-of-pocket costs spent more than 20 percent of their income on acute care services and prescription drugs, but when long-term care costs were included 30 percent spent that amount.[18] Using data on disabled elderly people living in the community from the 1982–1984 National Long-Term Care Survey and matching medicare part A and B records, the authors calculated the cumulative impact of out-of-pocket spending for acute care services, prescription drugs, home care, and nursing home care services. They found that when home care expenses were added to acute care and prescription drug expenses, the proportion of elderly persons with out-of-pocket expenses above 20 percent of their income rose from 20 percent to 24 percent. With the inclusion of nursing home expenses, the proportion who were catastrophic spenders rose to 30 percent. Nursing home use was a particularly strong predictor of catastrophic spending—80 percent of those who used nursing home care spent more than 20 percent of their income on out-of-pocket acute and long-term care costs.

Two additional studies of out-of-pocket spending for home care have relied on measures of average spending by elderly persons. Liu, Manton, and Liu, analyzing data from the 1982 Long-Term Care Survey, reported that disabled, community-based elderly persons spent an average of $164 monthly on out-of-pocket home care payments ($1,968 per year).[19] Furthermore, they found that though out-of-pocket costs for the majority of elderly home care users were $40 or less per month in 1982, about 10 percent spent ten times that amount. Using a sample of the entire elderly population from the 1987 National Medical Expenditure Survey, Altman and Walden estimated that annual out-of-pocket spending on home care averaged $937 for individuals ages 65 to 74, $1,598 for ages 74 to 84, and $1,850 for ages 85 and older.[20] Although neither study characterizes out-of-pocket spending for home care as catastrophic, both provide evidence that home care expenses contribute significantly to out-of-pocket expenditures for elderly persons.

The general finding that long-term care use (particularly nursing home stays) substantially increases out-of-pocket health care expenditures for older Americans is not surprising given the current system of long-term care financing. Elderly persons have a considerable risk of becoming impoverished when faced with a lengthy nursing home stay. Wiener and colleagues found that less than 10 percent of elderly persons in the United States could afford to pay for a year of nursing home care solely out of income.[21] The breadth and extent of out-of-pocket spending for long-term care therefore warrants further investigation and particular attention within the broader study of catastrophic out-of-pocket health care spending by the elderly population.

Defining Catastrophic Expenditures

No single definition of catastrophic out-of-pocket health care expenditure has been adopted by researchers. Some have used absolute dollar amounts, such as $5,000 per year.[22] Others have chosen a definition that accounts for differences in ability to pay by measuring out-of-pocket expenses that exceed a certain percent of household or per capita income—generally 10 to 20 percent for studies of acute care spending.

Wyszewianski suggests that an important first step in defining cat-astrophic health care spending is to distinguish between "high-cost" cases and "financially catastrophic" cases—the latter referring to out-of-pocket costs relative to an individual's ability to pay (generally measured as a percentage of income).[23] Failure to present catastrophic costs relative to ability to pay can lead to an incomplete picture of the dynamics of out-of-pocket spending for long-term care. Enormous bills associated with nursing home or home care would be cata-strophic for almost everyone, but even small bills can be devastating to people of limited means. Thus, absolute costs that are manageable for some people may prove ruinous for others.

Selecting a definition of catastrophic out-of-pocket expenses will shape the public policy options chosen to remedy the problems associ-ated with high out-of-pocket spending by elderly persons. In general, focusing on the reduction of total out-of-pocket expenditures for elderly long-term care users by creating an out-of-pocket spending ceiling or cap may primarily benefit upper-income persons who have money to spend on nursing home care. However, such a policy may neglect the needs of those with lower incomes who face impoverish-ment at spending levels well below the cap. Conversely, raising the personal needs allowance for medicaid nursing home patients may not have a large impact on reducing overall levels of out-of-pocket ex-penditures, but it may help significant numbers of people, particularly low-income persons who are institutionalized for short periods.[24]

The desire to protect elderly Americans from the financial burdens of long-term care embodies two distinct goals. One is to protect them from using up their life savings simply because they end up in a nursing home or need extensive home care. At present, the long-term care system contrasts radically with the principles of the medicare program. Although reducing out-of-pocket expenditures for acute health care services has been a central feature of the medicare program since its inception, no comparable program exists for elderly Americans with long-term care needs. A nonmeans-tested approach is of primary importance to those in the middle- and upper-income groups who have significant assets to protect. This is related to the similar but distinct goal of helping elderly persons avoid dependence on welfare (that is, medicaid) after a lifetime of financial indepen-dence. Although highly rated by elderly Americans, protecting the assets of this population is probably the most controversial goal of long-term care financing. Granted, there are problems with the current system, but some question whether helping elderly people preserve financial assets to be passed on to adult children is an appropriate goal of public policy. What are savings for, they ask, if not for care needed toward the end of life?

In determining what level of long-term care expenditures should be considered financially catastrophic for elderly persons, three additional issues should be addressed. First is the question of how to account for the ordinary living expenses associated with long-term care—for example, room and board for nursing home patients. These costs are generally included in total nursing home expenses, even though they represent ordinary living expenses paid out of pocket by elderly persons living at home. It is therefore appropriate to increase the level of expenditures used to define a financially catastrophic long-term care burden compared with a financially catastrophic acute care burden.[25] Similarly, defining what services should be counted in determining out-of-pocket home care costs can be tricky. For example, services that enable disabled elderly persons to function independently in the community may include certain ordinary living expenses that nondisabled individuals use as well. Distinguishing between home care services that substitute for ordinary living expenses (such as housekeeping or chore services) and those that represent the true added costs of home care may vary from person to person, depending on economic status, level of impairment, and type of home care services they receive.[26]

A second issue related to the development of a catastrophic out-of-pocket spending threshold is the question of how the assets of elderly persons should be treated, particularly for the majority who own their own homes. If assets are excluded from ratios of out-of-pocket spending to financial status, then those with substantial assets but relatively low income may appear to be worse off than they actually are. Including a measure of net worth based on assets as well as income would provide a more complete picture of how the burden of catastrophic health care expenditures is distributed among the elderly population, but defining this measure is complicated by the type of assets elderly persons hold. For example, though home ownership is common among older people, houses represent highly illiquid assets that demand special consideration.[27]

Finally, a carefully defined unit of observation is a necessary component of a well-defined measure of catastrophic out-of-pocket expenses. Wyszewianski notes that individual income reported on a per capita basis may underestimate the ability to pay for households with two or more incomes.[28] Although it is probably reasonable to assume that married couples share their resources, family income that includes multiple generations may overestimate ability to pay if there are no controls for household size and little information about how financial resources are shared.

In sum, although defining a catastrophic out-of-pocket long-term care spending threshold raises some issues similar to those in studies of catastrophic acute care spending, we would argue that the distinctions between acute and long-term care warrant a higher threshold for long-term care spending. The definition of a catastrophic expense reflects historical circumstances and public attitudes toward protection of the assets of elderly Americans, as well as more mundane issues related to the measurement of such assets.[29] Under these circumstances, reasonableness rather than precision is the goal.

METHODS

To investigate the distribution and relative impact of catastrophic long-term care expenses on elderly Americans, this study used the Brookings–ICF Long-Term Care Financing Model. The model was originally developed in 1986 and 1987 and substantially refined and updated in 1988 and 1989. It provides a way of simultaneously projecting many characteristics of the older population that will affect their need for and use of long-term care, together with the financial resources they will likely have to pay for it.[30]

The Brookings–ICF Long-Term Care Financing Model is a microsimulation model that starts with a sample of actual people and simulates what happens to each of them individually. The model begins with a nationally representative sample of the adult population, including a data record for each person's age, sex, income, assets, and other relevant characteristics. It then simulates changes in the population from 1986 through 2020, indicating for each person both general changes (such as age and economic status) and those specific to long-term care (such as onset and recovery from disability, use of health care services, and method of payment for them).

Structure of the Model

There are six major components of the Brookings–ICF Long-Term Care Financing Model.

Representative population database. The model starts with a population database, the 1979 Current Population Survey (CPS), which contains a representative sample of 28,000 adults of all ages. The 1979 CPS provides information on income, assets, family structure, and earning histories, including social security earnings.

Income simulator. The model simulates labor force activity, income, and marital status for each person using a modified version of Lewin-VHI's Pension and Retirement Income Simulation Model (PRISM). Using data from the 1985 National Nursing Home Survey and the 1984 Survey of Income and Program Participation, the model also simulates housing and financial assets for elderly persons.

Disability rates for elderly persons. Using probability estimates derived primarily from the 1982–1984 National Long-Term Care Survey and the 1982 New Beneficiary Survey, disability rates for elderly persons are derived. The model assigns one of four disability levels to each person at age 65 and then simulates a disability level for each year thereafter. Annual changes vary by age, marital status, and prior level of disability.

Use of long-term care services. For each year of the simulations, the model selects those people who would need to enter nursing homes, then determines their length of stay and whether they are discharged or die while in residence. The model uses nursing home admission probabilities estimated from longitudinal data from the 1982–1984 National Long-Term Care Survey.

Sources and levels of payment. The fifth part of the model simulates the sources of payment and the level of expenditures for every person receiving nursing home or home care services. This is based on data from the 1985 National Nursing Home Survey, the 1984 National Long-Term Care Survey, and Health Care Financing Administration (HCFA) data on medicare and medicaid. Incorporated into the model are eligibility requirements for medicare, medicaid, and other public programs.

Aggregate expenditures and service use. Finally, the model accumulates medicare, medicaid, private insurance, and other payer and out-of-pocket expenditures for the simulated cases each year.

Model Assumptions

In the base case chosen for this analysis, changes in the population were simulated with the assumption that current public programs and private funding mechanisms will remain constant. Because all projections depend on assumptions about future trends, the choice of parameters regarding death and disability rates, for example, greatly affect the results.

Assumptions about death and disability. The projections are based on the Social Security Administration (SSA) mid-range II-B assumptions,[31] which assume substantial improvements in longevity over time. Disability rates are assumed to remain constant over time but vary by age, gender, and marital status. In controlling for these variables, it is assumed that the population becomes neither sicker nor healthier over time.

Economic assumptions. Economic assumptions also follow the Social Security Administration's mid-range projections. Over the long run, inflation is assumed to be about 4 percent per year. Real wage growth reflects actual rates until 1986 and then follows SSA projections, which vary between 1.0 and 2.4 percent annually. The model follows the labor force participation forecasts of the Bureau of Labor Statistics through the year 2000, which project substantially more women in the work force.

Long-term care use. Nursing home admission rates are kept constant throughout the projection period, implying that the supply of nursing home beds will increase as necessary to accommodate more admissions from the growing elderly population. Thus, the model does not assume that demand for nursing home care use in the future will be any more or less constrained by bed supply than it is now.

Reimbursement rates. Payment rates for nursing home and home care vary by source of payment—medicare, medicaid, private payer, and other payer—but all are assumed to increase by 5.5 percent a year.[32]

Public program eligibility requirements. Program benefits and eligibility rules are assumed to remain constant, except for inflation. For medicaid beneficiaries, the spousal impoverishment provisions of the Medicare Catastrophic Coverage Act of 1988 are simulated.

Benchmarking adjustments. Expenditures for medicare and medicaid nursing home and home care are benchmarked against HCFA program data for 1993.

Baseline Projections

The model begins the simulation with a nationally representative sample of 28,000 adults using individual records from the May 1979 Current Population Survey Special Pension Supplement. To reduce random variation, the database is run through the model twice. To smooth year-to-year variability of the estimates, results are presented as five-year averages. The final output from the model provides detailed information for each person age 65 and older for each year from 1986 to 2020 on measures such as age, marital status, disability, amount and sources of income, assets, use of nursing home and home care services, and payment sources for these services.

Using a Monte Carlo simulation technique, the model simulates changes in status for each person in each year of the projection period based on demographic and economic characteristics. Each change in status (such as marriage, admission to a nursing home, or death) is called an event.

The model simulates events by drawing a random number between zero and one and comparing it to the predetermined probability of that event occurring for a person with particular sociodemographic characteristics. For example, the annual probability of death for an eighty-five-year-old woman requiring help with two or more of the activities of daily living (ADLs) who is not in a nursing home is 0.03. In other words, 3 out of every 100 such women are expected to die each year. If the random number drawn by the model is less than or equal to 0.03 for this particular woman, she is assumed to die in that year; if it is between 0.03 and 1.0, she is assumed to continue to live.

Definitions of Catastrophic Expenditures

Tables and figures showing projected changes in absolute out-of-pocket expenditures are provided for 1993 to 2018. All spending projections are in constant 1993 dollars and are based on spending over the duration of a nursing home admission. Nursing home stays interrupted by hospital admissions or short stays at home were added together to create a single episode. Lifetime financial burdens were not used because of the conceptual difficulties in developing an appropriate measure.[33]

Three types of catastrophic measures are presented in this analysis, and all are based on nursing home stays. The first approach is based on the number of medicaid-financed patients. Unlike medicare, which provides coverage without regard to income, medicaid eligibility is means tested. To qualify for medicaid, an elderly person must first use up virtually all of his or her assets (a process known as "spending down") and must contribute all income to pay for nursing home services, except for a small personal needs allowance (usually $30 per month). In 1993, the maximum amount of assets that could be retained was $2,000 for an unmarried individual. Thus, the number of nursing home patients who received medicaid at any point during the year is a rough approximation of the number of persons who incur catastrophic expenses.

A second measure of catastrophic expenditures examines absolute expenses for community-based and nursing home care. Defining a high-cost expenditure threshold is an arbitrary process. This study chose to define $20,000 as high-cost care—roughly the median annual family income among elderly persons projected for the year 2008, the midpoint in our projected time span. Using this threshold, we estimated the percent of elderly nursing home users who spend $20,000 or more out-of-pocket per admission.

The third approach to defining catastrophic care is based on the ratio of out-of-pocket expenses relative to the income and assets of elderly persons. In acute care studies, it is commonly argued that catastrophic spending occurs when people spend 10 percent or more of their income for health care.[34] In this study, we define catastrophic costs as out-of-pocket expenses that are more than 40 percent of income and assets. More precisely, the spending ratio used to define a population of elderly persons who spent 40 percent or more on nursing home care consists of a numerator equal to the out-of-pocket contributions made by an individual for the entire length of stay, and a denominator equal to the income that individual would have received during a nursing home stay, plus his or her assets. Measures of income and assets used in this ratio are based on joint holdings for married persons and individual holdings for single persons. Sources of income include social security, pensions, supplemental security income (SSI), individual retirement accounts (IRAs), wages, and asset earnings. Assets include the net value of fixed and interest-earning assets less liabilities, such as loans and credit card bills. Following medicaid eligibility rules, primary motor vehicles were excluded from calculation of net assets. Home equity was included as part of the denominator in some of the simulations. The home equity measure subtracts mortgages held on any real estate property owned jointly for married individuals and held individually for unmarried individuals.

RESULTS

Table 8-1 provides a percentage breakdown of aggregate elderly out-of-pocket spending for nursing home care in 1993 and 2018 illustrating the association between out-of-pocket spending and gender, marital status, age, income, discharge status, and length of stay. Spending distributions change over time for age, marital status, and income groupings but remain fairly stable for the other three categories. Elderly persons over age 85 account for an increased proportion of total nursing home out-of-pocket expenditures among this population, rising from about 44 percent of total expenditures in 1993 to 49 percent of total expenditures in 2018. This shift toward increased spending for older elderly persons as a group over time reflects the predicted increase in the number and proportion of the oldest-old in the general population. The aging of America is also likely to affect increases in aggregate out-of-pocket nursing home spending by unmarried elderly persons, rising from 64 percent in 1993 to almost 72 percent in 2018, because older elderly individuals are less likely to be married.

The most dramatic change over time is in the distribution of out-of-pocket spending by elderly admissions in the lowest and highest

TABLE 8-1. *Out-of-Pocket Spending for Nursing Home Care, 1993 and 2018[a,b]*

Percent (unless otherwise noted)

Out-of-pocket nursing home expenses	1993	2018
Total out-of-pocket spending (billions of 1993 dollars)	$ 28.0	$ 67.2
All elderly admissions	100.0	100.0
Men	32.7	34.1
Women	67.3	65.9
Age		
65–74	20.1	19.9
75–84	36.1	31.2
85+	43.8	48.9
Marital status		
Married	35.9	28.3
Unmarried	64.1	71.7
Discharge status		
Deceased	81.2	80.9
Alive	18.8	19.1
Annual income (1993 dollars)[c]		
$0–7,499	10.8	5.1
7,500–14,999	29.7	19.6
15,000–19,999	12.4	11.3
20,000–29,999	21.1	18.8
30,000–49,999	11.3	22.7
50,000+	14.6	22.5
Length of stay		
1–30 days	0.3	0.3
31–60 days	0.7	0.7
61–90 days	1.2	0.8
91–364 days	7.3	7.8
1–2 years	11.0	9.0
2–3 years	13.2	14.6
3–5 years	18.3	19.7
5+ years	48.0	47.0

Source: Brookings–ICF Long-Term Care Financing Model. The year 1993 represents the five-year average for the period 1991–95; 2018 represents the five-year average for the period 2016–20.

a. Out-of-pocket spending includes both income and assets, measured in constant 1993 dollars.

b. All measures in this table refer to the cohort of elderly individuals (age 65 and older) admitted to a nursing home in the period 1991–95 or the period 2016–20. Spending distributions represent the share of out-of-pocket spending accounted for by the group. For example, in 1993, 26 percent of all persons in the sample who were admitted to nursing homes were married, but they accounted for 35.9 percent of out-of-pocket spending.

c. Sources of income include social security, pensions, supplemental security income (SSI), individual retirement accounts (IRAs), wages, and asset earnings. Annual income is measured jointly for married persons, individually for unmarried persons.

income groups. For example, the proportion of out-of-pocket spending for elderly persons in the lowest income bracket (up to $7,499) decreases by half, from 10.8 percent in 1993 to 5.1 percent in 2018, whereas the proportion of out-of-pocket spending attributable to higher income admissions who earn $30,000 to $49,000 doubles, from 11.3 percent in 1993 to 22.7 percent in 2018. This shift in the distribution of out-of-pocket spending by income groups reflects rising incomes among elderly Americans.

Among the six population characteristics in table 8-1, the widest disparity within a category is for out-of-pocket spending by discharge status. Elderly persons who die while in nursing homes account for more than 80 percent of total out-of-pocket nursing home spending among this population in 1993 and 2018, compared with those who are discharged alive, who account for the remaining 20 percent of aggregate out-of-pocket spending. The distribution of out-of-pocket spending for nursing home care is also substantially different for elderly men and women and for married and unmarried individuals. Women account for about two-thirds of out-of-pocket spending for nursing home care in 1993 and 2018, and unmarried admissions account for about the same proportion in both years.

Other characteristics also exhibit consistent within-group differences over time. As table 8-1 shows, the proportion of out-of-pocket spending for nursing home care rises with age, with the largest proportion attributable to elderly persons age 85 or older (44 percent in 1993 and 49 percent in 2018). When elderly residents are grouped by length of nursing home stay, the bulk of out-of-pocket spending is incurred by those who spend more than five years in nursing homes. These long-term admissions account for almost half of all spending (48 percent of aggregate out-of-pocket spending in 1993 and 47 percent in 2018).

These demographic differences reflect the typical profile of elderly nursing home users, who are predominantly female and unmarried.[35] Likewise, use of nursing home care rises with age.[36] As for the relationship between discharge status and nursing home use, those individuals who die while in nursing home care are significantly more likely to have experienced longer nursing home stays than are those who are discharged alive.[37]

Out-of-pocket spending by elderly Americans for nursing home care continues to dwarf spending for home and community-based services through 2018. As figure 8-1 shows, annual out-of-pocket spending for elderly nursing home users will rise from $28,100 in 1993 to $43,900 in 2018, an increase of 56 percent. During the same period, average out-of-pocket spending for users of home and community-based services (home care and other noninstitutional long-term care) will grow from $1,600 in 1993 to $2,400 in 2018, a 50 percent increase. With out-of-pocket spending for nursing home care and community-based care expected to increase at about the same rate over the next twenty-five years, the disparity between institutional and noninstutitional spending will remain constant.

Overall increases in out-of-pocket spending for long-term care services through 2018 likely reflect both increasing income and assets of elderly persons in general as well as price increases for long-term care services that exceed the general inflation rate.

FIGURE 8-1. *Average Out-of-Pocket Spending per Long-Term Care Admission, Selected Years, of All Elderly Persons*[a]

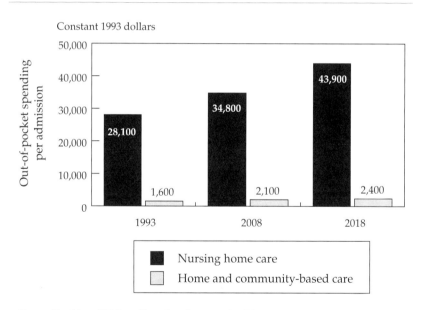

Source: Brookings–ICF Long-Term Care Financing Model.

[a] Admission cohort includes all elderly individuals (age 65 or older) admitted in that year. The year 1993 represents the five-year average for the period 1991–95, 2008 the five-year average for the period 2006–10, and 2018 the five-year average for the period 2016–20. Average out-of-pocket spending includes both income and nonhousing assets.

Catastrophic Measures: Number of Medicaid Nursing Home Patients

The number of elderly nursing home residents who receive medicaid at any time during the year is projected to increase from 1.4 million in 1993 to 2.0 million in 2018 (figure 8-2), while the percentage of nursing home residents dependent on medicaid will decline slightly, from 61 percent in 1993 to 56 percent in 2018 (table 8-2). Because medicaid eligibility requirements were held constant for the simulation period, rising income and assets of elderly persons may account for these proportionate decreases.

Catastrophic Measures: Absolute and Relative Out-of-Pocket Nursing Home Costs

Turning to measures of absolute and relative catastrophic out-of-pocket expenses, table 8-3 presents the proportion of elderly nursing home admissions reaching out-of-pocket spending thresholds in 1993, 2008, and 2018. In absolute terms, the proportion who spend

FIGURE 8-2. *Number of Elderly (Age 65+) Medicaid Nursing Home Patients, 1993, 2008, and 2018*[a]

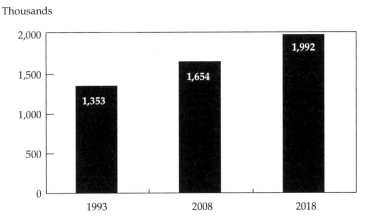

Thousands

Source: Brookings–ICF Long-Term Care Financing Model.
[a]Number of patients financed by medicaid at any time during the year. The year 1993 represents the five-year average for the period 1991–95, 2008 the five-year average for the period 2006–10, and 2018 the five-year average for the period 2016–20.

TABLE 8-2. *Elderly Medicaid Nursing Home Patients, 1993, 2008, and 2018*[a]

Year	Number	Percent of all elderly nursing home patients
1993	1,352,673	61
2008	1,653,896	56
2018	1,991,819	56

Source: Brookings–ICF Long-Term Care Financing Model. The year 1993 represents the five-year average for the period 1991–95, 2008 the five-year average for the period 2006–10, and 2018 the five-year average for the period 2016–20.

a. Number and percent of all nursing home patients (age 65 or older) who are financed by medicaid at any time during the year.

TABLE 8-3. *Absolute and Relative Measures of Catastrophic Out-of-Pocket Spending by Elderly Nursing Home Admissions, 1993, 2008, and 2018*[a]

Catastrophic measure	Percent of all elderly admissions		
	1993	*2008*	*2018*
Absolute measure (out-of-pocket spending per admission)			
Percent who spend $20,000 or more	27	28	33
Relative measures (out-of-pocket spending per admission)[b,c]			
Percent who spend ≥40% of income and nonhousing assets	36	36	39
Percent who spend ≥40% of income and total assets	23	22	23

Source: Brookings–ICF Long-Term Care Financing Model. The year 1993 represents the five-year average for the period 1991–95, 2008 the five-year average for the period 2006–10, and 2018 the five-year average for the period 2016–20.

a. Admission cohort includes all elderly individuals (age 65 or older) admitted in that year.

b. The spending ratio has as its numerator out-of-pocket expenses for nursing home care for the entire length of stay; the denominator is equal to the income that the individual would have received had he or she not entered the nursing home, plus his or her family's assets (measured jointly for married individuals).

c. Sources of income include social security, pensions, supplemental security income (SSI), individual retirement accounts (IRAs), wages, and asset earnings. Assets include the net value of interest earning assets less liabilities, such as loans and credit card bills. The primary motor vehicle was excluded from the calculation of net assets. Home equity (market value net of mortgages held on the property or properties) is included in the measure of total assets.

$20,000 or more per admission (in constant 1993 dollars) increases slightly, from 27 percent in 1993 to 33 percent in 2018. Using the two relative measures, the proportion of elderly persons who spend at least 40 percent of their income and nonhousing assets on out-of-pocket nursing home expenses rises moderately, from 36 percent in 1993 to 39 percent in 2018.[38] Alternatively, when home equity is included in the relative measure of out-of-pocket spending, the proportion of elderly nursing home admissions meeting the catastrophic spending threshold of 40 percent shows almost no change over the simulation period 1993 to 2018, holding steady at about 23 percent of admissions.[39]

Two observations are relevant to the estimates presented in table 8-3. First, there is relative stability among all three catastrophic measures over time. Although the price of nursing home care will likely rise faster than the general inflation rate, the predicted increase in the elderly population's income and assets appears to cancel out the impact of increasing age on catastrophic out-of-pocket spending on nursing homes.

Second, including home equity in the measurement of elderly assets substantially reduces the proportion of elderly persons with catastrophic out-of-pocket nursing home expenses throughout the simulation period. Although more than one-third of elderly admissions face out-of-pocket expenses equal to 40 percent or more of their income and nonhousing assets, less than one-quarter of elderly admissions are projected to face that level of out-of-pocket spending relative to their total income and assets, including home equity (table 8-3). About three-quarters of elderly persons own a home,[40] which explains the reduction in catastrophic spending when home equity is included in the measure of assets. Thus, adding home equity to the relative measure of elderly income and assets reduces the proportion of elderly Americans projected to face catastrophic out-of-pocket nursing home expenses.

Out-of-Pocket Spending by Subgroups of Elderly Admissions, 1993

In table 8-4, the admission cohort, which includes all elderly individuals who were admitted to nursing homes in 1993, is disaggregated by demographic and income groups to allow for comparisons across measures of catastrophic out-of-pocket spending. For example, a higher proportion of married (34 percent) than unmarried elderly

TABLE 8-4. *Measures of Catastrophic Out-of-Pocket Spending, 1993*[a]

Measure	Total admissions 1993	Catastrophic measures (percent)		
		Absolute[b] ($20,000+)	Ratio I[c] (nonhousing assets)	Ratio II[d] (including home equity)
All elderly admissions	998,510	27	36	23
Men	301,784	26	30	16
Women	696,726	27	39	27
Age				
65–74	155,620	31	30	19
75–84	410,185	22	30	19
85+	432,705	29	44	29
Marital Status				
Married	258,922	34	20	7
Unmarried	739,588	24	41	29
Discharge status				
Deceased	676,242	33	41	27
Alive	322,268	12	26	16
Annual family income				
(1993 dollars)				
$0–7,499	267,389	12	45	29
7,500–14,999	365,955	26	46	29
15,000–19,999	119,009	26	25	18
20,000–49,999	196,043	39	21	13
50,000+	50,114	58	2	1
Nonhousing family assets				
(1993 dollars)				
$0–9,999	537,021	23	51	33
10,000–29,999	102,610	26	31	13
30,000–59,999	88,097	24	23	19
60,000–119,999	104,761	30	22	15
120,000+	166,021	39	6	5
Length of stay				
1–30 days	251,273	<1	5	2
31–60 days	106,972	<1	10	7
61–90 days	75,612	<1	7	7
91–364 days	208,995	8	35	16
1–2 years	87,453	57	59	38
2–3 years	73,903	57	70	46
3–5 years	81,912	71	78	56
5+ years	112,390	87	80	61

Source: Brookings–ICF Long-Term Care Financing Model. The year 1993 represent the five-year average for the period 1991–95.

a. All measures in this table refer to the cohort of elderly individuals (age 65 and older) admitted to a nursing home in 1991–95.

b. The absolute spending measure refers to the percent of admissions who spend $20,000 or more out of pocket.

c. Ratio I = percent of admissions with out-of-pocket expenses equal to at least 40 percent of their relative income and nonhousing assets. The spending ratio sets the numerator equal to out-of-pocket expenses for the entire length of stay; the denominator equals the income the individual would have received had he or she not entered the nursing home, plus his or her family's non-housing assets (measured jointly for married individuals, individually for unmarried individuals).

d. Ratio II = percent of admissions who spend at least 40 percent of their relative income and total assets out of pocket. Spending ratio numerator was calculated as in note c. The denominator includes all sources listed in note c plus home equity (market value net of mortgages held on the property or properties).

persons (24 percent) will spend $20,000 or more per admission. However, when out-of-pocket spending is measured relative to income and nonhousing assets (table 8-4, column 2), unmarried individuals are about twice as likely as those who are married to spend more than 40 percent of their income and nonhousing assets on nursing home care (41 percent of unmarried versus 20 percent of married persons admitted). Likewise, when home equity is included in the measure of assets, the proportion of unmarried elderly persons with catastrophic expenses (table 8-4, column 3) is about four times greater than the proportion with catastrophic expenses who are married (29 percent of unmarried versus 7 percent of married persons admitted). This result is probably explained by the higher average income and assets married elderly persons have relative to those who are unmarried and their consequently greater ability to pay out of pocket for long-term care services.

A comparison of out-of-pocket spending by income and asset groups provides the most dramatic illustration of how choosing a measure of catastrophic spending makes a significant difference in how such spending is portrayed. For example, using the absolute out-of-pocket measure, $20,000 or more per stay in 1993, the proportion of elderly persons who incur out-of-pocket costs at this level increases as annual family income increases—from 12 percent with annual incomes under $7,500 to 58 percent with incomes of at least $50,000 per year. In contrast, using either of the relative measures of catastrophic spending from table 8-4 (including or excluding home equity), the proportion of elderly people admitted to nursing homes incurring catastrophic expenses relative to their income and assets decreases as income increases. Although 45 percent of those elderly persons with incomes under $7,500 are projected to spend more than 40 percent of their income and nonhousing assets out of pocket, only 2 percent of those with incomes of at least $50,000 per year will incur out-of-pocket expenses at that level (table 8-4, column 2). Similarly, when home equity is included in the assets held by elderly people, the proportion at the catastrophic spending level drops from 29 percent of those with annual income less than $7,500 to just 1 percent of those with annual income of at least $50,000.

A second measure of financial status is nonhousing family assets, which provides a broader picture of financial status than just income. As is true for the measurement of annual income, assets are measured jointly for married individuals. Table 8-4 shows those individuals with nonhousing assets totaling less than $10,000 are substantially more likely to face catastrophic out-of-pocket spending burdens under the relative spending measures than are elderly with greater wealth. More than half of all admitted patients in the lowest asset category (less than $10,000) face catastrophic spending burdens relative to their assets, compared with less than 10 percent of those whose assets total $120,000 or more.

Two additional points should be noted concerning comparisons of catastrophic spending by income and assets. First, including home equity in the measure of assets would not completely eliminate the problem of catastrophic expenses, even for wealthier elderly persons. In 1993, 15 percent of elderly nursing home users with assets between $60,000 and $119,000 and 5 percent of those with total assets of $120,000 or more would face catastrophic out-of-pocket expenses relative to their income and total assets.

The second point concerns how the impact of including home equity in the calculation of net income and assets for elderly nursing home users is spread among elderly persons of varying income and asset levels. By far, the greatest change is demonstrated for those in the lower brackets. Without home equity, just over half (51 percent) of elderly admissions whose nonhousing assets total less than $10,000 face relative catastrophic expenses in 1993. Yet when home equity is included in the calculation of family financial resources, the proportion of those in the lowest asset group who face catastrophic expenses drops to 33 percent. Likewise, for those individuals with nonhousing assets of $10,000 to $29,000, the percent of admitted patients with catastrophic out-of-pocket expenditures declines by more than half, from 31 percent when only nonhousing assets are included, to just 13 percent when home equity is added to assets. In sum, home ownership makes a significant difference for low-income admissions.

Discharge status and length of stay demonstrate the greatest consistency across alternative measures of catastrophic spending. Table 8-4 shows that whether absolute or relative measures of catastrophic spending are used, nursing home patients who die before they are discharged are about twice as likely to incur catastrophic expenses compared with those discharged home from care. Similarly, as lengths of stay increase, the proportion of elderly persons who meet or exceed absolute and relative catastrophic spending thresholds increases. Those individuals who are institutionalized for three years or more have at least a 60 percent chance of incurring catastrophic expenses. In contrast, 10 percent or less of elderly individuals admitted for less than 91 days are projected to incur catastrophic expenses, whether out-of-pocket costs are measured either in constant absolute dollars or relative to their income and assets.

Out-of-Pocket Spending by Subgroups of Elderly Patients, 2018

Disaggregated estimates of out-of-pocket nursing home expenses in 2018 are provided in table 8-5, which (like table 8-4) provides estimates for various elderly subgroups under absolute and relative definitions of catastrophic out-of-pocket spending. In most cases, the subgroup changes follow the direction of change in the aggregate measure. For instance, the proportion of admissions spending more than $20,000 increases slightly, from 27 percent in 1993 to 33 percent in 2018. Likewise, in all cases save one, the estimates for absolute out-of-pocket spending remain constant or increase moderately for all elderly subgroups. The lone exception is for elderly persons with minimum annual incomes of $50,000 or more. The proportion with catastrophic spending in this group declines from 58 percent in 1993 to 48 percent in 2018—a change probably explained by rising elderly incomes and assets, which may shield the highest-income subgroup from the effects of an aggregate increase in levels of absolute spending. In other words, because the proportion of elderly admissions in the highest-income category more than doubles (from about 5 percent in 1993 to 11 percent in 2018), it would take a huge increase in the number of high-income admissions spending more than $20,000 to be reflected in proportional measures.

The second and third columns displayed in table 8-5 show the proportion of nursing home admissions in 2018 with out-of-pocket nursing home expenses equal to at least 40 percent of their income and assets. For the most part, the direction and magnitude of change over time is similar for elderly subgroups as in the aggregate. The slight aggregate increase (from 36 percent in 1993 to 39 percent in 2018) in the proportion of those with out-of-pocket expenses equal to at least 40 percent of their income and nonhousing assets is reflected in modest increases projected by the model for most elderly subgroups (ratio I, tables 8-4 and 8-5). Likewise, the catastrophic measure that includes home equity (holding steady at 23 percent in 1993 and

TABLE 8-5. *Measures of Catastrophic Out-of-Pocket Spending, 2018*[a]

		Catastrophic measures (percent)		
Measure	Total admissions 2018	Absolute[b] ($20,000+)	Ratio I[c] (nonhousing assets)	Ratio II[d] (including home equity)
All elderly admissions	1,591,822	33	39	23
Men	455,432	38	35	20
Women	1,136,390	31	41	24
Age				
65–74	268,512	39	41	21
75–84	554,918	32	35	21
85+	768,392	32	41	26
Marital Status				
Married	364,501	40	24	6
Unmarried	1,227,321	31	44	28
Discharge status				
Deceased	1,015,672	41	46	28
Alive	576,150	20	28	15
Annual family income (1993 dollars)				
$0–7,499	207,898	16	55	37
7,500–14,999	490,537	30	54	33
15,000–19,999	213,228	33	39	21
20,000–49,999	512,443	39	26	15
50,000+	167,716	48	5	4
Nonhousing family assets (1993 dollars)				
$0–9,999	731,360	24	59	35
10,000–29,999	175,939	29	41	16
30,000–59,999	121,844	22	26	10
60,000–119,999	178,159	33	23	13
120,000+	384,520	44	12	11
Length of stay				
1–30 days	409,349	<1	4	1
31–60 days	181,935	<1	7	4
61–90 days	91,001	<1	8	2
91–364 days	333,905	20	51	19
1–2 years	156,694	59	62	37
2–3 years	117,252	82	68	45
3–5 years	119,717	82	79	60
5+ years	181,969	98	81	61

Source: Brookings–ICF Long-Term Care Financing Model. The year 2018 represent the five-year average for the period 1991–95.

a. All measures in this table refer to the cohort of elderly individuals (age 65 and older) admitted to a nursing home in 2016–20.

b. The absolute spending measure refers to the percent of admissions who spend $20,000 or more out of pocket (1993 dollars).

c. Ratio I = percent of admissions with out-of-pocket expenses equal to at least 40 percent of their income and nonhousing assets. The spending ratio sets the numerator equal to out-of-pocket expenses for the entire length of stay; the denominator equals the income the individual would have received had he or she not entered the nursing home, plus his or her family's nonhousing assets (measured jointly for married individuals, individually for unmarried individuals).

d. Ratio II = percent of admissions who spend at least 40 percent of their income and total assets out of pocket. The spending ratio numerator was calculated as in note c. The denominator includes all sources listed in note c plus home equity (market value net of mortgages held on the property or properties).

2018) is reflected in minor changes in subgroup estimates for 1993 and 2018 (ratio II, tables 8-4 and 8-5).

CONCLUSION

As a group, elderly persons who use nursing home care currently have considerable financial risk exposure and will continue to be burdened with substantial out-of-pocket payments for institutional long-term care services in the future. The three measures of catastrophic expenses used here indicate that the proportion of elderly nursing home users facing catastrophic out-of-pocket expenses will remain fairly stable over the twenty-five-year period 1993 to 2018. First, more than half of all elderly nursing home patients will continue to rely on medicaid financing over the next twenty-five years. Second, about one-third of elderly nursing home patients will incur out-of-pocket expenses of $20,000 or more per stay through 2018. Third, by 2018, nearly four in ten elderly patients admitted to nursing homes will encounter out-of-pocket expenses equal to or exceeding 40 percent of their relative incomes and nonhousing financial assets.

The stability of these measures over time indicates that rising incomes and assets among elderly Americans will not reduce the proportion of those in nursing home care who will face catastrophic expenses over the next twenty-five years. Thus, adopting a wait-and-see approach to the problem of financial impoverishment resulting from high out-of-pocket nursing home expenses is not likely to alleviate the burden of high out-of-pocket, long-term care costs. In short, without a change in public policy, nursing home stays will continue to impoverish elderly patients.

Further analysis of catastrophic spending estimates for elderly persons in nursing home care revealed consistent spending patterns over time among groups with similar characteristics. Two of the most obvious trends involve length-of-stay patterns and family income and assets. As nursing home stays increase beyond 90 days, the proportion of elderly admissions who will encounter catastrophic out-of-pocket expenses rises dramatically. For stays of 90 days or less, no more than 10 percent of those admitted will spend more than $20,000 per stay or more than 40 percent of their income and assets. Yet for prolonged stays of three years or more, more than half of all those admitted to nursing home care will encounter catastrophic out-of-pocket expenses.

Lower-income elderly persons shoulder a disproportionate share of catastrophic expenses compared with their wealthier counterparts. Well over 40 percent of all elderly nursing home admissions with incomes of less than $15,000 per year spent 40 percent or more of their combined relative income and nonhousing assets on nursing home care in 1993. In contrast, that year only 2 percent of those with annual incomes of $50,000 or more faced catastrophic expenses equal to or greater than 40 percent of their combined assets and income.

Public policy recommendations derived from this analysis should recognize that targeting spending for low-income elderly persons who are admitted to care and for those with prolonged nursing home stays may help to significantly reduce the rate of financial impoverishment in these two groups. However, it is not clear that one solution can be found that would reduce the burden of catastrophic spending for both groups. For example, it is possible that providing coverage for long-term nursing home stays would substantially reduce the proportion of elderly persons with large out-of-pocket expenses. Yet even short-term nursing home stays may pose a substantial burden on those who are poor or near-poor. Similarly, a relatively modest liberalization of medicaid eligibility rules would likely reduce the burden for poor and near-poor individuals but would not necessarily help those with substantial assets.[41]

We have also explored here the relationship between catastrophic out-of-pocket spending and elderly income and assets, including home equity. It is evident from this analysis that including home equity in the measure of assets held by elderly Americans substantially reduces the proportion admitted to nursing homes encountering catastrophic out-of-pocket expenses, now and in the future. What is not apparent is whether home equity should be treated as just any other asset. Although medicaid has traditionally excluded the principal residence from consideration in determining a person's spend-down qualifications, recent federal legislation requires states to attempt to recover the cost of care from the estates of medicaid recipients.[42] The question is whether public policy should allow special consideration for family homes, both in terms of symbolic importance and their role (particularly among those with modest assets) in assuring greater financial stability for future generations.

The desire to shield elderly persons from financial impoverishment resulting from high out-of-pocket spending for long-term care is tempered by concerns about the use of public funds to protect private assets. At the center of the debate is how a balance can be achieved between what elderly Americans can reasonably be expected to pay for such care from their own resources (either out of pocket or through private insurance) and what portion should be considered a public responsibility.

NOTES

1. Recent data suggest that what progress medicare had made in helping elderly Americans pay for routine medical care is now being outstripped by inflation in the health care sector and sharply increased cost sharing, resulting in higher out-of-pocket expenses for elderly beneficiaries. See, for example, AARP/Public Policy Institute, *Coming Up Short: Increasing Out-of-Pocket Health Spending by Older Americans* (Washington: American Association of Retired Persons, 1994); Marilyn Moon, *Medicare Now and In the Future* (Washington: Urban Institute Press, 1993), chapter 1; and *Families United for Senior Action, Health Cost Squeeze on Older Americans: A Report* (Washington: Families USA Foundation, February 1992).

2. Estimates from the Brookings–ICF Long-Term Care Financing Model.

3. Unmarried medicaid nursing home patients, for example, may retain only about $2,000 in nonhousing assets and must contribute all of their income, except for a small personal needs allowance (usually $30 per month), to help pay for their nursing home use. Congressional Research Service, *Medicaid Source Book: Background Data and Analysis (A 1993 Update)*, Committee Print, prepared for the Subcommittee on Health and the Environment of the House Committee on Energy and Commerce, 103 Cong. 1 sess. (January 1993), p. 203.

4. The remaining 1 percent is attributable to other state and local payers, charity care, and out-of-pocket expenditures by persons other than the recipient of care.

5. Estimate from the Brookings–ICF Long-Term Care Financing Model.

6. Authors' estimates, based on data from the Office of National Cost Estimates, Health Care Financing Administration.

7. Peter Kemper and Christopher M. Murtaugh, "Lifetime Use of Nursing Home Care," *New England Journal of Medicine*, vol. 324 (February 28, 1991), pp. 595–600.

8. Pamela Farley Short and others, "Public and Private Responsibility for Financing Nursing Home Care: The Effect of Medicaid Asset Spend-down," *Milbank Quarterly*, vol. 70, no. 2 (1992), pp. 277–98.

9. Leon Wyszewianski, "Financially Catastrophic and High-Cost Cases: Definitions, Distinctions, and Their Implications for Policy Formulation," *Inquiry*, vol. 23 (Winter 1986), pp. 382–94.

10. Mary Grace Kovar, "Expenditures for the Medical Care of Elderly People Living in the Community in 1980," *Milbank Quarterly*, vol. 64, no. 1 (1986), pp. 100–131.

11. Judith Feder, Marilyn Moon and William Scanlon, "Medicare Reform: Nibbling at Catastrophic Costs," *Health Affairs*, vol. 6, no. 4 (1987) pp. 5–19; Leon Wyszewianski, "Families with Catastrophic Health Care Expenditures," *Health Services Research*, vol. 25, no. 5 (1986), pp. 617–34.

12. Rose M. Rubin and Kenneth Koelln, "Out-of-Pocket Health Expenditure Differentials Between Elderly and Non-Elderly Households," *Gerontologist*, vol. 33 (October 1993), pp. 595–602.

13. Feder, Moon and Scanlon, "Medicare Reform: Nibbling at Catastrophic Costs," exhibit 1.

14. Korbin Liu, Maria Perozek, and Kenneth Manton, "Catastrophic Acute and Long-Term Care Costs: Risks Faced by Disabled Elderly Persons," *Gerontologist*, vol. 33 (June 1993), pp. 299–307; Theresa A. Coughlin, Korbin Liu, and Timothy D. McBride, "Severely Disabled Elderly Persons with Financially Catastrophic Health Care Expenses: Sources and Determinants," *Gerontologist*, vol. 32 (June 1992), pp. 391–403; Thomas Rice, "The Use, Cost, and Economic Burden of Nursing Home Care in 1985," *Medical Care*, vol. 27 (December 1989), pp. 1133–47; Thomas Rice and Jon Gabel, "Protecting the Elderly against High Health Care Costs," *Health Affairs*, vol. 5 (Fall 1986), pp. 5–21.

15. Rice and Gabel, "Protecting the Elderly Against High Health Care Costs."

16. Rice, "The Use, Cost, and Economic Burden of Nursing Home Care in 1985."

17. Coughlin, Liu, and McBride, "Severely Disabled Elderly Persons."

18. Liu, Perozek, and Manton, "Catastrophic Acute and Long-Term Care Costs," table 3.

19. Korbin Liu, Kenneth G. Manton, and Barbara Marzetta Liu, "Home Care Expenses for the Disabled Elderly," *Health Care Financing Review*, vol. 7 (Winter 1985), pp. 51–58.

20. Barbara M. Altman and Daniel C. Walden, "Home Health Care: Use, Expenditures, and Sources of Payment," AHCPR Pub. No. 93-0040, *National Medical Expenditure Survey Research Findings 15* (Rockville, Md.: Agency for Health Care Policy and Research, U.S. Public Health Service, April 1993).

21. Raymond J. Hanley, Joshua M. Wiener, and Katherine M. Harris, "The Economic Status of Nursing Home Users," in Joshua M. Wiener and others,

Long-Term Care: Service Use and Trends, report to the Health Care Financing Administration (Brookings, 1994), p. 21.

22. Howard Birnbaum, *The Cost of Catastrophic Illness* (Lexington, Mass.: Lexington Press, 1978).

23. Wyszewianski, "Financially Catastrophic and High-Cost Cases."

24. A comparison of public and private long-term care financing options and their impact on out-of-pocket expenses for elderly people is provided in Joshua M. Wiener, Laurel Hixon Illston, and Raymond J. Hanley, *Sharing the Burden: Strategies for Public and Private Long-Term Care Insurance* (Brookings, 1994).

25. Although hospital patients also receive room and board, these ordinary living expenses represent a much smaller proportion of the total cost of an acute care stay. In addition, because lengths of stay are shorter for acute care, patients generally do not give up their private residences for the duration of their stay, as an elderly person facing a long nursing home stay might do.

26. The following example helps to illustrate the difficulty of defining the true added costs of long-term care: A seventy-five-year-old single person who lives at home has hired a housekeeper to come in once a week for the past 15 years. In the past year, the person suffered a broken hip and now finds it difficult to stand for long periods of time. This person may increase the housekeeper's hours, or alternatively, may maintain the same schedule but ask the housekeeper to perform a different mix of tasks to compensate for the new level of impairment. Should this individual's expenditure for housekeeping services be considered home care or an ordinary living expense? If the housekeeper's payment is credited to home care, then the individual effectively reduces his or her ordinary living expenses by that amount. Obviously, such a detailed analysis of out-of-pocket expenditures is not practical in a large-scale investigation. This example illustrates why, compared to acute care, a higher out-of-pocket spending threshold is justified in the analysis of out-of-pocket expenses for home care services as well as for nursing home care.

27. For a discussion of home equity conversions, see Alice M. Rivlin and Joshua M. Wiener, with Raymond J. Hanley and Denise Spence, *Caring for the Disabled Elderly: Who Will Pay?* (Brookings, 1988).

28. Wyszewianski, "Financially Catastrophic and High Cost Cases," p. 386.

29. From a conceptual standpoint, an alternative approach to defining a financially catastrophic burden would be to calculate the value of a typical market basket of goods (food, shelter, utilities, entertainment, normal medical expenditures, etc.) that would constitute a normal lifestyle for an elderly person. In turn, this market basket could be used to measure the relative impact of acute and long-term care costs on the ability to maintain a normal lifestyle. One could then be more explicit about the relative burden

imposed by out-of-pocket medical care costs. However, measurement problems (including achieving a reasonable definition of a "normal" lifestyle that accounts for geographic and cultural differences among the elderly population) are considerable.

30. For a more detailed explanation of the Brookings–ICF Long-Term Care Financing Model, see Wiener and others, *Sharing the Burden,* chapter 2 and appendix A.

31. *1988 Annual Report of the Board of Trustees of the Federal Old-Age and Survivors Insurance and Disability Insurance Trust Funds* (Washington, 1988).

32. This assumption presumes that nursing home and home care prices will continue to increase in the future to keep pace with projected wage and fringe benefit growth in the rest of the economy. This projected rate of growth is based on the 1989 Social Security Administration Office of the Actuary's long-run assumption that the consumer price index will increase at 4.0 percent a year, real wages at 1.3 percent a year, and fringe benefits at 0.2 percent a year.

33. Although a measure of nursing home costs over an individual's lifetime is an appealing approach, it poses difficulties when attempting to define a catastrophic spending threshold. For example, suppose an individual has two nursing home stays—one of short duration, one of a much longer duration with a number of years between the two stays. Should his or her lifetime expenditures be compared to the individual's net worth at the time of the first stay, the second stay, or some combination of the two? It is not clear which measure would provide the clearest picture of the relative impact of catastrophic costs.

34. Both studies of acute care out-of-pocket costs and proposals for reducing acute care catastrophic spending among elderly people have used percent-of-income measures in the range of 10 to 20 percent of income. Wyszewianski, "Families with Catastrophic Health Care Expenditures," p. 619.

35. Christopher M. Murtaugh, Peter Kemper, and Brenda C. Spillman, "The Risk of Nursing Home Use in Later Life," *Medical Care,* vol. 28 (October 1990), pp. 952–62.

36. Steven E. Feinleib, Peter J. Cunningham, and Pamela Farley Short, "Use of Nursing and Personal Care Homes by the Civilian Population, 1987," AHCPR Pub. No. 94-0096, National Medical Expenditure Survey Findings 23 (Rockville, Md.: Agency for Health Care Policy and Research, August 1994); Esther Hing, "Use of Nursing Homes by the Elderly: Preliminary Data from the 1985 National Nursing Home Survey," *Advance Data No. 135* (National Center for Health Statistics, May 14, 1987).

37. Denise A. Spence and Joshua M. Wiener, "Nursing Home Length of Stay Patterns: Results from the 1985 National Nursing Home Survey," *Gerontologist,* vol. 30, no. 1 (1990), pp. 16–20.

38. For purposes of this study, a ratio of out-of-pocket expenses to income and assets of elderly persons was calculated in which the numerator is set equal to out-of-pocket spending per admission and the denominator is the income that the individual would have earned if he or she had not been institutionalized, plus net family assets. A catastrophic ratio is defined as 0.4 or greater—that is, elderly admissions whose out-of-pocket expenses equal or exceed 40 percent of their income and assets measured relative to their length of stay.

39. The home equity measure includes the family nonhousing assets and the estimated market value of all real estate properties (including principal residence, vacation property, rental property, and other) less outstanding mortgages. As was true for the measure of nonhousing assets, home equity was measured jointly for married elderly couples and individually for unmarried elderly persons, and a spending ratio of 0.4 or more was considered catastrophic.

40. Joint Center for Housing Studies, *State of the Nation's Housing* (Harvard University, 1993), p. 27.

41. For a comparison among public and private sector initiatives designed to reduce the burden of catastrophic long-term care spending for elderly Americans who use nursing home care, see Wiener and others, *Sharing the Burden.*

42. Omnibus Budget Reconciliation Act of 1993, P. L. 103-66, August 10, 1993. Although more than half of all states have existing asset recovery programs, OBRA 93 mandates their operation.

PART 4
Home and Community-Based Care

Chapter 9

KORBIN LIU, JEAN HANSON, AND
TERESA COUGHLIN

Characteristics and Outcomes of Persons Screened into Connecticut's 2176 Program

Recent proposals to expand home and community-based care (HCBC) used degrees of physical and cognitive disability as criteria to be met for eligibility for services. The proposals also directed benefits toward the most severely disabled individuals. The Health Security Act, for example, specified dependencies in three or more activities of daily living (ADLs—for example, bathing or dressing) as one criterion for eligibility for expanded HCBC services. Other proposals required either two or three ADL dependencies.[1]

Supporting research has provided estimates of the number of persons who would be eligible under different proposals and of expected program costs according to the specific HCBC program implemented.[2] Much less information currently exists, however, on how many people eligible by virtue of their disability would not eventually receive services from the program. The reasons why people would not participate, or are restricted from participating, may range from their having formal service needs exceeding a program's allowable cost limits to their personal preferences for entering nursing homes.

Information about those people who would not receive services could help produce better estimates of the potential number of users

We are grateful to Myra Kerr and Joan Quinn of Connecticut Community Care, Inc. (CCCI), for enabling us to analyze CCCI data and providing continuing consultation about Connecticut's medicaid home and community-based care program. We also thank John Marcotte and Doug Wissoker of the Urban Institute for their advice and support on statistical methods used in the research.

from the eligible population. The reasons for nonparticipation could also help clarify which features of the programs may present barriers to receipt of services. Finally, the outcomes of different groups of people who were initially assessed as eligible for HCBC services can be illuminated. Do recipients of program-funded services differ from nonrecipients in tendency to enter nursing homes, likelihood of remaining in the community, and death rate?

This chapter uses data from the state of Connecticut to analyze the characteristics and outcomes of persons screened into Connecticut's medicaid 2176 waiver program. This program targets persons at high risk of institutionalization and aims to substitute home and community-based care for nursing home care.

Because not all persons screened into the program actually received services, the focus of our analysis was on comparing persons who became clients of the program with others who did not become clients. We grouped persons who did not receive services into the following three categories: an individual whose cost of care exceeded program-established cost caps; an individual or family who refused the care plan offered or withdrew from the assessment process; or an individual who was expected to be placed in an institution. We addressed two questions about program participants and persons who did not receive services. First, how did persons who did not receive program services differ from participants in the program? Second, are there differences between the participants and nonrecipients in terms of eventual nursing home use or death?

Our analysis of persons screened into a medicaid 2176 waiver program is specific to Connecticut. Although Connecticut's program and residents are not necessarily representative of other states, the information gleaned may have general implications for other HCBC programs.

BACKGROUND ON HCBC AND CONNECTICUT'S PROGRAM

Home and community-based care is an important type of long-term care for disabled elderly persons because most of them live in the community rather than in institutions. HCBC can be provided either formally by paid caregivers or informally by family and friends. Although informal caregivers provide most HCBC for disabled elderly persons, an increasing number of these individuals are receiving help from paid caregivers. A recent study found, for example, that the proportion of disabled elderly persons living in the community who used paid HCBC increased from 27 percent in 1982 to 35 percent in 1989.[3] Reflecting this trend, expenditures for HCBC have been growing rapidly. Since 1988 national expenditures for HCBC more than tripled, reaching $33 billion in 1993.[4] A large proportion (22 percent) of national HCBC expenditures was paid by medicaid, the federal-state program for low-income persons.

Medicaid has three main HCBC programs—personal care, home health care, and waiver programs—which differ in design and focus. Home health care is a mandatory medicaid benefit and is structured much like medicare's home health care benefit in that it has a strong medical orientation. The personal care program is an optional service under medicaid and consists of help with activities such as bathing, dressing, and eating, and help with housekeeping duties such as meal preparation and shopping. In 1993, thirty-two states offered personal care to their residents.[5]

States can also apply to the federal government for authorization to provide HCBC through various waiver authorities.[6] Waiver programs are generally targeted to persons who would otherwise receive medicaid services in a nursing facility. Prompted by concern that medicaid had too strong of an institutional bias, the first of the community-based waivers was established in the Omnibus Budget Reconciliation Act of 1981 and called the Medicaid Home and Community-Based Services program. Less formally, it has become known as the "2176 waiver program" (after the section in OBRA 81) or the 1915(c) program (after the section of the Social Security Act).[7] Connecticut's HCBC program is an example of a medicaid HCBC waiver program.

Through this waiver, states are allowed to provide a broad range of home and community-based care services for elderly persons, mentally retarded individuals, and other chronically ill persons. Services provided in 2176 programs must be budget neutral; that is, the state must demonstrate that the average per capita cost with the waiver does not exceed the average per capita cost without it.

Waiver programs offer states numerous advantages, perhaps the most important being that waiver programs greatly limit states' risk. For example, under waiver programs, states can offer services to residents only in a specific geographic area or be restrictive in their criteria for eligibility (for example, targeting only persons at risk of being institutionalized). Another important advantage is that states are allowed to apply the more generous institutional financial eligibility standards rather than the stricter medicaid income standards usually applied to persons living in the community. Waiver programs thus enable states to provide HCBC to persons who may not otherwise qualify for medicaid.

A recent survey of medicaid HCBC programs found that among the forty-five responding states, most 1915(c) waiver programs that serve elderly persons are offered statewide.[8] About half of the waiver programs used the highest financial eligibility standard allowed under the waiver authority. (At present, states are allowed to extend eligibility to persons with incomes up to 300 percent of the supplemental security income [SSI] level, which was about $15,600 in 1993). The waiver programs provide a wide variety of services, including respite care, homemaker, personal care, transportation, and nursing.

The survey also showed that states employ various types of cost containment measures to ensure the budget neutrality of their waiver programs. Virtually all state programs employ ceilings, or caps, on the amount of allowable services. Such caps are usually tied to a percentage of the state's medicaid nursing home payment rate, and many cost caps are set at 100 percent of nursing home rates. Cost caps may be applied to each client or are averaged across all care plans in an agency's caseload. Of all programs using cost caps, 80 percent apply the cost cap to each care plan.[9] States using this method believe that it provides greater program cost control than allowed by the averaging method. To allow programs to serve persons with very high care costs, many of these states have policies that permit case managers to request state approval to exceed individual caps.

Connecticut's 2176 program provides medicaid-funded home and community-based services to individuals 65 years of age and older who would have otherwise been accepted for medicaid-funded skilled nursing facility services. The program applies to elderly medicaid recipients or those who would become medicaid recipients within 180 days after being admitted into a nursing facility. To qualify for the 2176 program, an elderly person must meet the income and asset rules applicable to an institutionalized medicaid applicant. The gross income limit is 300 percent of SSI income level, and the asset limit for an unmarried applicant is $2,000.

The Connecticut program is intended to be a straight entitlement in which all eligible persons are accepted. The program targets clients through a two-step process. First, persons qualify if hospital personnel indicate that they are likely to be discharged to a nursing home or if nursing home staff identify them as likely candidates for admission within sixty days. Until recently, Connecticut was among a small number of states that required nonhospitalized persons seeking HCBC services to first apply to nursing homes and be put on waiting lists. Second, a uniform health screen is applied to determine whether an elderly person needs a nursing home level of care and whether institutionalization would be long term (that is, more than ninety days); persons in need of short-term nursing home care do not qualify for HCBC services.

The uniform health screen is completed by hospital personnel or by medicaid staff nurses from the Connecticut Department of Social Services. The screen collects information including dependencies in ADLs or instrumental activities of daily living (IADLs—for example, shopping or meal preparation), cognitive status, and profiles of informal care. The department reviews the screen to determine "level of care" eligibility for the program and to refer appropriate clients to a case manager for an assessment of their service needs. The screen is also used to authorize level of care required by elderly medicaid clients or applicants who are admitted directly to a nursing home. The standards for potential placement were approximately equivalent to two or more ADLs out of five possible, four or more IADLs out of eight possible, or six or more errors out of ten on mental status questions.

Full assessment and case management services are provided in Connecticut by Connecticut Community Care, Inc. (CCCI). CCCI personnel conduct a full assessment of service needs, using a more extensive instrument than the health screen described previously. Based on the results of the assessment, individualized plans for community-based social and medical services are developed including, but not limited to, 2176 program services. The plan specifies the type, frequency, and cost of all services required including informal care. The case manager is required to involve informal support and pursue other funding sources before relying on 2176 program funds.

Once the care plan is completed, the case manager must determine whether it meets two cost limits, which compare state funds for 2176 services to costs of nursing home care. First, state costs for community-based "social" services cannot exceed 60 percent of the weighted average rate for nursing home care. Social services include adult day care, homemaking, companionship, chores, emergency response systems, meals, counseling, and financial management.

Second, the state's cost for the client's total plan of care (medical plus social services) cannot exceed the state costs of nursing home care; medical services include professional health services (for example, skilled nursing) and home health aide care. In general, medical services involve "hands-on" care (including ADL assistance), in contrast to assistance with nonpersonal care needs such as chores and companionship.

Like many other states, Connecticut's cost cap is equivalent to 100 percent of average nursing home care costs; in Connecticut that amount is approximately $3,000 a month. It is applied on a person-specific basis. The state does permit temporary increases in costs as a result of special circumstances, such as when the spouse caregiver of a program client is temporarily in the hospital. Informal care is determined through extensive discussions with potential clients and their families, with assessment of current care contributions as an initial basis for amount available. If case managers determine that available informal care and formal care under the cost cap cannot meet the needs of the potential clients, those clients are restricted from participation in the 2176 program but are provided assistance with placement in a nursing home.

For persons who do not exceed the cost cap, the state's expected cost for a client is derived by deducting the client's average applied income contribution from the weighted average monthly rate for nursing home care. The applied income is equivalent to the balance of an individual's gross income after deducting the amount equivalent to 200 percent of the federal poverty level; the applied income requirement does not apply to persons who qualify for medicaid based on the usual community income standard.

After the assessment, eligible persons are offered a choice: a plan of community care or assistance to obtain placement for institutional care. If they choose to participate, services generally commence promptly after the assessment. It is also important to note that some persons withdraw from the assessment and the process of formulating a care plan before their completion. Other persons may have intended to enter nursing homes in the first place, but they required an assessment that served as a "preadmission screen" before admission to a nursing home could occur. Because the state also performs preadmission screening, not all persons subject to this procedure are referred to CCCI for assessments. Moreover, persons assessed by CCCI for the purpose of preadmission screening are not identified as such.

DATA SOURCES AND METHODS

This study used data from three sources. The first source was the assessment by CCCI that determines whether people meet program eligibility criteria and whether they can be adequately served by the 2176 program. A standardized assessment instrument is used to collect information on prospective clients' personal characteristics, including demographic, functional and health status, sources of informal care, and financial status. Questions on demographic characteristics include age, sex, race, marital status, and living arrangement. Health and functional status questions refer to medical conditions and dependencies in ADLs and IADLs. The five core ADLs in our analysis were bathing, dressing, getting in and out of bed, using the toilet, and eating. Prospective clients are also asked who helps them with performing IADLs and ADLs, with what frequency they are helped, and how the helper is related to them (for example, spouse or child).

The assessment data also contain information on the outcome of the interview: whether the person was admitted, not admitted, or eligible but not admitted. If the person is not admitted, the case manager also specifies the reason for nonadmission.

The second data source was the state of Connecticut's Consolidated Master Death File. This file contains detailed information on all persons who died in Connecticut including date of death, place of death, and cause of death. The third data source was Connecticut's Nursing Home Inventory, which contains information on all persons who use nursing homes in the state. Data elements in the file include date of nursing home admission and date of discharge. Selected information from the Nursing Home Inventory, the death file, and CCCI assessment data was merged to create the analysis file for this study.

We constructed the merged file to provide longitudinal information on outcomes of all persons screened by CCCI, regardless of whether they became clients of the 2176 program. We used the file to determine how characteristics of those persons were associated with their risk of eventual nursing home admission and death.

We obtained data on all persons referred to the 2176 program who were assessed for the first time by CCCI between January 1, 1988, and December 31, 1990. A total of 5,275 persons met this criterion, of whom 3,619 were program participants and 1,656 were not. Cases with missing data on key items and cases with incorrect information were excluded from the analysis file, along with cases in which assessment and outcome data could not be matched. After editing, we derived a final analysis sample of 4,707 persons of whom 3,257 were participants and 1,450 were not. We tracked all sample persons through September 30, 1991.

Reasons for Not Being Clients

CCCI recorded a broad range of reasons why persons did not become clients of the 2176 program. These reasons included client or family refusal of services after care plans were established, client family withdrawal of application during the assessment process, preference for placement in nursing homes, and ineligibility because cost of care plans exceeded 60 percent of social services or 100 percent of total HCBC service costs. We grouped the reasons into three general categories: costs of HCBC services exceeded program established limits; client or family chose not to participate; and expected placement for institutional care. The last category includes persons who were assessed in hospital units as being expected to have permanent placement in long-term care units and persons who opted to go to nursing homes after the assessment. The logic of the groupings reflects, respectively, the program's decision that costs for particular individuals were too high, the individuals' or their families' decision not to participate, and the individuals' apparent predisposition for nursing home care. A fourth category was client death, which occurred after an assessment, but before provision of services or final determination of medicaid eligibility.

Informal Care and Living Arrangement

We developed a hierarchical classification of informal care and living arrangement, which would reflect the likely primary caregiver as well as strength of an individual's informal care network. In this classification, persons were placed into four possible categories. The first category consisted of persons who were living with their spouses. We reasoned that this arrangement also reflected a situation in which informal caregiving was relatively strong and constant. Persons not living with their spouses, but living with a child, were placed in the second category. The third category consisted of persons who lived neither with spouse nor child but who had a child as the primary caregiver. The final category contained all persons who did not fall into any of the prior three groups. We reasoned that persons in this last category had a relatively weak informal care situation.

ANALYSES OF THE DATA

We conducted descriptive and multivariate analyses of the data. The dependent variables in each of our multivariate analyses were categorical measures. In the first analysis, we examined individuals who screened into the program to determine the relationship between personal characteristics and their likelihood of being in one of several categories, either participants or subgroups of persons who did not receive services, by the reasons described previously. In the second analysis, we estimated the relationship between personal characteristics and risk of nursing home admission or death. In both cases, the dependent variable was constructed as discrete categories.

As a consequence of the qualitative nature of the dependent variables, logistic regression models were used.[10] This model has the following functional form:

$$P_i = 1 \div [1 + e^{-(\alpha + \beta X_i)}]$$

The model can be written as:

$$\log \left(\frac{P_i}{1 - P_i} \right) = \alpha + \beta X_i$$

In this model P_i is defined as the probability that individual i had the outcome (for example, was a participant; went to a nursing home), α is an intercept term, X_i contains a set of explanatory variables, and β contains associated parameters.

A binomial logistic regression model was used when the dependent variable had only two possible outcomes (for example, nursing home admission/death, no nursing home admission/death). When the dependent variable had more than two possible outcomes, a multinomial logistic regression model was used. This was the case when we estimated the relationship between personal characteristics and whether individuals became participants or a member of one of the categories of persons who did not receive services. In logistic regression, the parameters are estimated by the maximum likelihood estimation method.

Results in the following section are presented in three forms—slope coefficients, odds ratios, and probabilities—which are functionally interrelated. As a consequence of the natural log transformation, the coefficients of the explanatory variables of logit models tend to be difficult to interpret. Whereas the slope coefficients gives the changes in the log odds ratio per unit change in the explanatory variable, it is often easier to speak in terms of the odds ratios or probabilities. In examining the effects of a personal characteristic on an outcome, the odds ratio presents the relative likelihood of a particular outcome given the presence of the characteristics relative to the absence of the characteristic. The odds ratio is independent of the levels of other characteristics in the model. We use this measure in reviewing the effects of the array of specific characteristics in the multivariate models. Probabilities, on the other hand, are a function of other variables in the model. We use predicted probabilities to illustrate the effects of combinations of characteristics on, for example, likelihood of being a participant relative to exceeding program allowable costs.

PROFILES OF PARTICIPANTS AND NONRECIPIENTS

In our analysis sample of 4,707 persons who were screened and found by the state to meet eligibility standards for nursing home admission, approximately 70 percent were participants, while the remaining persons were classified into one of four groups representing people who did not participate or were restricted from participating (table 9-1). The largest of these groups was persons who exceeded the program's allowable cost caps; the 727 persons in this group constituted 15 percent of the total sample and half of all persons who were not participants in the program. Six percent (n = 205) of the sample were persons who withdrew from the assessment process or refused care plans, and 8 percent (n = 375) were persons who were expected to be placed in institutions. The remainder of the sample was made up of persons who died shortly after the assessment (n = 63).

Table 9-1 also presents the characteristics of participants and each category of persons who did not receive services. The mean values indicate the proportion of persons in each sample with a particular characteristic. For example, .70 (or 70 percent) of the participants were female.

Exceed Cap

Small differences were found in demographic characteristics between participants and those persons who did not become participants because their resource needs exceeded the program cap. One exception was that a higher proportion of participants (70 percent) were female, in contrast to 66 percent of persons exceeding cap who were female.

Large differences between the two groups were found, however, in their informal care and living arrangements. A large proportion of the participants (49 percent) lived with spouse or child. In contrast, only 31 percent of those persons exceeding the cap had such living arrangements. And 39 percent of the participants had four or more informal caregivers, in contrast to only 13 percent of persons exceeding the cap who had that many informal caregivers. About half of the participants had cardiological or musculoskeletal conditions, whereas only about 40 percent of the persons exceeding the cap had such problems. A relatively small proportion of both groups had neurological difficulties.

Large differences in functional status were also found between the two groups. For example, 42 percent of the participants had three or more ADL dependencies, whereas 78 percent of persons exceeding the cap were disabled at this level. Similarly, 34 percent of participants had some cognitive impairment—based on less than six correct answers (out of ten) on mental status questions—whereas more than half of persons exceeding the cap had cognitive impairments. A much smaller proportion of the participants (37 percent) were incontinent compared with people exceeding the cap (52 percent).

TABLE 9-1. *Characteristics of Participant and Nonrecipient Samples*

Variable	Participants (n = 3,257)		Exceeded cap (n = 727)		Withdrew or refused (n = 285)		Expected institutional placement (n = 375)		Death (n = 63)	
	Mean	Standard deviation	Mean	Standard deviation	Mean	Standard deviation	Mean	Standard deviation	Mean	Standard deviation
Demographic										
Greater than age 85[a]	.27	.44	.29	.45	.24	.42	.32	.47	.33	.48
Between the ages of 75 and 84	.46	.49	.45	.50	.44	.50	.43	.50	.40	.49
Female	.70	.45	.66	.47	.62	.49	.69	.46	.49	.50
White	.90	.29	.90	.30	.90	.29	.93	.25	.94	.25
Informal support arrangement										
Living and primary caregiver arrangement[a]										
Lives with spouse	.25	.43	.14	.35	.21	.41	.17	.37	.29	.46
Lives with child	.24	.42	.17	.38	.24	.43	.19	.40	.20	.41
Child considered primary care person	.32	.47	.28	.45	.24	.45	.34	.47	.35	.48
Number of informal supporters[a]										
Two supporters	.23	.42	.26	.44	.28	.37	.27	.44	.19	.40
Three supporters	.19	.39	.13	.33	.17	.40	.15	.36	.22	.42
Four or more supporters	.39	.49	.13	.34	.20	.49	.20	.39	.29	.46
Health conditions										
Has cardiological difficulties	.52	.50	.42	.49	.41	.49	.47	.50	.44	.50
Has musculoskeletal difficulties	.48	.50	.37	.48	.40	.49	.40	.49	.35	.48
Has neurological difficulties	.13	.34	.15	.36	.12	.32	.12	.33	.13	.34

Functional status

Has difficulties with one or two ADLs[a]	.46	.50	.17	.37	.38	.49	.33	.47	.11	.32
Has difficulties with three or four ADLs	.30	.46	.44	.50	.32	.47	.37	.48	.46	.50
Has difficulties with five ADLs	.12	.33	.34	.48	.14	.35	.20	.40	.43	.50
Incontinence	.37	.48	.61	.49	.37	.48	.44	.49	.68	.47
MSQ less than 4[a]	.21	.40	.35	.48	.25	.43	.28	.45	.48	.50
MSQ 4–6	.13	.34	.21	.41	.14	.34	.16	.37	.13	.36
Major life crisis (past year)										
Illness	.61	.49	.41	.49	.42	.49	.42	.49	.66	.48
Other (relocation, spousal death, and so on)	.31	.46	.21	.41	.19	.40	.23	.42	.14	.35
Medicaid in community	.31	.46	.38	.49	.28	.45	.37	.48	.27	.45

Source: Urban Institute analysis of Connecticut Community Care, Inc., data, Connecticut's Consolidated Master Death File, and Connecticut's Nursing Home Inventory.

a. Reference categories/omitted categories are the following: (1) between the age of 65 and 74; (2) lives with individual other than child or spouse or lives alone, primary care person other than child; (3) zero or one informal supporter; (4) does not have difficulties with activities of daily living (ADLs); and (5) mental status quotient (MSQ) score greater than six correct.

A higher proportion of participants had a serious illness (61 percent) or other major life crisis (31 percent) in the past year than did persons exceeding the cap (41 percent and 21 percent, respectively). Finally, a slightly smaller proportion of participants (31 percent) were medicaid eligible for community benefits than were nonparticipants (38 percent).

Withdrew or Refused

In contrast to the group of people who exceeded the program cap, persons who withdrew from the assessment process, or refused the care plans after they were completed, were more similar in characteristics to the participants. Demographically this group contained a smaller proportion of females than did the participants (62 percent versus 70 percent). This group had almost as large a proportion living with spouse or child as did the participants (45 percent versus 49 percent). However, participants had twice the proportion of persons with four or more informal supporters (39 percent versus 20 percent) as did persons who withdrew or refused services.

Participants and persons who withdrew or refused were also very similar in functional status. For example, 42 percent of the participants had 3 or more ADL dependencies, whereas this nonparticipant group had 46 percent of persons with that level of ADL dependency. No difference was found in the proportion of persons who were incontinent, and differences in mental status quotient (MSQ) scores were minor.

As with the persons who exceeded the cap, persons who withdrew or refused had a small proportion of persons with major life crises in the past year. A smaller proportion of such persons were on medicaid, however, than either the participants or persons whose needs exceeded the program cap.

Expected Institutional Placement

Persons identified by CCCI case managers as likely for nursing home placement were demographically quite similar to participants, although a higher proportion of them were over age 85 than the participants (32 percent versus 27 percent). A smaller proportion of the expected nursing home patients lived with spouse or child (36 percent) than did the participants (49 percent). Like the preceding groups of persons who did not become clients of the 2176 program, a relatively small proportion of them (20 percent) had four or more informal supporters. This finding is consistent with earlier research indicating that limitations in available informal caregivers are positively associated with nursing home use.

In contrast to the participants, the group of persons who were expected to be institutionalized had higher proportions of persons with three or more ADLs, persons who were incontinent, or persons with cognitive impairments. These results are consistent with prior research indicating the positive association between level of disability and risk of nursing home placement. Although this group of nonparticipants had a smaller proportion of persons with a major life crisis in the past year than did the participants, it contained a higher proportion of persons on medicaid than did the participants.

Deaths

A small number of persons screened into the 2176 program died shortly after the assessment. In contrast to the participants, this group contained a higher proportion of persons over 85 years of age (33 percent versus 27 percent) and a smaller proportion of females (49 percent versus 70 percent). Although some differences existed between the two groups in informal support and living arrangement, the most notable differences appeared to be in the area of functional status. About 89 percent of persons who died had three or more ADL dependencies, and 43 percent had five ADL dependencies. In contrast, only 42 percent of participants had three or more ADL dependencies, and only 13 percent had five ADL dependencies. Persons who died had a slightly higher proportion of persons who had a major illness in the past year than did the participants (66 percent versus 61 percent). Differences between the two groups in the proportion of persons on medicaid appeared to be small.

CHARACTERISTICS AND LIKELIHOOD OF PARTICIPATION

To identify the independent effects of personal characteristics on being a 2176 program participant or being a nonrecipient, by reason category, we conducted a multinomial logistic regression analysis in which we tested whether having a certain characteristic affected the likelihood of a person being in one of the nonclient groups relative to being a participant. The explanatory variables were the same ones described in table 9-1. Table 9-2 presents the estimated effects of the independent variables for each subgroup of nonclients. The odds ratio (OR) is also presented when a coefficient was statistically significant at the .05 level. The OR reflects the relative likelihood of being in a subgroup relative to being a program participant if a person possessed the personal characteristic. For example, persons who had three to four ADLs were 5.23 times more likely than persons with fewer than three ADLs (the reference category) to have exceeded the program cap than to be a participant. The following compares each of the nonclient subgroups with participants.

Exceeded Cap

In comparing persons whose care needs exceeded the program cap with participants, we found that almost all of the characteristics in table 9-2 are statistically significant predictors. Many of the relationships reflect the distributions in table 9-1. Especially notable are variables reflecting the effects the availability of informal care and degree of disability on the likelihood of persons exceeding the cap. In general persons with relatively strong informal care arrangements were more likely to be a participant than to exceed the program cap. For example, in contrast to the reference category for living/caregiving arrangement—persons not living with spouse or child and not having a child as primary caregiver—persons living with a child were only one-fifth (OR = .20) as likely to exceed the cap as persons in the reference category. The estimates also show the importance of number of informal caregivers. For example, a person with four or more informal caregivers (that is, "Support 4") was only 21 percent (OR = .21) as likely to have exceeded the cap as someone with only one or no informal caregiver (the reference category).

In contrast to the increasing strength of living and caregiving arrangement in predicting a lower likelihood of exceeding the program cap, increasing levels of disability tended to raise the likelihood of exceeding the cap. A person with three to four ADLs was more than five times more likely (OR = 5.23) to have exceeded the cap than persons with less than three ADLs (the reference category). Persons with five ADLs were ten times (OR = 10.36) more likely to have exceeded the cap than persons with fewer than three ADLs. These results might be expected because, all other things being equal, persons with higher levels of disability would require more paid help, and their expected costs would be, in turn, more likely to exceed the program's allowable cost cap.

We also found that persons who were medicaid eligible in the community had a greater likelihood (OR = 1.37) of not being a participant of the program. A partial explanation for this result is that community medicaid-eligible persons, who were also entitled to other medicaid-financed home and community-based care, had the option to choose alternative programs that might have offered a greater quantity of some services than available through the 2176 waiver program.

Withdrew or Refused

The characteristics that differentiated people who withdrew from the application process or refused the care plan from participants were mainly demographic or related to caregiving and living arrangements. For example, persons who were living with spouse were half (OR = .49) as likely to withdraw or refuse than to enroll in the 2176 program. Similarly, persons who had four or more informal supporters, in contrast to persons with one or no informal caregivers, were less likely (OR = .39) to withdraw or refuse participation in the program.

An interesting finding in this comparison between participants and persons who withdrew from the assessment process or refused care plans was that functional status was not a significant predictor. This finding suggests that disability level, if used independently to target persons for participation in a 2176 program, may not be effective. Besides differences in caregiving and living arrangements, other factors, such as personal preferences, unmeasured financial resources, desire to enter nursing homes, or alternative home and community-based care programs (for example, medicaid personal care), may be important in determining whether an individual or his family chooses to participate in a 2176 program.

TABLE 9-2. *Likelihood of Exceeding Cap, Withdrawing or Refusing, Expected Institutionalization or Death, for Nonrecipients of Services in the 2176 Program, by Personal Characteristics*

Characteristic[a]	Exceeded cap (n = 727)		Withdrew or refused (n = 285)		Expected institutional placement (n = 375)		Death (n = 63)	
	Estimate	Odds ratio	Estimate	Odds ratio	Estimate	Odds ratio	Estimate	Odds ratio
Intercept	-.71	.49	-.51	.60	-1.11	.32	-4.41	.01
Greater than age 85[b]	-.16	...	-.47	.62	.08	...	.03	...
Between the ages of 75 and 84	-.14	...	-.31	.73	-.05	...	-.26	...
Female	-.27	.76	-.36	.69	-.14	...	-.93	.39
Informal support arrangement								
Living and primary caregiver arrangement[b]								
Lives with spouse	-1.99	.14	-.71	.49	-1.01	.36	-.90	.40
Lives with child	-1.60	.20	-.31	...	-.85	.42	-.64	...
Child considered primary care person	-.44	.64	-.49	.61	-.11	...	.58	...
Number of informal supporters[b]								
Two supporters	-.69	.50	-.26	...	-.50	.60	-.87	.42
Three supporters	-1.04	.35	-.46	.62	-.72	.48	-.43	...
Four or more supporters	-1.58	.21	-.94	.39	-1.14	.31	-.77	.46
Health conditions								
Has cardiological difficulties	-.23	.79	-.37	.68	-.09	...	-.20	...
Has musculoskeletal difficulties	-.34	.70	-.18	...	-.27	.75	-.39	...
Has neurological difficulties	.06	...	-.14	...	-.07	...	-.16	...

Functional status

Has difficulties with three or four ADLs	1.65	5.23	.25	· · ·	.73	2.07	2.01	7.5
Has difficulties with five ADLs	2.34	10.36	.34	· · ·	1.04	2.84	2.68	14.7
Incontinence	.42	1.52	-.04	· · ·	.06	· · ·	.39	· · ·
MSQ less than 4[b]	.45	1.57	.04	· · ·	.24	· · ·	.78	2.18
MSQ 4-6	.62	1.85	-.01	· · ·	.25	· · ·	.25	· · ·

Major life crisis (past year)

Illness	-.73	.48	-.63	· · ·	-.69	.49	.41	· · ·
Other (relocation, spousal death, and so on)	.07	· · ·	-.34	· · ·	· · ·	· · ·	-.78	.46
Medicaid in community	.31	1.37	-.16	· · ·	.22	· · ·	-.14	· · ·

Source: Urban Institute analysis of Connecticut Community Care, Inc., data, Connecticut's Consolidated Master Death File, and Connecticut's Nursing Home Inventory.

a. Characteristic is significant at the .05 level when odds ratio is presented.

b. Reference categories/omitted categories are the following: (1) between the age of 65 and 74; (2) lives with individual other than child or spouse or lives alone, primary care person other than child; (3) zero or one informal supporter; (4) less than 2 activities of daily living (ADLs); and (5) mental status quotient (MSQ) score greater than six correct.

Expected Institutional Placement

Characteristics that differentiated persons who were expected to be placed in institutions from participants were mainly informal support arrangements and ADLs. For example, persons who lived with spouses were only 36 percent as likely to be expected to be placed in nursing homes than to be participants in the 2176 program. In general, the findings indicated that strength of the caregiving and living arrangement was negatively associated with persons being in the expected institutional placement category, relative to being program participants. Similarly, we found that higher ADL dependencies increased the likelihood of persons expecting institutional placement rather than being a participant in the program. Interestingly, persons with a major illness in the past year were less likely to be in the institutional placement category than to be a participant. This finding suggests that persons in this category were more likely to enter nursing homes because of chronic conditions and disability rather than an acute medical problem.

Deaths

Consistent with the descriptive findings in table 9-1, the most important characteristics distinguishing persons who died from participants were high levels of disability. Persons with five ADLs, for example, were almost fifteen times more likely to have died than to have enrolled in the 2176 program. Persons with severe cognitive impairment were also more likely to have died than to have become program participants.

Hypothetical Scenarios

To illustrate the effects of personal characteristics on the expected placement of persons by subgroups, we derived predicted distributions by combinations of characteristics. We present four hypothetical scenarios (table 9-3). One scenario represents an individual with "strong (informal care) support" and is characterized by living with spouse and by having four or more informal supporters. In contrast to the observed 69 percent (.69) of participants, persons with these characteristics were predicted to have an 88 percent (.88) likelihood of

TABLE 9-3. *Predicted Distributions of Participant and Nonrecipient Groups, by Hypothetical Scenario*[a]

Scenario	Participation	Exceeded cap	Withdrew or refused	Expected institutional placement	Deaths
Observed/unadjusted	.69	.16	.06	.08	.01
Strong support					
Support = 4					
Lives with spouse	.88	.04	.03	.04	.01
Strong need					
Activities of daily living (ADL) = 5					
Mental status quotient (MSQ) < 4					
Incontinent	.44	.38	.04	.09	.05
Strong support and need					
ADL = 5					
Incontinent					
Support = 4					
Lives with spouse	.78	.10	.04	.06	.02
Nursing home risk					
Greater than age 85					
Caregiver neither spouse nor child					
Incontinent					
ADL = 5	.33	.50	.04	.10	.03

Source: Urban Institute analysis of Connecticut Community Care, Inc., data, Connecticut's Consolidated Master Death File, and Connecticut's Nursing Home Inventory.

a. Predicted distributions based on presence of characteristic and all other characteristics held constant.

being a program participant. Correspondingly, the proportion who exceeded the cap was lowered to one-fourth of the observed (.04 versus .16), while the proportion who refused and withdrew, or were expected to be institutional placements, were also reduced below the observed proportions.

Persons with "strong needs" had a much lower predicted proportion of participants (.44) than the observed, with correspondingly higher proportions exceeding cap (.38 versus the observed .16). When both "strong need and support" characteristics were present, persons were slightly more likely to be program participants than the overall average (.78 versus .69). Finally persons with several nursing home risk factors had the smallest proportion participating (.33) and the highest proportion exceeding the program's cost cap (.50 versus .16 for the overall average).

In sum, we found that many people referred to CCCI were quite disabled and did not become participants in Connecticut's home and community-based care program. Living and caregiving arrangements and level of disability had strong, independent effects on the likelihood of program participation. High levels of disability and relatively weak informal care resources characterized persons who did not receive services under this program because they exceeded the program cost cap. The characteristics of persons who were expected to be institutionalized were similar to those of persons exceeding the cost cap. However, persons who refused services or withdrew from the assessment process were more like the participants, who tended to have lower disability levels and stronger informal care situations.

DIFFERENCES IN OUTCOMES

We analyzed data on differences in nursing home admission and deaths between participants and the different categories of persons who did not receive 2176 services. We included in this analysis only persons for whom data were available that enabled us to observe their risk for at least a twelve-month period. Hence, sample sizes in this analysis are slightly different than those in table 9-1. The cumulative percentages, by month after assessment, of nursing home admissions for participants and persons in the other categories are presented in table 9-4. By twelve months after assessment, for example, 22 percent of the participants had been admitted to a nursing home. In contrast, more than twice as many (52 percent) of persons exceeding the program cap and those expected to be institutionalized had been admitted to a nursing home. Persons who withdrew from the assessment process or refused care plans, however, had twelve-month nursing home admission rates that were more comparable to those of participants.

For all groups, the highest incidence of nursing home admission occurred within the first three months of assessment. Some of the persons who were not enrolled in the 2176 program were probably

TABLE 9-4. *Cumulative Percentages, by Month after Assessment, of Nursing Home Admission for Participant and Nonrecipient Groups*

Month after assessment	(1) Participants (n = 3,160)	(2) Exceeded cap (n = 719)	Difference between cols. 1 and 2[a]	(3) Withdrew or refused (n = 279)	Difference between cols. 1 and 3	(4) Expected institutional placement (n = 372)	Difference between cols. 1 and 4[a]
One	3	21	18*	10	7	29	26*
Three	10	42	32*	19	9	42	32*
Six	16	48	32*	24	8	48	32*
Nine	19	51	32*	27	8	51	32*
Twelve	22	52	30*	29	7	52	30*

Source: Urban Institute analysis of Connecticut Community Care, Inc., data and Connecticut's Nursing Home Inventory.

* Significant at the .05 level.

a. Persons who could not be followed for at least twelve months after their assessment for the 2176 program, because of data limitations, were excluded from this analysis.

ready to enter nursing homes but could not do so until they had the CCCI assessment, which served as the preadmission screening required by medicaid. Some people in the "expect institutional placement" category were most likely to be candidates for preadmission screening, and others were in nursing homes when the assessments were conducted. People in the "exceeded cap" category had three-month nursing home admission percentages similar to those in the "expected institutional placement" category; the small first-month difference between the two might have been more attributable to the latter having been in nursing homes at the time of assessment.

For each subgroup, a large number of persons were not admitted to nursing homes by twelve months after assessment by CCCI. Particularly interesting are persons in the "expected institutional" placement category who were in institutional units at the time of the assessment or who expressed desire to be institutionalized after the assessment was completed. It was beyond the scope of this study to determine the reasons behind the unexpected findings, but improvements in functional status or unanticipated increases in availability of home care could have contributed to their not being admitted to nursing homes.

Nursing Home Admission or Death

Cumulative percentages of persons who went to nursing homes or died at various times after the assessment are presented in table 9-5. Among the participants, 41 percent died or went to a nursing home within one year after assessment. In contrast, persons exceeding cap and those expected to be institutionally placed had a 50 percent higher likelihood of experiencing one of these outcomes over a twelve-month period. The experience of persons who withdrew from the assessment process or refused their care plans were similar to participants in terms of their outcomes over a twelve-month period. Overall, the results on nursing home admission and death indicate that many persons who were referred to CCCI for assessment, regardless of whether they enrolled in the 2176 program, were very sick or disabled.

The findings for the subgroups tended to be similar in pattern to those in table 9-4, but the percentages were higher in all cells because of the measurement of the dual outcomes of nursing home admission

TABLE 9-5. *Cumulative Percentages, by Month after Assessment, of Nursing Home Admission or Death, for Participant and Nonrecipient Groups*

Month after assessment	(1) Participants (n = 3,160)	(2) Exceeded cap (n = 719)	Difference between cols. 1 and 2[a]	(3) Withdrew or refused (n = 279)	Difference between cols. 1 and 3	(4) Expected institutional placement (n = 372)	Difference between cols. 1 and 4[a]
One	6	26	20*	12	6	34	28*
Three	17	53	36*	27	10	53	36*
Six	28	62	34*	34	6	60	32*
Nine	35	67	32*	39	4	64	29*
Twelve	41	68	27*	42	1	65	24*

Source: Urban Institute analysis of Connecticut Community Care, Inc., data, Connecticut's Consolidated Master Death File, and Connecticut's Nursing Home Inventory.

*Significant at the .05 level.

a. Persons who could not be followed for at least twelve months after their assessment for the 2176 program, because of data limitations, were excluded from this analysis.

or death. An interesting question raised by the findings in table 9-4 is the whereabouts of the one-third of persons in the exceeded cap and expected institutional placement categories who were neither in nursing homes nor recorded as having died within one year of the assessment. Although some may have received assistance from other medicaid-financed home care programs (for example, home health care), it would be important in future research to determine how all of the people in that subgroup met their long-term care needs while residing in the community.

Effects of Personal Characteristics

To estimate the extent to which the observed differences in outcomes between participants and other subgroups occurred because of differences in the distribution of observed characteristics, we standardized the distributions of characteristics of each group on a regression model predicting the likelihood of admission to a nursing home or death within twelve months of their assessment.[11] The results indicate the extent to which differences in nursing home admission or in death risks between participants and other subgroups may have been due to differences in their personal characteristics.

Results of this standardization indicate that the differences in personal characteristics only partially explained the differences in the observed twelve-month nursing home admission/death risks between participants and persons in those other groups (table 9-6). For example, the observed twelve-month probability of participants (41 percent) was considerably lower than that of people who had exceeded the program cap (68 percent). If the participants possessed the observed characteristics of the people who exceeded the cap, their predicted probability (49 percent) would still be considerably lower than that of the people who had actually exceeded the cap. Similar results are seen in comparisons that use predicted probabilities based on the characteristics of persons expected to be institutionalized. The observed differences between participants and persons who withdrew or refused was small, and the effect of the standardization was not notable.

The findings from this analysis indicate that factors other than those identified in this study differentiate the nursing home admission or death outcomes of participants and persons who did not receive program services because they exceeded program allowable

TABLE 9-6. *Actual and Predicted Probability of Nursing Home Admission or Death over a Twelve-Month Period*

Item	Participants	Exceeded cap	Withdrew or refused	Expected institutional placement
Predicted probability for participants based on characteristics of subgroup[a]	.41	.49	.43	.45
Actual probability of each group	.41	.68	.42	.65

Source: Urban Institute analysis of Connecticut Community Care, Inc., data, Connecticut's Consolidated Master Death File, and Connecticut's Nursing Home Inventory.

a. Mean characteristics of each subgroup were standardized on the logistic regression model of participants predicting nursing home admission or death in twelve months. The model variables and means for subgroups are the same as those in table 9-1.

costs or were expected to be placed in nursing homes. These factors are apparently not simple to identify and were probably not measurable based on data from the assessments used to develop care plans.

In sum, this section presented findings indicating that persons who did not become participants in the 2176 program had higher risks of institutionalization and death than participants in the program. Differences in personal characteristics of the subgroups did not explain most of the differences in outcomes. The particularly high incidence rates of admission to nursing homes in the first three months after assessment suggest that many were on the verge of going to nursing homes and could not be diverted. Although the HCBC program might have delayed institutionalization for some, it is more likely that the assessment process separated people by their predisposition for entering nursing homes.

DISCUSSION

We studied persons who were screened into Connecticut's 2176 waiver program to determine differences in characteristics and outcomes of those who were participants and others who did not become clients of the 2176 program. The findings from this study have implications for proposals to expand home and community-based care.

They also provide insight on the interplay between home and community-based care and nursing home use.

Most proposals focus eligibility on the most severely disabled persons (for example, two or more ADLs or three or more ADLs) who tend to be at high risk of being institutionalized. Most proposed (and existing) programs also include, as a practical matter, some means for controlling program costs. Often this is accomplished by placing a cap on the amount of services that an eligible individual might receive. Our findings indicate that targeting eligibility to the most severely disabled, while containing costs with caps on amount of services allowed, presents a paradox. Despite the goal of most home and community-based care programs to target the most severely disabled, who tend to be at highest risk of entering nursing homes, many of those persons would have service costs that exceed program cost caps and, consequently, were restricted from participating in the 2176 program.

Our findings also showed that regardless of the severity of their disability, persons screened into the Connecticut 2176 program were more likely to become participants of the program if they had relatively strong informal care, in terms of primary caregivers and numbers of informal helpers. The strength of the informal care network functioned, in effect, to limit formal care costs to amounts that did not exceed the program cap.

As in many other states, the amount of the cost cap for the 2176 program in Connecticut is the average nursing home payment rate. The application of Connecticut's cap essentially provides a "level playing field" between community-based and nursing home care. As long as their formal care costs do not exceed the program cost cap, persons meeting income and disability criteria have access to medicaid-funded HCBC or nursing home care. Those who exceed the cap do not have the option of medicaid-financed HCBC. Both groups naturally also have the option of finding some other means to receive community-based care. Findings from our analysis indicate that in the sample of persons screened into the 2176 program each of three avenues was chosen by some individuals.

Despite the apparent lack of choice of persons who exceeded the cost cap, nursing home care may well be the appropriate option for most of them. Individuals whose formal care requirements exceeded nursing home costs tended to have weaker informal care networks, while requiring extensive assistance for dependencies in many ADLs, including nonschedulable ones, such as using the toilet and getting in and out of bed. Such needs are often equivalent to twenty-four hours of supervision, which is extremely costly if, for example, done primarily by formal sources of care.[12] Moreover, such persons are likely to be at high risk of injury or contracting other acute conditions that may require hospitalization or other medical care. Risk of inconstancy in supervision or personal care in home care presents the possibility that, for many persons in this situation, nursing homes may be the most appropriate setting for receiving long-term care.

Finally, because persons not enrolled in the 2176 program were much more likely to use nursing homes or die shortly after assessment, the process of care planning appeared to help define people in terms of who can remain in the community under the cost cap and ADL requirements and others who were more suited to enter nursing homes. The line between home and community-based care and nursing home care, however, may be very fine because substantial nursing home use was found for program participants as well as for each subgroup of persons who did not receive program services. The determination of eligibility and the management of HCBC services seem to require some difficult decisionmaking by case managers. This notion supports the importance of human judgment as a complement to established eligibility and service criteria.

In conclusion, whether some severely disabled persons eligible for the HCBC program can reside in the community or go to a nursing home depends, in part, on the amount of services that programs are able to afford. Theoretically, any disabled person can receive sufficient community-based services in order to remain in the community. For some, however, the costs can be substantial. An important question regarding future developments in HCBC programs is how much society is willing to pay for the very costly individuals when, given fiscal realities and limitations in informal care, nursing home care may be the less costly (and perhaps higher quality-of-care) solution for many of them.

NOTES

1. Melvina Ford and others, "Summary Comparison of Major Health Care Reform Bills," *CRS Report for Congress,* 94-71 EPW (Washington: Congressional Research Service, 1994).

2. Department of Health and Human Services, Office of the Assistant Secretary for Planning and Evaluation, *Cost Estimates for the Long-Term Care Provisions under the Health Security Act* (March 1994).

3. Korbin Liu and Kenneth G. Manton, "Changes in Home Care Use by Disabled Elderly Persons: 1982–1989," *CRS Report for Congress*, 94-398 EPW (Washington: Congressional Research Service, 1994).

4. Department of Health and Human Services, *Cost Estimates for the Long-Term Care Provisions.*

5. Teresa A. Coughlin, Leighton Ku, and John Holahan, *Medicaid since 1980: Costs, Coverage, and the Shifting Alliance between the Federal Government and the States* (Washington: Urban Institute Press, 1994).

6. There are several important waiver authorities including the 1915(e) waiver for "boarder babies," the 1915(c) model waivers and the 1115(a) waiver. Here we limit our discussion to the 1915(c) waiver program.

7. The other main waiver authority is referred to as the "1915(d) waiver program." Unlike the 1915(c) program, the 1915(d) program is targeted expressly to elderly persons who are at risk of institutional placement. At present, Oregon is the only state that has implemented a 1915(d) waiver program.

8. Donna Folkemer, "State Use of Home and Community-Based Services for the Aged under Medicaid: Waiver Programs, Personal Care, Frail Elderly Services and Home Health Services," Working Paper 9405 (Washington: American Association of Retired Persons, 1994).

9. Diane Justice, "Case Management Standards in State Community-Based Long-term Care Programs for Older Persons with Disabilities," *CRS Report for Congress*, 94-419 EPW (Washington: Congressional Research Service, 1993).

10. Gujarati Damodar, *Basic Econometrics* (McGraw-Hill, 1988); and Alfred Demaris, "Logit Modeling: Practical Applications," Sage University Paper Series on Quantitative Applications in the Social Sciences, 07-86 (Newbury Park, Calif.: Sage Publications, 1992).

11. For each subgroup, we multiplied the means for each variable (table 9-1) against the corresponding coefficient in a logistic regression model predicting nursing home/death risks of participants. The sum of the products was exponentiated to obtain odds, which were subsequently converted to predicted probabilities.

12. For example, the cost of twenty-four-hour assistance from home health aides in Connecticut is estimated at approximately $100,000 a year.

Chapter 10

SHARON K. LONG

Combining Formal and Informal Care in Serving Frail Elderly People

Home and community-based care programs seek to delay or eliminate the need for nursing home care by providing services in the community to individuals at high risk of institutionalization. Most home care is provided informally (unpaid) by family and friends; it is—to the public—an inexpensive part of the support system that allows elderly persons to remain in the community. Community-based formal (paid) care is intended to reduce nursing home admissions both by providing services to the elderly individual and by easing the burden of caregiving on the individual's informal caregivers. Although some level of displacement is intended, community care could be very expensive if it substituted for substantial shares of existing informal care.

Designing policies that meet the needs of elderly persons in the community in the face of limited public resources requires a better understanding of the use of formal and informal care. The available research provides mixed evidence that formal care is a substitute for informal care. With the exception of a single study, early work found little, if any, displacement of informal care by formal care.[1] However, many studies relied on small sample sizes or limited measures of caregiving, such as number of types of care or number of visits, instead of hours of care.[2] More recent work provides greater evidence that formal care offsets some informal care, although, again, the measures of caregiving were limited.[3]

In this chapter I examine the relationship between formal and informal care for a sample of low-income frail elderly persons who enrolled in a community-based care management program in Connecticut. Although not representative of the broader elderly population, information from this study could provide insights that have implications for similar programs targeted to low-income elderly populations at risk of institutionalization. However, different program objectives, eligibility criteria, or cost-containment procedures could produce different outcomes from those reported here. Like much of the earlier research, the cross-sectional data used in this study permit an assessment of the tradeoffs between formal and informal care, not of the change in informal care as a result of the introduction of formal care services.[4] This study extends previous research by including a measure of the price of formal care, measuring hours of informal and formal care, and using a sample of more than 4,000 disabled elderly individuals.

ANALYSIS SAMPLE

Connecticut Community Care, Inc. (CCCI), is a statewide, private, nonprofit organization that provides assessment and case management services and coordinates health and social services that allow dependent persons to remain in the community. During the period covered by this study (1990–92), CCCI administered two major public programs targeted to low-income frail elderly persons at risk of institutionalization: the Promotion of Independent Living Program and the Preadmission Screening and Community Based Services Program (PAS/CBS), Connecticut's medicaid 2176 waiver program. Under both programs, clients contributed toward the cost of their care. In 1992 the two programs were merged into the newly named Connecticut Home Care Program for Elders.

The publicly funded programs administered by CCCI aimed to substitute home and community-based care for nursing home care. Under the combined program, assistance was available to medicaid recipients and those who would become medicaid recipients within 180 days after being admitted into a nursing facility. To qualify, an elderly person had to meet the income and asset limits for an institutionalized medicaid applicant and to incur costs for community-based care below certain thresholds: (1) the costs for social services (such as adult day care, homemaker, companionship, chores, meals, counseling, and financial management) could not exceed 60 percent of the weighted average rate for nursing home care; and (2) the total cost of the plan for care (medical plus social services) could not exceed the state's cost of nursing home care (approximately $3,000 per month). These cost-containment procedures acted to restrict participation in the program mostly to individuals with strong informal care networks (which reduced the need for and, thus, cost of formal care). As reported by Korbin Liu, Jean Hanson, and Teresa Coughlin in chapter 9, individuals with severe disabilities who required extensive assistance generally exceeded nursing home costs, unless they had very strong informal care networks.

If the needs of the potential client could not be met within the cost caps, the individual was not enrolled in the program and instead was assisted with nursing home placement. For such individuals, institutional care would be less costly than community-based care. Individuals who met the cost caps were offered the choice of community-based care or assistance with nursing home placement, because some applicants were seeking a required preadmission screening for nursing home admission. The analysis in this chapter was restricted to those who entered the community-based care program.

The sample of elderly persons who applied to and were admitted into the program was not representative of the elderly population in general. In particular, those who sought a care management program likely had care arrangements that were under stress. Those accepted into the program had to meet the program's cost-containment requirements, which was less likely for someone with greater disability and a more fragile informal care network. The program served a relatively narrow subset of the community-based frail elderly population, as it targeted benefits to those who were most disabled yet could be affordably served within the community. The relationship between formal and informal care within this population was of policy interest, having relevance for other home and community-based care programs geared to such populations. Relative to the characteristics of the broader population of home health and hospice patients in the United States, as indicated in the 1992 National Home and Hospice Care Survey, the sample for this study was older (age 80 versus age 70), more likely to be female (77 versus 67 percent), less likely to be married (19 versus 33 percent) or never married (7 versus 12 percent), and somewhat more impaired (1.8 versus 1.7 activities of daily living [ADLs] that required assistance).

DATA

The key element of CCCI care management was the assessment, which was used to identify the needs of the elderly individual, determine who could best meet those needs (family, friends, or formal caregivers), and determine whether the impaired person should remain at home or move to more appropriate surroundings. The assessment included information on demographic and social characteristics, functional and health status, sources of informal care, and financial status.

For those who remained in the community, a case manager developed a care plan in consultation with the elderly individual, the family, and others involved in the person's care. The care plan provided a comprehensive inventory of all sources of formal and informal caregiving available to the individual. At least every thirty days the client was contacted by the case manager and the care plan was reviewed; at a minimum of every six months a reassessment was completed, with the care plan changed as needed. The care plan included information on the frequency, number of hours, and types of formal and informal care, such as adult day care, bath aide, chores, companion, homemaker, supervision, medications, home health aide, nursing services, skilled therapies, respite care, emergency response systems, and transportation.

This study used both the initial assessment and initial care plan data for individuals age 65 or older who entered CCCI between January 1990 and December 1992. Because entry into CCCI was likely to have been precipitated by a change in the client's circumstances, the relationship between formal and informal care was examined five months after admittance to the program.[5] The formal and informal care arrangements that were analyzed in this chapter reflected those developed by the CCCI case manager through discussions with the elderly individual and her or his informal care network. The case manager took into consideration the availability, willingness, and ability of potential informal caregivers in developing a care plan to meet the needs of the elderly individual within the cost constraints of the program.

An important issue that arose in using these data was the possibility of misreporting of informal care. First, estimating the number of hours spent in informal care, especially for those living with the elderly individual, can be very difficult for the caregivers. Second, because formal care was paid for, the number of hours spent likely were recorded with a high level of accuracy by the case manager, while informal caregiving hours, for which no payment was made, might not have been recorded as carefully. For example, if the family provided care in excess of that agreed to under the care plan, that information would not be captured in the data recorded by the case manager.

Measures of informal caregiving in the CCCI assessment (which sought information from the elderly individual on her or his informal caregivers) and the case manager's care plan were roughly consistent. Nevertheless, the hours of informal care recorded by the case manager were likely subject to measurement error.[6] To the extent that those errors in measurement were correlated with the variables in the model, the estimates obtained were biased.

CONCEPTUAL MODEL

The analysis relied on a simple conceptual model of caregiving that assumed that the two sources of care—formal and informal—were determined jointly. Informal care was assumed to influence the level of formal care, and formal care was assumed to influence the level of informal care. In the simplest framework, a system of two equations emerged:

$$F = a_F I + X_F' B_F + e_F \qquad (1)$$

$$I = a_I F + X_I' B_I + e_I \qquad (2)$$

F is hours of formal care; I, hours of informal care; X, vectors of explanatory variables (for example, need for care, the price and availability of care, income, and sociodemographic characteristics); a and B, coefficients to be estimated; and e, error terms.

Displacement of informal by formal care would imply that, in equation (2), the amount of informal care (I) would fall as the amount of formal care (F) increased, corresponding to the coefficient a_I less than 0. In contrast, a finding of a_I greater than or equal to 0 would imply supplementation of care; an increase in formal care would not be offset by a reduction in informal care. As a result, the total level of assistance provided to the elderly person would rise, or be supplemented, by the full increase in formal care.

The conceptual model is a fully simultaneous model in which the endogenous variables—formal and informal care—appear as explanatory variables as well.[7] Two issues must be addressed in estimating this model. First, a simultaneous equations estimator must be used because ordinary least squares estimates are inconsistent in the presence of endogenous explanatory variables. Second, the estimation approach must incorporate the censoring of the dependent variables—hours of care were observed only for those who received the particular type of care. In the sample for this paper, 78 percent of the elderly individuals received informal care, while 94 percent received formal care.[8]

To address these issues, a simultaneous equations estimator based on two-stage least squares was used.[9] Because of the censoring of hours of informal care, the equation for informal care was estimated using a simultaneous equations estimator—instrumental variables—within a censored regression or tobit model. The formal care equation was estimated using instrumental variables and ordinary least squares because that variable was subject to relatively little censoring. This two-stage estimation framework provided consistent estimates of the parameters of the formal and informal care equations.[10]

One drawback of the estimation framework was the possibility of high intercorrelation or multicollinearity between the instrumental variables and the explanatory variables in the model, because the instrumental variables were constructed from regressions on all of the explanatory variables included in the model. High levels of multicollinearity would result in imprecise estimates of the parameters because of the large variances of the estimators.

An alternative approach to the direct estimation of the structural model was to estimate the reduced form of the simultaneous model. That framework, which specified the endogenous variables as functions of only exogenous or independent variables, did not require identification of the model and, because no endogenous variables were on the right-hand side of the equations, was more straightforward to estimate than the simultaneous equations model. In addition, the estimation of the model was not subject to the impacts of multicollinearity that could arise in estimating a two-stage model. The reduced-form estimates for the model also provided an indication of the consistency of the findings from the two-state model.

MODEL SPECIFICATION

The levels of formal and informal care depended on the individual's health status and need for care, the price and availability of care, income, and sociodemographic characteristics. Numerous variables were included in the models (table 10-1).[11]

Informal and formal care were measured as the number of hours of care provided over a month. The care measures included home health aides, personal and bath aides, help with chores, homemakers, supervision, socialization, adult day care, and respite care. Skilled medical care—skilled nursing; skilled physical, speech, and occupational therapy; and counseling—was excluded because CCCI did not record the number of hours of care for those services and because the reduction in informal care associated with an increase in less-skilled formal care arguably was of most concern from a policy prospective. Replacing informal medical care with formal skilled medical care was likely to be a desirable outcome and was consistent with current public programs. Medicare and medicaid generally covered medical care (including home health aides), but not personal care services and supportive services.

The hours of care variables were in log form to adjust for the skewed nature of the distribution—a small share of cases received high levels of care.[12] The mean hours of care of the logged variables corresponded to 51.4 hours per month of formal care and 25.3 hours of informal care.

Skilled medical care was included as a predetermined variable in the model under the assumption that a sequential decisionmaking process was followed in caregiving. That is, a decision was made on skilled medical care first, then on the sources of other care. The level of skilled medical care received by the elderly person was taken as given in the decision on informal and formal care for other types of care.[13] Skilled medical care was measured as the log of the number of visits for skilled nursing, skilled therapy, and counseling over the month. For this sample, the mean of the logged variable corresponded to 1.8 visits per month.

Health status was measured as the number of limitations in ADLs and instrumental activities of daily living (IADLs). The ADLs included getting in and out of bed, bathing, dressing, using the toilet, and eating; the IADLs, housework, medications, meal preparation,

TABLE 10-1. *Definitions and Means for Variables Included in the Models*

Explanatory variable	Empirical measure	Variable name	Informal care	Formal care	Mean (standard deviation)
			Included in the equation		
Endogenous variables	Log of hours of informal care per month (nonpaid care provided by family, friends, and others)	Log hours of informal care		X	3.23[a] (2.19)
	Log of hours of formal care per month (paid care provided by contracted provider)	Log hours of formal care	X		3.94[a] (1.47)
Skilled medical care	Log number of skilled medical care visits for skilled nursing, skilled therapy, and counseling	Log skilled medical care visits	X	X	1.02 (1.16)
Health status	Number of activities of daily living (ADLs)— transferring, bathing, dressing, toileting, and eating— with which had difficulties	ADL scale	X	X	1.81 (1.48)
	Number of instrumental activities of daily living (IADLs)—housework, medications, meals, money management, telephoning, and shopping—with which had difficulties	IADL scale	X	X	4.30 (1.37)
Price of care	Log of average cost per hour for homemaker visits[b]	Log price of formal care		X	2.57 (0.02)
	On medicaid (1 = yes, 0 = no)	On medicaid		X	0.40 (0.49)
Availability of care	Married (1 = yes, 0 = no)	Now married	X		0.19 (0.40)
	Never married (1 = yes, 0 = no)	Never married	X		0.07 (0.25)

TABLE 10-1. *(continued)*

Income and wealth	Annual income greater than $10,000 (1 = yes, 0 = no)	Income > $10,000	X	X	0.17 (0.38)	
Recent life changes	Major life change associated with illness in past year (1 = yes, 0 = no)	Major illness	X	X	0.60 (0.49)	
	Major life change associated with the death of relative or significant other, family discord or trouble, marital status, or financial status in past year (1 = yes, 0 = no)	Major life change	X	X	0.36 (0.48)	
Individual characteristics	Age (years)	Age	X	X	79.59 (6.76)	
	African American or Hispanic (1 = yes, 0 = no)	Minority	X	X	0.14 (0.34)	
	Female (1 = yes, 0 = no)	Female	X	X	0.77 (0.42)	
	Region of state— northwest, southwest, south central, eastern, and north central (1 = yes, 0 = no)[c]	Region A Region B Region C Region D Region E	X	X	0.18 0.22 0.16 0.21 0.23	

Source: Urban Institute analysis of Connecticut Community Care, Inc., data.
N = 4,068.
a. Mean log hours of informal care corresponded to 25.3 hours of care; mean log hours of formal care corresponded to 51.4 hours of care.
b. The price of formal care for the individual was proxied as the average price of care paid to providers of homemaker services by Connecticut Community Care, Inc.
c. The northwest region was Waterbury, Danbury, and Winsted; southwest, Norwalk, Bridgeport, and Stamford; south central, New Haven, Derby, and Orange; eastern, Norwich, Putnam, and New London; and north central, Hartford, West Hartford, New Britain, and Enfield.

money management, telephoning, and shopping. Individuals with greater limitations on ADLs and IADLs likely had increased use of both formal and informal care. Individuals within the sample needed help with an average of 1.8 (of 5) ADLs and 4.3 (of 6) IADLs.

A critical issue in the estimation of a system of simultaneous equations is the identification of the equations. One or more exogenous variables must distinguish a particular equation from the other equations in the system to estimate the parameters of that equation. For this analysis, the identifying variables were those associated with the price and availability of care. Thus the price of formal care had a direct impact on the use of formal care and affected informal care hours via the level of formal care. Participation in the medicaid waiver program was expected to reduce the price of formal care because benefits were more comprehensive than those available through either private insurance or medicare.

Price of formal care was proxied as the average price paid to providers of homemaker services by CCCI five months after the date of the individual's enrollment in CCCI. The price paid to providers reflected the price paid by CCCI and was not necessarily the price paid by a particular elderly individual. I did not have information on the cost borne by each elderly individual (which would vary depending on whether home health care was subsidized and, if subsidized, the form of that subsidy—for example, public program or private insurance) or on the elderly individual's actual out-of-pocket expenditures.[14] All individuals contributed to the cost of the program. The price of formal care was about $13 an hour on average for the sample. Forty percent of the sample was on medicaid at the time of enrollment into CCCI.

In a similar manner, the availability, or price, of informal care was assumed to have a direct impact on hours of informal care, while affecting formal care only indirectly via the level of informal care. The two most common proxies used in the literature for the potential supply of informal caregivers were marital status and the number of children. In this chapter, the availability of informal care was measured by two dummy variables indicating that the elderly person (1) had never married (as a proxy of whether the individual had children) or (2) was currently married. Those who had never married (7 percent of the sample) were expected to have fewer potential informal caregivers (as they were less likely to have children), while those who were married (19 percent of the sample) had at least one potential informal caregiver—their spouse. The omitted category consisted of widowed, divorced, and separated individuals.

A preferred specification of the model would have included a direct measure of the number and characteristics of the elderly individual's children, as children are an important source of informal caregiving. Although CCCI's database had information on who provided care for the elderly individuals (including their children), it did not have information on the composition of the elderly individual's family. As a result, whether the individual had children could not be directly controlled, so only a rough proxy for a key explanatory variable—the price of informal care—was used.[15]

Direct measures of living arrangements were not included because evidence existed that living arrangements were endogenous to the caregiving decision—the elderly person could move in with caregivers or the caregivers could move in with the elderly person to facilitate caregiving arrangements. Earlier research suggested that living arrangements were a key component of caregiving arrangements, with decisions on living arrangements and caregiving determined simultaneously.[16] While the CCCI data provided information on current living arrangements, I did not have information on the individual's living arrangement options (particularly, whether they had children with whom they could live). Thus I could not analyze the simultaneous choice of living arrangement and caregiving arrangements.

Information on income from the CCCI database was limited to categorical measures. As a result, income was measured in the model using a categorical variable indicating that the individual had annual income greater than $10,000. Seventeen percent of the sample fell in this category.

Because the sample was made up of elderly individuals who applied for and had been accepted into a care management program, two variables were included in the model as controls for recent changes in circumstances that could cause care arrangements to be in flux: (1) a dummy variable indicating that the individual had a major illness over the past year and (2) a dummy variable indicating that the individual experienced a major life change associated with the death of a relative or significant other, family discord, marital status, or financial status over the past year. Sixty percent of the sample had a major illness and 36 percent another major life change over the preceding year. About 70 percent of the sample had either a major illness or other major life crisis over the past year.

Age, race, ethnicity, and gender were included to control for tastes and preferences. Age also provided an additional measure of disability, as frailty tended to increase with age. Not surprisingly, the sample members were older (age 80 on average) and female (77 percent). Relatively few of the sample members were either African American or Hispanic (14 percent).

A series of dummy variables for region within the state (northwest, southwest, south central, eastern, and north central) were included to control for area characteristics that could affect caregiving, such as the availability of formal care providers.

RELATIONSHIP BETWEEN FORMAL AND INFORMAL CARE

In the sample of low-income, frail elderly persons enrolled in a community-based care program, a statistically significant displacement of informal care by formal care took place, although the magnitude of offset was not large (table 10-2). The coefficient on the log of hours of formal care (–0.54) implied that a 10 percent increase in hours of formal care would be accompanied by an 5.4 percent decline in hours of informal care.[17] For an individual receiving the average levels of formal and informal care, an increase in formal care of two hours would result in a reduction of about one-half hour of informal care.

The reduced-form estimates provided additional support for some displacement of informal care by formal care (table 10-3). To understand the relationship between formal and informal care, the coefficient on the price of formal care in the informal care equation is of most interest. If formal care displaced informal care, the use of informal care should increase with the price of formal care. The coefficient on the price of formal care was 11.2 and was statistically significant. The reduced-form model, like the simultaneous equations model, provided evidence of informal care dropping with the falling price of formal care.

Regarding the relationship of formal and informal care among those with greater levels of disability, an increase in formal care was associated with an increase in informal care for the most impaired elderly persons (those with three or more ADL limitations). According to these estimates (table 10-4), a 10 percent increase in formal care implied about a 5 percent increase in informal care. In contrast, for the less impaired elderly individuals in the sample, a 10 percent increase

TABLE 10-2. *Two-Stage Least Squares Estimation Results*

	Equation	
Explanatory variable	Informal care (standard error)	Formal care (standard error)
Log hours of care		
Formal	−0.539[b]	—
	(0.222)	
Informal	—	−0.359[b]
		(0.154)
Constant	0.789	−4.585
	(0.653)	(6.208)
Log skilled medical care visits	0.110[b]	0.228[a]
	(0.046)	(0.032)
Activities of daily living (ADL)		
scale	0.286[a]	0.259[a]
	(0.058)	(0.040)
Instrumental activities of daily		
living (IADL) scale	0.618[a]	0.427[a]
	(0.116)	(0.083)
Now married	0.291[c]	—
	(0.175)	
Never married	−0.499[b]	—
	(0.233)	
Log price of formal care	—	2.505
		(2.417)
On medicaid	—	0.284[a]
		(0.095)
Income > $10,000	−0.031	0.219[a]
	(0.141)	(0.998)
Major illness	−0.146	−0.134[c]
	(0.110)	(0.074)
Major life change	0.229[c]	0.486
	(0.120)	(0.080)
Age	0.008	0.003
	(0.008)	(0.005)
Minority	0.085	0.027
	(0.152)	(0.105)
Female	0.187	0.169[b]
	(0.135)	(0.084)
Region A	−0.347[c]	0.161
	(0.200)	(0.135)
Region B	0.751[a]	0.296[b]
	(0.221)	(0.148)

TABLE 10-2. *(continued)*

Region C	$(0.328)^c$	−0.044
	(0.191)	(0.131)
Region D	0.020	0.264^b
	(0.158)	(0.106)
Likelihood ratio test		
(degrees of freedom)	1,147.56 (16)	1,215.86 (16)
Mean of dependent variable	3.23	3.94

Source: Urban Institute analysis of Connecticut Community Care, Inc., data.
N = 4,068.
a. Significant at the .01 level.
b. Significant at the .05 level.
c. Significant at the .10 level.

TABLE 10-3. *Reduced-Form Model Estimation Results*

	Equation	
Explanatory variable	Informal care (standard error)	Formal care (standard error)
Constant	-28.954^a	5.684^b
	(5.151)	(2.591)
Log skilled medical care visits	−0.039	0.240^a
	(0.037)	(0.019)
Activities of daily living (ADL) scale	0.165^a	0.203^a
	(0.034)	(0.017)
Instrumental activities of daily living (IADL) scale	0.484^a	0.256^a
	(0.037)	(0.019)
Now married	0.445^a	-0.278^a
	(0.112)	(0.057)
Never married	-0.530^a	−0.005
	(0.162)	(0.081)
Log price of formal care	11.181^a	−1.406
	(2.009)	(1.010)
On medicaid	-0.271^a	0.373^a
	(0.095)	(0.048)
Income > $10,000	-0.185^c	0.287^a
	(0.112)	(0.056)
Major illness	−0.077	-0.106^b
	(0.085)	(0.043)

TABLE 10-3. *(continued)*

Major life change	0.201[b]	−0.025
	(0.085)	(0.043)
Age	0.008	−0.010
	(0.006)	(0.003)
Minority	0.040	0.006
	(0.123)	(0.062)
Female	0.135	0.081
	(0.104)	(0.052)
Region A	−0.497[a]	0.334[a]
	(0.129)	(0.064)
Region B	0.724[a]	0.033
	(0.117)	(0.060)
Region C	0.431[a]	−0.200[a]
	(0.129)	(0.066)
Region D	−0.100	0.296[a]
	(0.122)	(0.061)
Likelihood ratio test		
(degrees of freedom)	1,175.32 (17)	1,224.79 (17)
Mean of dependent variable	3.23	3.94

Source: Urban Institute analysis of Connecticut Community Care, Inc., data.
N = 4,068.
a. Significant at the .01 level.
b. Significant at the .05 level.
c. Significant at the .10 level.

in formal care would result in a 9 percent reduction in informal care. For the most impaired elderly persons, formal care supplemented informal care. Given the cap on program expenditures under the medicaid waiver program, this finding suggested that those with high ADL limitations (and, most likely, a high level of need for services) must have a strong informal caregiving network to be able to stay within the program cap and remain in the community. For individuals with high ADLs who did not have a strong informal caregiving network, the costs of formal care to meet their needs were more likely to put them over the expenditure cap and result in a nursing home entry (and exclusion from the database used in this study). Thus the individuals with high ADLs included in this sample were a subset of the most disabled elderly persons.

TABLE 10-4. *Estimated Elasticities of Substitution by Disability Status*

Disability status	Estimated elasticity of substitution of formal for informal care
Number of activity of daily living (ADL) limitations per individual	
Less than three	−0.86[a]
Three or more	0.51[b]

a. Significant at the .01 level.
b. Significant at the .05 level.

OTHER FINDINGS

In presenting the other findings of the model, I focus on the results from the simultaneous equations model (table 10-2).

Health Status. Not surprisingly, poor health—as measured by the number of limitations on ADLs and IADLs—was a significant determinant of hours of both informal and formal care. Both informal and formal care increased with disability.

Informal and formal care also increased with the level of skilled medical care received by the elderly individual. The need for skilled medical care was an additional indicator of disability.

Availability of Informal Caregivers. As expected, the greater availability of informal caregivers, as proxied by the marital status dummy variables, had a significant relationship with hours of informal care. An individual who had never married (and, presumably, had fewer potential caregivers) received less informal care, while a married individual (whose spouse was a possible caregiver) received more informal care.

Price of Formal Care. Given the possibility of formal caregiving as a replacement for informal care, individuals were expected to be responsive to changes in the price of formal care. To the contrary, the coefficient on price in the formal care equation was positive, although not statistically significant. Because the variable for medicaid participation (an indicator of a lower price for care) was statistically significant, the coefficient on price of care could be a reflection of the poor quality of the proxy for the price of care. The price data reflected the average price paid to providers of homemaker services in the market and not necessarily the cost to the elderly individual. The coefficient on price of care in the formal care equation was negative, although not statistically significant, in the reduced-form model. Medicaid participation, which reduced the cost of formal care, was associated with significantly higher levels of formal care.

Income. As economic theory would predict, demand for formal care was higher for those with higher income, suggesting that formal care is a normal good—more formal care is purchased as income increased.

Recent Life Changes. A major illness over the past year was associated with significantly lower levels of formal care, while other major life changes were associated with significantly higher levels of informal care. The negative relationship between a major illness and formal care usage could reflect the CCCI cap on spending for formal care, in that such individuals were likely to be receiving high levels of skilled formal care (and, thus, could not also receive high levels of other formal care and remain in the program). Overall, these findings suggested that changes in individual circumstances before CCCI program entry had significant impacts on caregiving arrangements under the program.

SUMMARY

In this chapter I have examined the relationship between formal and informal care for a sample of low-income frail elderly persons who enrolled in a community-based care management program. Although not generalizable to the broader elderly population, the findings could be useful to policymaking because of their relevance to programs targeting similar populations at risk of institutionalization. For this population, I estimated statistically significant displacement of informal care by formal care, although the magnitude of that displacement was not large. For an individual receiving the average levels of formal and informal care, an estimated increase in formal care of two hours would result in a reduction of about one-half hour in informal care. Thus, even with the offset in informal care, the total quantity of care provided to the average individual would increase, or be supplemented, by one and one-half hours. In this case, 75 percent of the increase in formal care hours supplemented the average individual's total quantity of care, while 25 percent displaced informal care.

The supplementation of the individual's total quantity of care, in conjunction with some displacement of informal care, was consistent with a home and community-based care program that provided assistance both to address the unmet needs of disabled elderly persons and to reduce the caregiving burden on informal caregivers. Under such a program, a partial offset in informal care in combination with an increase in formal care was an intended outcome. Given that disabled elderly persons studied here applied for a case management program (presumably, in part, because their informal caregiving network was under stress), the estimated displacement in informal care was not large relative to the increase in formal care (and the associated increase in the total quantity of care).

Several limitations to this study suggested that the findings should be interpreted conservatively. First, the care plan data represented the care arrangements reported by the case manager. Those data could underrepresent the levels of care provided by the informal care network.

Second, caregiving arrangements are made by the elderly individual, his or her informal caregiving network, and, for a CCCI enrollee, the case manager. Because only limited information was available on the potential network of caregivers from the CCCI data, the model of informal caregiving did not include all of the variables that were likely to have an important role in the decisionmaking process, most notably, the number and characteristics of the elderly individual's children.

Third, the caregiving arrangements for the sample of frail elderly persons likely were in flux because they had recently chosen to enroll in a care management program. As a result, the cross-sectional analysis reported here might not reflect the long-term relationship between formal and informal care. Given the improvements in the data entry procedures since CCCI began its data collection effort, the follow-up care plan data collected by CCCI could be used to examine the stability of the informal and formal caregiving relationship over time.

Finally, I have examined the use of informal and formal care by elderly individuals within the community, taking their living arrangements as given. Although the estimation issues are complex, an analysis of the joint decisions on caregiving and living arrangements (including nursing home entry) is needed.[18]

NOTES

1. Evidence that formal care was a substitute for informal care was found by Vernon L. Greene, "Substitution between Formally and Informally Provided Care for the Impaired Elderly in the Community," *Medical Care*, vol. 21, no. 6 (June 1983), pp. 609–19. Studies finding little or no displacement included Amanda Smith-Barusch and Leonard S. Miller, "The Effect of Services on Family Assistance to the Frail Elderly," *Journal of Social Services Research*, vol. 9, no. 1 (Fall 1985), pp. 31–46; Jon B. Christianson, "The Effect of Channeling on Informal Caregiving," *Health Services Research*, vol. 3, no. 1 (April 1988), pp. 99–117; Ira Moscovice, Gestur Davidson, and David McCaffrey, "Substitution of Formal and Informal Care for the Community-Based Elderly," *Medical Care*, vol. 26, no. 10 (October 1988), pp. 971–81; Perry Edelman and Susan Hughes, "The Impact of Community Care on Provision of Informal Care to Homebound Elderly Persons," *Journal of Gerontology:Social Sciences*, vol. 45, no. 2 (March 1990), pp. S74–S84; and Raymond J. Hanley, Joshua M. Wiener, and Katherine M. Harris, "Will Paid Home Care Erode Informal Support?," *Journal of Health Politics, Policy, and Law*, vol. 16, no. 3 (Fall 1991), pp. 507–21.

2. For example, Greene, "Substitution between Formally and Informally Provided Care for the Impaired Elderly in the Community"; Moscovice, Davidson, and McCaffrey, "Substitution of Formal and Informal Care for the Community-Based Elderly"; Edelman and Hughes, "The Impact of Community Care on Provision of Informal Care to Homebound Elderly Persons"; Smith-Barusch and Miller, "The Effect of Services on Family Assistance to the Frail Elderly"; and Hanley, Wiener, and Harris, "Will Paid Home Care Erode Informal Support?"

3. More recent work providing evidence that formal care displaced some informal care included Sharon L. Tennstedt, Sybil L. Crawford, and John B. McKinlay, "Is Family Care on the Decline? A Longitudinal Investigation of the Substitution of Formal Long-Term Care Services for Informal Care," *Milbank Quarterly*, vol. 71, no. 4 (1993), pp. 601–24; and Susan L. Ettner, "The Effect of the Medicaid Home Care Benefit on Long-Term Care Choices of the Elderly," *Economic Inquiry*, vol. 32 (January 1994), pp. 103–27. The paper by Tennstedt, Crawford, and McKinlay focused on a limited set of types of care,

264 : Formal and Informal Care in Serving Frail Elderly People

not the full array of caregiving activities. Ettner used the number of caregiving "activity-days" received per week.

4. An exception to the use of cross-sectional data was Tennstedt, Crawford, and McKinlay, "Is Family Care on the Decline?," in which data collected periodically from 1984 to 1991 were used to examine the prevalence of substitution over time. Rates of substitution of formal for informal care of 14 to 20 percent were estimated over the period.

5. The data for this study were available from a newly automated database developed by Connecticut Community Care, Inc. (CCCI). Because of some confusion about the data to be included in that file, case managers in some CCCI offices did not add updated care plan data to the file for some periods. When the missing data were discovered, CCCI took steps to reconstruct the missing data for those still active in the program in 1993. Because of high levels of missing updated care plan data for the study sample, this study focused on the period immediately following admission to the program. An attempt to focus on those CCCI regions with good follow-up data resulted in very small sample sizes for the analysis.

6. Comparing these figures with the Channeling experiment, a ten-site test of public financing of home care as a substitute for nursing home care, I found that, on average, my sample had higher levels of formal care use (51.4 versus 31.4 hours per month) and much lower levels of informal care use (25.3 versus 167.3 hours per month). These differences reflected variations in the populations studied and the data collection methods. Although similar in several respects to the sample of this chapter, the Channeling sample was more likely to be married and male and tended to be substantially more disabled. These differences suggested both greater need for care and more potential informal caregivers for the elderly persons in that sample. The data used in the Channeling experiment were obtained from interviews with the disabled elderly person (or proxy) and the primary informal caregiver. In contrast, this study relied on information recorded in the care plan by the case manager. The level of informal care recorded by the case manager, like that reported by the caregivers themselves, was subject to measurement error. For a description of the Channeling experiment, see Peter Kemper and others, "The Evaluation of the National Long-Term Care Demonstration," *Health Services Research*, vol. 23, no. 1 (April 1988), pp. 1–174.

7. For a discussion of simultaneous equations models, see William H. Greene, *Econometric Analysis* (Macmillan, 1990), pp. 591–660.

8. The care measure used here excluded skilled medical care, such as skilled nursing; skilled occupational, physical, and speech therapies; and counseling.

9. The method used was developed in Forrest Nelson and Lawrence Olson, "Specification and Estimation of a Simultaneous Equation Model with Limited Dependent Variables," *International Economic Review*, vol. 19 (1978), pp. 695–710.

10. The estimation approach was described in William H. Greene, *LIMDEP: User's Manual and Reference Guide* (Bellport, N.Y.: Econometric Software, 1993), pp. 636–37. The two-step procedure for estimating the parameters of the model was as follows. Step 1: Estimate the reduced-form for formal care by ordinary least squares and the reduced-form for informal care by tobit regression. Compute the predicted values for formal and informal care to be used as instrumental variables. Step 2: Estimate the structural equations using the predicted values. Again, the formal care equation was estimated by ordinary least squares, and the informal care equation via tobit regression. Compute the correct standard errors based on the asymptotic covariance of the estimates.

11. Individuals who were in the hospital, in a long-term care facility, or comatose at the month of analysis were excluded from the study. Individuals who were discharged from the program were also excluded, as were those with missing or bad data. The bad or missing data exclusion reduced the sample by 3.4 percent.

12. For example, some elderly individuals in the sample received twenty-four-hour supervision. Because the log of zero is not defined, the hours of care measure was increased by 1 to permit the taking of logs.

13. Alternatively, it can be argued that the provision of skilled medical care was not independent of the provision of unskilled care. Medical personnel could assist with nonmedical needs or unskilled caregivers could identify a need for skilled care. Under that model, care of elderly persons was the joint product of skilled and unskilled care from both informal and formal sources.

14. Under all programs administered by CCCI, clients contributed toward the cost of their care. For those with limited out-of-pocket costs for formal care, the price of formal care would be a factor in determining whether their care exceeded the program's cost cap and, therefore, whether they were ineligible for the assistance.

15. The CCCI assessment did collect information from the elderly individuals on how often they saw their children. A constructed variable that assumed that the "don't know" and "not applicable" responses to that question indicated individuals who did not have children yielded similar results to the model presented here. The "never married" variable was preferred as a proxy for individuals who did not have children because missing responses to the question underlying the constructed measure likely were correlated with receipt of assistance from children.

16. See, for example, Beth J. Soldo, Douglas A. Wolf, and Emily M. Agree, "Family, Households, and Care Arrangements of Frail Old Women: A Structural Analysis," *Journal of Gerontology:Social Sciences*, vol. 45, no. 6 (November 1990), pp. S238–S249; Peter Kemper, "The Use of Formal and

Informal Home Care by the Disabled Elderly," *Health Services Research,* vol. 27, no. 4 (October 1992), pp. 421–51; and Sharon L. Tennstedt, Sybil Crawford, and John B. McKinlay, "Determining the Pattern of Community Care: Is Coresidence More Important Than Caregiver Relationship?," *Journal of Gerontology:Social Sciences,* vol. 48, no. 2 (March 1993), pp. S74–S83.

17. Within the log-log specification estimated here, the coefficient on hours of care could be interpreted directly as an elasticity.

18. A recent first effort to estimate such a model found little displacement of informal care by formal care either directly or through changes in living arrangements as a result of a public community-based care program. See Liliana E. Pezzin, Peter Kemper, and James Reschovsky, "Does Publicly Provided Home Care Substitute for Family Care? Experimental Evidence with Endogenous Living Arrangements," Working Paper (Rockville, Md.: Agency for Health Care Policy and Research, August 1994).

Chapter 11

JENNIFER SCHORE

Regional Variation in the Use of Medicare Home Health Services

Recent growth in the use of the medicare home health benefit has been disproportionate to growth in other sectors of the medicare budget.[1] Some increase was expected because of the expanded role of home health care in providing postacute care in the wake of prospective payment for medicare-covered hospitalizations. The wider availability of home health care, following the clarifications of medicare regulations in response to the 1988 *Duggan v. Bowen* lawsuit, was also expected to result in greater use of the benefit. Nonetheless, the extraordinary growth that has occurred in the use of the benefit and in home health care as an industry has caught the attention of policymakers.

Moreover, great regional variation in the levels of care that home health care patients receive has led to questions about whether more or less home health care than appropriate is provided in some areas. Investigating the sources of this variation is important because they affect approaches that might be taken to reduce the variation. For example,

—If regional variation occurs because of the provision of unnecessary care in some regions, the medicare program might be able to generate substantial savings by cutting back on the provision of unnecessary care. However, if regional variation occurs because of underprovision of care that leads to adverse patient outcomes, savings might be produced by improving the quality of care, thereby limiting adverse outcomes and reducing the use of other services.

—Medicare's regional home health fiscal intermediaries (FIs) have come under periodic criticism for inconsistent interpretation of medicare regulations. If regional variation in home health services use results from differences in FI practice, procedures to increase consistency might be needed once again.

—If regional differences in the use of the medicare home health benefit occur because of differences in the availability of alternatives to home health care, then assessing which types of care are most cost effective and which could be implemented in high-use regions is important. The availability and use of such care could then be promoted. These alternatives include residential services (such as nursing homes, assisted living facilities, and foster care) and community-based care (such as medicaid home health, medicaid home and community-based waiver programs, other public programs, and privately funded services).

In this chapter, I address two primary questions: why the use of home health care varies so widely across regions; and whether a corresponding variation occurs across regions in patient outcomes, suggesting that lower levels of care lead to poorer outcomes or that higher levels lead to better outcomes. I address these questions by constructing and analyzing a database of Health Care Financing Administration (HCFA) administrative and other secondary data that describes patients before, during, and immediately after home health care episodes. The database also includes information on the agencies providing care and the service environments of counties in which the agencies are located.

This study must be viewed as preliminary. Its goal was to identify associations among use of home health services, potential patient outcomes, and characteristics, rather than to determine the specific reasons underlying regional variation. Moreover, secondary data, such as those used in this study, are limited because they provide only crude descriptions of home health care patients, agencies, and service environments. With these caveats, however, this study provides a reasonable starting point for investigating the questions at hand.

BACKGROUND

Between 1980 and 1993, expenditures for the medicare benefit increased fifteenfold, and the number of beneficiaries using home health services tripled (table 11-1). This growth reflects a 132 percent increase in the proportion of beneficiaries using home health care, as well as a 29 percent increase in the medicare rolls. The sizable increase in users was accompanied by an even larger increase in the number of visits provided per user (nearly 150 percent). At the same time, the home health care industry experienced enormous growth,

TABLE 11-1. *Medicare Home Health Care Use and Expenditures, 1980–93*

Item	1980	1985	1990	1993
Medicare expenditures on home health care (millions of dollars)	662	1,773	3,714	9,726
Percentage home health care expenditures of total medicare expenditures	2.0	2.8	3.7	6.4
Number of beneficiaries using home health care (millions)	.96	1.59	1.97	2.87
Percentage home health care users of all medicare beneficiaries	3.4	5.1	5.7	7.9
Average number of visits provided per home health care user	23	25	36	57
Average charge per visit provided (dollars)	33	51	69	81

Sources: Charles Helbing, Judith Sangl, and Herbert Silverman, "Home Health Agency Benefits," *Health Care Financing Review*, 1992 annual supplement (1993), pp. 125–48, for 1980, 1985, and 1990 statistics; Katherin Levit and others, "National Health Expenditures, 1993," *Health Care Financing Review*, vol. 16 (Fall 1994), pp. 247–94, for total medicare expenditures ($151.1 billion) used to compute percentage of 1993 medicare expenditures; and personal communication with the staff of the Health Care Financing Administration's Office of Research and Demonstration for 1993 home health statistics.

with the number of medicare-certified home health agencies more than doubling, from just under 3,000 in 1980 to 7,000 at the end of 1993.

Changes in the definition of the home health care benefit have played a key role in the increase in its use. Since the benefit's inception in 1965, coverage regulations have shifted away from the view of home health care as providing strictly limited posthospital care and toward it as providing home-based acute care more generally. Later, this view of home health services expanded to include the ongoing provision of services to beneficiaries with chronic illnesses and skilled care needs. The first shift came in 1980, when the Omnibus Reconciliation Act eliminated the original requirement that a beneficiary have a prior hospitalization of at least three days and removed the one-hundred-visit limit on annual home health use.

The implementation of medicare prospective payment for inpatient hospital care in 1983 was expected to lead to a major increase in the use of home health and other postacute services, as patients were discharged from the hospital "quicker and sicker." An increase in the review and denial of medicare home health claims in the mid-1980s may have temporarily dampened the effect of prospective payment on use of home health services, however. Yet the high claim denial rates eventually led to a 1988 lawsuit (*Duggan* v. *Bowen*) that opened the way for more liberal interpretation of benefit coverage requirements. As a result, HCFA clarified home health regulations in 1988 and 1989. The clarifications stated that use of the home health care benefit could no longer be denied solely on the basis of a beneficiary's chronic disease or need for long-term services if the patient also had skilled care needs.

Not only have the use of and spending for medicare home health care grown faster than almost any other sector of medicare services,[2] but the amount of care rendered to patients receiving home health services has exhibited marked variation across geographic regions. For example, among home health care episodes that started in 1990 and 1991, the mean number of visits per episode varied from twenty-five in western states to approximately fifty in the southern and southwestern states.[3] Similarly, in 1990, sixty-three visits were rendered per person served in the East South Central states, compared with twenty-three in the Pacific states.[4] The same pattern occurred in 1991.[5]

OVERVIEW OF THE STUDY

To explore potential sources of regional variation in medicare home health use, the database constructed for this study was based on a nationally representative, 10 percent random sample of beneficiaries who used home health care in 1990, 1991, or 1992. The unit of observation was a home health care episode. A standard definition of episode was used to overcome agency differences in admission and discharge practices, defining episodes as periods covered by strings of consecutive medicare home health claims that were preceded and followed by at least a thirty-day hiatus in claims.[6] Medicare claims data describing the home health episodes were merged with data from a variety of HCFA files and the Area Resource File (ARF). The database consisted of 634,844 home health episodes that started in 1990, 1991, or 1992. The analysis of home health use measures was based on the 398,522 episodes that started in 1990 and 1991, however. (Measures based on episodes beginning in 1992, particularly late

1992, were subject to a high degree of truncation).[7] Episodes were categorized by the geographic region in which the agency was located; the nine regions used are those routinely reported by HCFA.[8]

The study first compared regional means and distributions of home health use measures (number of visits per episode, episode length, and visits per episode day); patient outcomes; and patient, agency, and county characteristics. We then estimated regression models to determine the extent to which differences in characteristics accounted for regional differences in home health care use. (Figure 11-1 summarizes the control variables used for the regression analysis.) We also estimated models to examine differences in patient outcomes after controlling for patient, agency, and county characteristics.

The study had three major limitations that underscore its preliminary nature. First, HCFA's administrative data and other secondary data provide only crude descriptions of home health care patients, agencies, and service environments. Many factors affecting use of home health services (for example, the functional status of patients, their adherence to prescribed treatments, availability and capability of informal caregivers, and other features of patients' home environment) can be measured only with primary data, if at all. Data on other factors, such as county-level home health capacity or availability of home and community-based services, would have enhanced the database but were not readily available. Second, the study identifies associations among use of home health services, potential patient outcomes, and patient, agency, and area characteristics from which conjectures are drawn about the causes of regional variation. The study does not purport to determine causality.

Finally, the study is particularly tentative in its conclusions about claims-based patient outcomes (whether the beneficiary returned to home health care, was admitted to a hospital, or died shortly after a study episode). These conclusions must be tentative because it is not possible to label an outcome measure based on secondary data as adverse or as resulting directly from home health care. For example, a hospital admission shortly after an episode of home health care could reflect poor-quality home health care or an appropriate decision on the part of an agency to move a patient to a higher level of care. Moreover, such a hospitalization could be unrelated to the care provided by the home health agency (for example, if the patient was not adhering to treatment recommendations, despite the agency's

FIGURE 11-1. *Summary of Control Variables for Regression Analysis*[a]

Patient characteristics
Gender
Race
Age
Principal condition (at episode start)
Comorbid conditions (at episode start)
Medicare service use and reimbursement (during the six months before episode)
  Inpatient
  Skilled nursing facility (SNF)
  Home health care
Whether patient had inpatient stay ending during 14 days before episode
Whether patient had SNF stay ending during 14 days before episode
Year of episode start

Environmental characteristics (for agency county)
Urban/rural status
Number of medicare SNF beds per 1,000 beneficiaries
Hospital occupancy rate
Number of hospital beds per 1,000 persons age 65 or older
Average inpatient length of stay
Proportions of hospitals with geriatric acute care, geriatric assessment, geriatric
  clinics, and home health agencies
Number of home health agencies per 10,000 beneficiaries
Number of physicians per 10,000 persons
Number of hospital-based RNs and LPNs per 10,000 persons
Number of hospital-based physical, occupation, and speech therapists per 10,000
  persons
Per capita income
Proportion of elderly population living in poverty
Average annual medicare reimbursement

Agency characteristics
Facility type
Profit status
Whether medicaid certified
Years in operation at episode start
Region of agency

a. See Jennifer Schore, "Patient, Agency, and Area Characteristics Associated with Regional Variation in the Use of Medicare Home Health Services" (Princeton, N.J.: Mathematica Policy Research, Inc., September 1994), appendix tables A.1 to A.17, for overall and regional means for the ninety-two control variables used in this study's regression analysis.

best efforts). Thus a higher incidence of "adverse" outcomes in areas with fewer visits per episode may reflect unmeasured differences in patient and area characteristics.

In the sections that follow, home health episodes are compared with the characteristics of patients, agencies, and service environments across regions. I then discuss the extent to which data assembled for the study explain regional variation in use of home health services on the basis of findings from the regression analyses. I conclude with an examination of the characteristics of unusually long home health episodes and a comparison across regions of the association between potential patient outcomes and home health care use.

HOME HEALTH EPISODES

Nationally, the mean number of visits rendered during medicare-covered episodes that started in 1990 or 1991 was forty-seven; mean episode length was ninety-four days (table 11-2). Consistent with earlier findings, many fewer visits were rendered, on average, by agencies in the Pacific region (Alaska, California, Hawaii, Oregon, and Washington) and Middle Atlantic region (New Jersey, New York, and Pennsylvania), with twenty-eight and thirty visits per episode, respectively. By contrast, many more visits were rendered by agencies in the East South Central region (Alabama, Kentucky, Mississippi, and Tennessee) and West South Central region (Arkansas, Louisiana, Oklahoma, and Texas), with ninety-five and sixty-four visits, respectively. This range in visits rendered reflects a more than 200 percent difference between the highest- and lowest-use regions.

Both the length of an episode and the number of visits rendered per day contribute to the number of visits rendered during an episode. Each could potentially account for part of the large regional variation observed in visits rendered per episode. The variation in visits rendered per episode day was relatively small, however, with a difference of just under 40 percent between the regions with the greatest and fewest numbers of visits per day. By contrast, enormous variation occurred across regions in mean episode length. Episodes averaged ninety-four days nationally. However, episodes in the East South Central region averaged 180 days, compared with just sixty in the Pacific region—a difference of 200 percent.

TABLE 11-2. *Visits Rendered and Episode Length, by Geographic Region*[a]

Item	New England	Middle Atlantic	East North Central	West North Central	South Atlantic	East South Central	West South Central	Mountain	Pacific	U.S. overall
Number of visits per episode										
Mean	55.8	30.4	36.1	33.6	51.7	94.6	64.2	42.6	27.5	46.5
Median	15	14	14	14	22	27	20	15	12	16
Mean number of visits per episode day	.57	.50	.44	.46	.61	.51	.54	.57	.50	.52
Episode length (days)										
Mean	95.3	66.3	93.9	83.4	94.2	180.3	121.3	77.1	59.7	94.1
Median	42	38	46	40	46	66	54	37	31	43
Episode length (percent distribution)										
1 to 30 days	38.3	41.1	34.7	40.0	34.2	24.7	31.2	42.9	49.5	37.2
31 to 60 days	26.4	33.0	30.0	28.9	31.4	21.1	26.4	27.5	28.4	29.1
61 to 90 days	10.5	9.6	10.2	9.1	10.1	10.3	10.3	9.6	7.9	9.7
91 to 180 days	12.3	9.6	12.6	11.3	11.9	15.0	13.0	10.1	8.0	11.3
181 to 365 days	5.8	3.8	6.3	5.6	6.1	10.7	9.2	5.4	3.4	6.0
More than 365 days	6.7	2.9	6.2	5.1	6.2	18.1	9.9	4.4	2.7	6.5
Number of episodes	27,798	67,409	60,355	24,244	80,636	34,850	38,556	14,943	49,731	398,522

Source: Mathematica Policy Research, Inc., analysis of data from Health Care Financing Administration, Bureau of Data Management and Strategy, Medicare 40 Percent Home Health Bill Records Files (1990–92).

a. This table is based on episodes starting in 1990 or 1991 to avoid the truncating of episodes starting in 1992. Episodes with end dates in December 1992 may have continued into 1993; there were 4,674 such episodes among those starting in 1990 (2.5 percent) and 9,910 among those starting in 1991 (4.6 percent).

Of the forty-seven visits rendered during a typical episode nationally, 64 percent were provided by skilled nurses, 20 percent by home
health aides, 15 percent by therapists (primarily physical therapists),
and only 1 percent by medical social workers (table 11-3). Although regional variation in the proportion of visits delivered by nurses was
moderate, differences between the East South Central and Pacific
regions in the proportions of therapist and home health aide visits were
striking. Home health aide visits made up 29 percent of episodes in the
East South Central region, but only 14 percent in the Pacific region.
Almost the reverse was true of therapist visits. Moreover, just over a
quarter of episodes in the East South Central region included any therapist visits, compared with just under half in the Pacific region.

HOME HEALTH CARE USERS, AGENCIES, AND COUNTIES

Medicare claims and eligibility data provided most of the study's variables
describing home health care patients: demographic and mortality information, use of medicare-covered services before and after home health
care episodes, and primary and secondary diagnoses at episode start.
Home health care plan data on some functional limitations and recommended treatments from HCFA's Regional Home Health Intermediary
database were available for a subsample of episodes. HCFA's Provider of
Services file data were used to describe the profit status and facility base
of home health agencies. The ARF provided data describing the county in
which the agency was located, including urban-rural status, proportion of
elderly persons living in poverty, skilled nursing facility (SNF) and hospital bed supply, and the supply of hospital-based nurses and therapists (as
a proxy for the supply of such professionals in home care).[9]

Home health care users in the two South Central regions emerged
as patients likely to have long-term needs. As noted, their home
health care episodes, analyzed in this study, were much longer than
average. They also had greater numbers of home health visits during
the six months prior to the episodes and were more likely to have
new episodes within thirty-one to sixty days after the episodes
studied (table 11-4). Patients in both South Central regions were
much more likely to have a principal diagnosis of diabetes or of hypertension or another cerebrovascular condition; patients in the East

TABLE 11-3. *Type of Home Health Care Visits Rendered, by Geographic Region*[a]

Item	New England	Middle Atlantic	East North Central	West North Central	South Atlantic	East South Central	West South Central	Mountain	Pacific	U.S. overall
Any visit (percentage)										
Skilled nurse	90.1	93.6	94.5	93.2	90.3	94.4	93.7	91.4	87.6	92.0
Home health aide	43.1	35.8	36.3	39.3	47.9	51.5	46.1	44.7	37.0	41.9
Therapist	35.2	35.7	29.2	25.6	35.6	26.7	25.8	40.9	46.2	33.8
Medical social worker	8.4	12.5	12.9	10.2	18.1	12.6	12.0	20.5	32.3	16.0
Percentage of visits										
Skilled nurse	61.9	67.0	69.5	68.7	59.8	59.9	63.9	59.8	59.2	63.5
Home health aide	21.3	16.2	16.1	17.9	22.6	29.2	23.9	19.6	14.3	19.7
Therapist	15.9	15.8	13.2	12.6	16.3	10.1	11.4	18.7	23.0	15.4
Medical social worker	0.6	0.9	1.1	0.8	1.1	0.6	0.7	1.7	3.4	1.2
Mean episode length (days)	95	66	94	83	94	180	121	77	60	94
Mean number of visits per episode	56	30	36	34	52	95	64	43	28	47
Number of episodes	27,798	67,409	60,355	24,244	80,636	34,850	38,556	14,943	49,731	398,522

Source: Mathematica Policy Research, Inc., analysis of data from Health Care Financing Administration, Bureau of Data Management and Strategy, Medicare 40 Percent Home Health Bill Records Files (1990–92).

a. This table is based on episodes starting in 1990 or 1991 to avoid the truncating of episodes starting in 1992. Episodes with end dates in December 1992 may have continued into 1993; there were 4,674 such episodes among those starting in 1990 (2.5 percent) and 9,910 among those starting in 1991 (4.6 percent).

South Central region (which had the higher home health use of the two regions) were also more likely to be incontinent or to suffer from malnutrition or shortness of breath. Patients in both regions were more likely to have venipuncture in their initial treatment plans, which could suggest that they were too frail or lacked the support to leave home for routine blood tests. Thus these patients emerge as chronically ill, frail, and in poor health. This picture is underscored by their above-average use of home health aide services during study episodes (noted in table 11-3) and their somewhat higher rates of mortality and hospital admission following home health care.

A very different profile of home health patients emerges in the Middle Atlantic and Pacific regions, where home health care use was lowest. Patients in the Middle Atlantic region were more likely to use home health services as postacute care, entering home health care within two weeks after a hospitalization. Patients in the Middle Atlantic and Pacific regions tended to be less likely to have diabetes, hypertension, or incontinence and were much less likely to have venipuncture in their treatment plans. Patients in the Pacific region received much more rehabilitative care and many more medical social services during home health than patients elsewhere (as noted in table 11-3). Patients in both regions had somewhat below-average rates of mortality and home health readmission following study episodes. Thus patients in these regions emerge as less frail and less chronically ill than their counterparts in the South Central regions.

The agencies serving patients in the high- and low-use regions also differed, as did the counties in which they were located. The agencies serving patients in the South Central regions were largely proprietary, whereas those serving patients in the Middle Atlantic and Pacific regions tended to be nonprofit. Patients in the South Central regions were served by home health agencies that tended to be located in relatively less populated counties and counties with above-average proportions of individuals with incomes below the poverty level, particularly among elderly persons. Patients in the Middle Atlantic and Pacific regions received services from agencies in relatively more populated counties and counties in which elderly residents had relatively higher incomes. Services that might function as alternatives to home health care might be more plentiful in areas such as the Middle Atlantic and Pacific regions, especially when compared with the poorer and less populated areas that dominate the South

TABLE 11-4. *Selected Characteristics of Home Health Care Users, Agencies, and Counties*[a]

Item	East South Central	West South Central	U.S. overall	Middle Atlantic	Pacific
Patient condition at episode start (percent)					
Diabetes (primary diagnosis)	11.4	9.7	7.0	5.8	4.6
Hypertension or other cerebrovascular disease (primary diagnosis)	8.3	8.0	5.2	4.1	3.3
Incontinence	6.5	3.2	2.1	0.7	2.1
Malnutrition/dehydration	6.8	6.0	5.2	4.0	4.7
Shortness of breath	45.8	13.7	29.8	30.1	30.5
Venipuncture in home health treatment plan	50.4	39.8	23.8	16.0	11.0
Prestudy episode medicare service use					
Number of home health visits in prior six months	9.1	7.6	5.7	4.3	4.1
Inpatient stay ending in prior two weeks (percent)	43.7	48.8	56.1	68.3	53.6
Poststudy episode outcomes (percent)					
Readmitted to home health between 31 and 60 days	19.3	13.5	11.0	8.9	8.4
Admitted to inpatient hospital within 30 days	26.0	23.8	22.4	22.8	19.6
Died within 30 days	16.3	13.6	12.4	10.7	11.6
County characteristics (percent)					
Episodes delivered by agencies in counties with less than 250,000 residents	55.4	49.8	33.9	12.3	18.5
Elderly persons living in poverty	21.4	18.6	12.4	10.3	7.6
Agency characteristics (percent)					
Episodes delivered by proprietary agencies	49.9	51.1	31.1	10.6	29.2
Sample size	52,830	64,395	634,844	106,349	77,667

TABLE 11-4. *(continued)*

Sources: Mathematica Policy Research, Inc., analysis of data from Health Care Financing Administration, Bureau of Data Management and Strategy, Medicare 40 Percent Home Health Bill Records Files (1990–92); Medicare National Claims History, Standard Analytical Files (1989–93); Medicare Provider of Services Files (1990–92); Area Resource File (1993); and Medicare Regional Home Health Intermediary Database (1991).

a. This table is based primarily on 634,844 episodes that started in 1990, 1991, or 1992. Regional patterns of visits rendered per episode and episode length are the same as those for 398,552 episodes that started in 1990 or 1991 (presented in table 11-2).

Poststudy episode outcomes are based on 383,938 episodes starting in 1990 or 1991 and completed prior to December 1992 to ensure that outcomes (for example, hospital admission) occurred following, rather than during, the home health care episode. Again, regional patterns for these episodes are the same as those for all episodes starting in 1990 or 1991.

Data on shortness of breath (dyspnea) and venipuncture were available for the subsample of episodes linked to 1991 Regional Home Health Intermediary database files. Linked subsample size is 156,798 for U.S. overall. Patterns of regional variation in visits rendered and episode length are the same for the linked subsample as for all episodes that started in 1990 or 1991.

Central regions. In fact, each state in the Pacific region spent more on home and community-based care per elderly resident in 1986 than did any of the East South Central states.[10]

POTENTIAL DETERMINANTS OF REGIONAL VARIATION

Regression models were estimated to determine the effects of patient, agency, and county characteristics on regional variation in home health services use. For each model, regression-adjusted, region-specific mean home health use was computed from coefficient estimates. A regression-adjusted, region-specific mean estimates a hypothetical average for a region, assuming the measured characteristics of the region were at national averages.[11] By contrast, unadjusted means account for a region's specific, possibly atypical, characteristics. Finally, the standard deviations of the adjusted and unadjusted region-specific means were computed as measures of regional variation.

A regression model of visits rendered per episode (controlling for the characteristics summarized in figure 11-1) showed, not surprisingly, that many of the characteristics distinguishing episodes in the highest- and lowest-use regions were also associated with statistically significant and substantial increases in visits rendered. These characteristics included having chronic illnesses, living outside a

TABLE 11-5. *Characteristics Strongly Associated with Number of Visits per Episode[a]*

Patient characteristic	County characteristics	Agency characteristics
Nonwhite +	Urban/rural status (relative to core counties in large metropolitan areas)[b]	Agency control (relative to nonprofit) Government – Proprietary +
Principal diagnosis groups (relative to diabetic care) All groups – except serious neuromuscular and degenerative diseases, stroke, urinary tract conditions (including incontinence), anemia, malnutrition/dehydration, ostomy care, care of complicated wounds (including amputations), and peripheral vascular diseases Comorbid conditions Neurological diseases + Incontinence + Secondary conditions complicating wound care + Prior service use Home health visits in the past six months +	Lesser metropolitan + Urbanized nonmetropolitan +	

Sources: Mathematica Policy Research, Inc., analysis of data from Health Care Financing Administration, Bureau of Data Management and Strategy, Medicare 40 Percent Home Health Bill Records Files (1990–92); Medicare National Claims History, Standard Analytical Files (1989–92); Medicare Provider of Services Files (1990–92); and Area Resource File (1993).

a. Estimation was carried out on a 5 percent random sample (19,764) of database episodes starting in 1990 or 1991 using tobit analysis. See Jennifer Schore, "Patient, Agency, and Area Characteristics," appendix B, table B.5A, for tobit coefficients and their probabilities. Characteristics represented by binary variables were listed here if they were statistically significant at the .05 level and they (1) had roughly a 10 percent or greater effect on the dependent variable (that is, were associated with an increase or decrease of five or more visits), or (2) were associated with a slightly smaller change but varied greatly across regions. Characteristics represented by continuous variables (for example, home health care visits before the study episode) were listed if they were statistically significant at the .05 level, and a one-standard deviation change in the variable was associated with an increase or decrease of 10 percent in the dependent variable. A + means an increase in the characteristic was associated with an increase in the dependent variable; a – means an increase in the characteristic was associated with a decrease in the dependent variable. For example, the greater the number of home health care visits the beneficiary received during the six months prior to the study episode, the more visits he or she was likely to receive during the study episode.

TABLE 11-5. *(continued)*

b. Urban/rural status categories come from the Department of Agriculture (as found in the Area Resource File) and are defined as follows:

Large metropolitan, core counties: core counties of greater standard metropolitan statistical areas (SMSAs) with population of 1 million or more

Large metropolitan, fringe counties: noncore counties of metropolitan areas with population of 1 million or more

Medium metropolitan: counties of metropolitan areas with population of 250,000 to 999,999

Lesser metropolitan: counties of metropolitan areas with population of less than 250,000

Urbanized nonmetropolitan: counties outside SMSAs with 20,000 or more residents commuting to urban areas

Less urbanized nonmetropolitan: counties outside SMSAs with 2,500 to 19,999 residents commuting to urban areas

Thinly populated: counties outside SMSAs with fewer than 2,500 residents commuting to urban areas

large metropolitan area, and receiving care from a proprietary agency (table 11-5).[12] Controlling for patient, agency, and county characteristics reduced the standard deviation of mean visits per episode across regions by about one-third (from twenty-one visits for unadjusted regional means to fourteen visits for regression-adjusted means) (table 11-6). Even after regression adjustment, however, the East South Central region still had the highest levels of home health care use, and the Pacific and Middle Atlantic regions still had the lowest. After analyzing three subsamples of episodes for which patients, at episode start, had the same general principal diagnosis (diabetes, serious cardiopulmonary disorders, and stroke or serious neuromuscular disorders), use levels in these regions were still above or below average. Moreover, region-specific models of home health care use indicated that roughly the same patient characteristics were associated with increased use overall and with increased use in individual regions. This suggests that large regional differences in home health care use do not result from gross differences in agency practice for a few specific conditions or types of patients.

Because medicare's regional home health FIs have been criticized repeatedly for inconsistent claims review, our research group was interested in assessing the role of FI practice in regional variation in home health services use.[13] However, our group's ability to assess the contribution of FI practice was limited to descriptive analysis by the high correlation between region and FI assignment. Descriptive findings suggest that FI practice did not play a major role in variation in the use of home health care. This assessment is based on the observation that average visits per episode and episode length were reasonably consistent across FIs within a region. For example, mean visits per episode and episode length were almost always well above average in the East South Central region, regardless of which FI processed the claims, while mean visits and episode length were almost always well below average in the Pacific region.

Our group concluded that data from the study database explained a substantial portion of regional variation. However, most of the variation must be explained by other factors, such as medical practice patterns, the supply of home health agency staff, the availability of home and community-based and residential alternatives to home health care, and difficult-to-measure patient characteristics (for example, adherence to recommended treatment regimens, functional status, availability of informal care, and preferences for informal versus formal or for community-based versus residential care).

CHARACTERISTICS OF LONG EPISODES

Regions with the highest mean number of visits also had the highest percentage of episodes lasting longer than a year. For example, in the high-use East South Central region, 18 percent of all episodes were longer than a year. By contrast, in the two lowest-use regions, the Middle Atlantic and Pacific, only 3 percent of episodes were longer than a year (table 11-2). Because the mean number of visits per day was almost identical for all three regions, episode length could be viewed as responsible for a large part of the regional variation in visits rendered. When, for expository purposes, episode length was included as a control variable in the model for number of visits per episode (described in tables 11-5 and 11-6), the standard deviation of the region-specific, regression-adjusted means was reduced by nearly another 50 percent (from 14 to 8). The contribution of episode length to regional variation in visits led us to look more closely at very long home health episodes and the patients who had them.

Seven percent of the episodes in the study database were longer than one year (table 11-7). Such episodes included an average of 295 visits and were roughly 20 months long, compared with 47 visits and roughly 3 months for episodes of any length. Moreover, for episodes longer than one year, 56 percent were ongoing in December 1992 (the end of data collection for the study). Thus the number of mean visits and episode length for these very long episodes were likely to be greatly understated.

TABLE 11-6. *Mean Home Health Care Visits per Episode, by Region*[a]

Region	Raw mean visits	Regression-adjusted mean visits	Percent change
East South Central	95	79	−17
West South Central	62	55	−11
South Atlantic	53	50	−6
New England	52	62	19
Mountain	45	49	9
East North Central	38	42	11
West North Central	33	40	21
Middle Atlantic	32	39	22
Pacific	27	37	37
Standard deviation	21	14	. . .
U.S. overall	47	47	. . .

Sources: Mathematica Policy Research, Inc., analysis of data from Health Care Financing Administration, Bureau of Data Management and Strategy, Medicare 40 Percent Home Health Bill Records Files (1990–92); Medicare National Claims History, Standard Analytical Files (1989–92); Medicare Provider of Services Files (1990–92); and Area Resource File (1993).

a. Estimation was carried out on a 5 percent random sample (19,764) of database episodes starting in 1990 or 1991 using tobit analysis.

TABLE 11-7. *Characteristics of Medicare Home Health Care Episodes Longer than One Year*[a]

Item	All episodes	Episodes longer than one year
Mean number of visits per episode	47	295
Mean episode length (months)	3	20
Percentage of episodes ongoing in December 1992	4	56
Percentage of episode visits, by discipline		
Skilled nurse	64	51
Therapist	15	4
Home health aide	20	44
Sample size	398,522	25,914

Source: Mathematica Policy Research, Inc., analysis of data from Health Care Financing Administration, Bureau of Data Management and Strategy, Medicare 40 Percent Home Health Bill Records Files (1990–92).

a. This table is based on episodes starting in 1990 or 1991 to avoid the truncating of episodes starting in 1992.

Care in very long episodes shifted away from nurses and therapists to home health aides. Among episodes longer than one year, skilled nurses provided 51 percent of visits, home health aides provided 44 percent, and therapists provided only 4 percent, compared with 64 percent, 20 percent, and 15 percent, respectively, for episodes of any length.

Regression analysis showed that patients with episodes longer than a year were characterized by their gender, age, certain diagnoses, and whether they started out using home health as postacute care. These patients were more likely to be female or to be younger than 65 (that is, permanently disabled according to medicare). They also tended to have chronic illnesses, such as diabetes or serious neuromuscular or degenerative diseases. They were less likely to have cancer or to have started out using home health services as postacute care.

From these results, patients with episodes longer than one year emerge as chronically ill or disabled. They tended to receive home health care for much longer than one year and to receive substantial assistance from home health aides, although they received very little rehabilitative care.

PATIENT OUTCOMES POTENTIALLY RELATED TO HOME HEALTH

Our second research question addressed the association between home health care use and patient outcomes. We found that patients using home health services in the low-use Pacific region had some of the lowest rates of home health care readmission, inpatient admission, and mortality during the period immediately following study episodes, while patients in the high-use East South Central region had some of the highest (table 11-4). Similarly, the Middle Atlantic region had lower rates for most patient outcomes, while the West South Central region had higher ones. (These patterns persisted in findings from regression analysis as well.) Differences in these patient outcomes for the high- and low-use regions led us to reject the hypothesis that low levels of home health care lead to poorer patient outcomes (or vice versa). The observed regional differences in outcomes probably reflect the relative pre-episode health of home health patients.

TABLE 11-8. *Use of Skilled Nursing Facilities (SNFs) Before and After Home Health Care Episodes*[a]

Percent

SNF use	East South Central	West South Central	U.S. overall	Middle Atlantic	Pacific
SNF stay ending two weeks before start of home health care	4.7	7.1	7.1	5.5	11.6
Admitted to SNF within 30 days of end of home health care	4.7	4.4	4.3	2.9	5.3

Sources: Mathematica Policy Research, Inc., analysis of data from Health Care Financing Administration, Bureau of Data Management and Strategy, Medicare 40 Percent Home Health Bill Records Files (1990–92); and Medicare National Claims History, Standard Analytical Files (1989–93).

a. The statistics on SNF use before home health care are based on 634,844 episodes that started in 1990, 1991, or 1992. Regional patterns of home health care visits rendered per episode and episode length are the same as those for episodes that started in 1990 or 1991 (presented in table 11-2).

The statistics on SNF use following home health care are based on 383,938 episodes starting in 1990 or 1991 and completed before December 1992, to ensure that SNF used occurred following, rather than during, the home health care episode. Again, regional patterns for these episodes are that same as those for all episodes starting in 1990 or 1991.

Patients in the Pacific region also had among the highest rates of SNF admission following home health care, as well as above-average use of SNFs immediately preceding home health care (table 11-8). SNFs may be relatively more widely used in this region. (Use of SNF care in the South Central and Middle Atlantic regions was near or below national averages.) SNF care has been found to substitute for home health care as postacute care and may have been one of the alternative sources of care available to frail patients in the Pacific region.[14]

CONCLUSION

In general, home health care agencies in the highest-use regions (East and West South Central) seem to be providing levels of care that are consistent with the needs of their relatively frail and chronically ill patients. Furthermore, the less costly care that may substitute for some home health care (for example, home and community-based services) may be in relatively short supply in these regions. The high rates of poverty among elderly persons in these regions suggest further that these beneficiaries may have few resources to purchase available services. Thus home health agencies in the regions may serve patients for as long as is justifiable.

By contrast, agencies in low-use regions such as the Pacific serve much less frail and chronically ill medicare beneficiaries. Besides evidence that home and community-based care may be in better supply in this region, our group's data showed levels of poverty among Pacific-region elderly persons to be much lower than average. Above-average use of SNF care was found among home health care patients in the Pacific region, both before and after home health care. In this region, alternatives to home health care may be more widely available, and elderly beneficiaries may be in a better position to purchase needed services. As a result, they may not rely so heavily on medicare home health services. Furthermore, the data suggest that low levels of home health care use in the Pacific region did not seem to lead to poorer patient outcomes (for those outcomes our group measured).

Characteristics of patients and areas clearly differ between the regions with the highest and lowest use of medicare home health services. Differences in the frailty and health status of home health care patients in the East South Central and Pacific regions lead us to speculate that many of the Pacific counterparts of the frail home health care patients in the East South Central region never enter home health care, possibly because they are served in other settings or by other programs. Beneficiaries in the Pacific who do enter home health care may move to other settings or programs after their pressing skilled needs end (or to SNFs, if their skilled needs are ongoing). Alternative care includes home and community-based services (for example, personal care, housekeeping, home-delivered meals, and transportation) and residential services (for example, nursing homes, assisted-living facilities, and foster care).

Future research would do well to examine to what extent the availability of services that may substitute for ongoing medicare home health accounts for regional differences in home health care use, whether this alternative care would be cost effective if implemented more widely in regions of the country with the highest home health care use, and whether it is feasible to implement alternative care in these regions.

The relatively higher penetration of health maintenance organizations (HMOs) in the Pacific region may also play a role in the lower levels of use among Pacific home health care patients, since studies have concluded that HMO enrollees receive less home health care than their fee-for-service counterparts.[15] We also recommend that future research examine to what extent the presence of HMOs accounts for regional differences in home health care use.

Because most of the regional variation in use of home health services was not explained by the study database, future research must also focus on the extent to which differences in agency staff supply, agency and physician practice patterns, and patient characteristics (other than those described by our group's data) explain the variation.

Since its inception in 1965, the medicare home health care benefit has been transformed from a short-term, postacute benefit to one that can cover care over the longer term. In some cases, home health services may be appropriate long-term care. In others, less costly care may exist that is at least as effective. As the need for long-term care increases in the coming decades, the importance of expanding the pool of knowledge surrounding these questions will grow commensurately.

NOTES

1. This chapter draws from Jennifer Schore, "Patient, Agency, and Area Characteristics Associated with Regional Variation in the Use of Medicare Home Health Services" (Princeton, N.J.: Mathematica Policy Research, September 1994). The report is available from the author on request.

2. Charles Helbing, "Medicare Program Expenditures," *Health Care Financing Review*, 1992 annual supplement (1993), pp. 23–54.

3. Jennifer Schore, Randall Brown, and Barbara Phillips, "Medicare Home Health Episodes 1990/1991: Distributions of Episode Length and Number of Visits Provided per Episode" (Princeton, N.J.: Mathematica Policy Research, January 1993).

4. Charles Helbing, Judith Sangl, and Herbert Silverman, "Home Health Agency Benefits," *Health Care Financing Review*, 1992 annual supplement (1993), pp. 125–48.

5. Christine Bishop and Kathleen Skwara, "Recent Growth of Medicare Home Health," *Health Affairs* (Fall 1993), pp. 95–110.

6. A thirty-day hiatus in claims was used to mark the end of one period of home health service provision and the start of a subsequent period. Thirty days was chosen in part because home health agencies typically submit claims to the Health Care Financing Administration monthly. HCFA's Per-

Visit Home Health Prospective Payment Demonstration also used the thirty-day gap definition to develop a case-mix adjuster for per episode prospective payment. Although other studies have used gaps of forty-five and sixty days to define episodes, the relatively shorter gap was believed to yield a more accurate case-mix adjuster. The thirty-day gap definition understates episode length relative to the other definitions and provides a conservative approach to examining episode length.

7. Thirty percent of episodes that started in 1992 were ongoing at the end of 1992, when the data collection period for the study ended. Even episodes that started in 1990 and 1991 were subject to some truncation. Among those starting in 1990, 2.5 percent were ongoing at the end of 1992. The comparable figure for episodes starting in 1991 was 4.6 percent. Separate descriptive analyses were not carried out for episodes starting in 1990 and 1991, but the analysis did control for year of episode start in the regression analysis.

8. States were assigned to geographic regions as follows:

— *New England*	Missouri	Louisiana
Connecticut	Nebraska	Oklahoma
Maine	North Dakota	Texas
Massachusetts	South Dakota	— *Mountain*
New Hampshire	— *South Atlantic*	Arizona
Rhode Island	Delaware	Colorado
Vermont	District of Columbia	Idaho
— *Middle Atlantic*	Florida	Montana
New Jersey	Georgia	Nevada
New York	Maryland	New Mexico
Pennsylvania	North Carolina	Utah
— *East North Central*	South Carolina	Wyoming
Illinois	Virginia	— *Pacific*
Indiana	West Virginia	Alaska
Michigan	— *East South Central*	California
Ohio	Alabama	Hawaii
Wisconsin	Kentucky	Oregon
— *West North Central*	Mississippi	Washington
Iowa	Tennessee	
Kansas	— *West South Central*	
Minnesota	Arkansas	

9. The Area Resource File did not contain recent data on the supply of non-hospital-based nurses and therapists. Levels of hospital-based professionals might correlate positively with levels of similar professionals working in home health care. However, if hospitals were appreciably more

(or less) desirable places to work than home health care agencies, the supply of hospital-based professionals might correlate negatively with the supply of similar professionals working in home health care. And if hospitals employ relatively more therapists and provide more therapy services, demand for therapy services from home health agencies might be lower.

10. Judith Feder, "Paying for Home Care," in Diane Rowlands and Barbara Lyons, eds., *Financing Home Care* (Johns Hopkins University Press, 1991).

11. The following regression model was used in this analysis:

$$(1) \qquad Y = b_1 R + b_2 P + b_3 E + b_4 A + e,$$

where Y is a measure of home health use (episode length in days, number of visits in an episode, or number of visits per episode day), R is a vector of regional binaries (plus an indicator of the year in which the episode began), P is a vector of patient characteristics, E is a vector of environmental characteristics, A is a vector of agency characteristics, b_i are vectors of regression coefficients, and e is a random error term.

The regression-adjusted mean for the South Atlantic region, the region excluded from the model, is:

$$(2) \qquad MEAN_{SA} = MEAN_{overall} - (b_1 * prop_1 + b_2 * prop_2 + \ldots + b_8 * prop_8).$$

For each of the eight included regions, the regression-adjusted mean is:

$$(3) \qquad MEAN_i = MEAN_{SA} + b_i,$$

where $i = 1, 8$ for each region, b_i is the marginal impact of region computed from logit coefficients or the actual tobit or ordinary least square (OLS) coefficients, and $prop_i$ is the proportion of episodes from each region.

To estimate the marginal impact that region i has on the probability of a binary outcome occurring (for example, being admitted to a hospital within thirty days after the end of a home health care episode), for each episode (based on a logit model) the predicted probability of the event occurring was computed, first assuming that it was provided by an agency in region i, and then assuming that it was provided by an agency in the reference region (South Atlantic). The differences between these two predicted probabilities were then averaged across all sample members to obtain the estimated effect of region i relative to the reference region.

The marginal impact of region on number of visits and length of episode was estimated by the coefficient obtained from a tobit model. This is not the usual approach for estimating the marginal effect of an independent variable on the dependent variable in this type of model. The usual application involves predicting the expected value for the dependent variable on the basis of the predicted probability that the dependent variable is zero, and a predicted value for the dependent variable given that it is greater than zero. Here, however, the tobit model was used only to account for the fact that some observations were truncated. Our research group wanted to estimate the effect of region on episode length and number of visits for the full episode, not simply the observed portion of that episode. The underlying "true" value of the dependent variable is the observed value for nontruncated episodes, and some value Y^* that is greater than the observed value for the truncated stays. The tobit coefficients estimated the effect of explanatory variables on the true value of the dependent variable, which is what we wanted.

12. None of the county-level supply measures from the ARF was statistically significant. In particular, SNF beds per beneficiary might not have been significant because this measure might have been dominated by beneficiary-level data on SNF use, or because the SNF bed measure was outdated, based on data from 1986. The variables measuring the supply of hospital-based nurses and therapists might not have been significant because they were not good proxies for the supply of similar home care professionals (see note 9).

13. General Accounting Office, *Medicare Home Health Services: A Difficult Program to Control* (Gaithersburg, Md., September 1981); General Accounting Office, *Medicare Need to Strengthen Home Health Care Payment Controls and Address Unmet Needs* (Gaithersburg, Md., December 1986); and General Accounting Office, *Medicare: Increased Denials of Home Health Claims during 1986 and 1987* (Gaithersburg, Md., January 1990).

14. Carl Neu, Scott Harrison, and Joanna Heilbrunn, "Medicare Patients and Postacute Care: Who Goes Where?" (Santa Monica, Calif.: RAND Corporation, November 1989).

15. Randall Brown and others, "Do Health Maintenance Organizations Work for Medicare?", *Health Care Financing Review*, vol. 15 (Fall 1993), pp. 7–24; and Peter Shaughnessy, Robert Schlenker, and David Hittle, "A Study of Home Health Care Quality and Cost under Capitated and Fee-For-Service Payment Systems" (Denver, Colo.: Center for Health Policy Research, February 1994).

Chapter 12

JOSHUA M. WIENER AND CATHERINE M. SULLIVAN

Long-Term Care for the Younger Population: A Policy Synthesis

Although attention to the deficiencies of the financing system and organization of long-term care for disabled elderly persons has increased, similar problems facing disabled persons under age 65 were
almost totally ignored by policymakers until recently. Moreover, although between one-third and two-thirds or more of the total disabled population is not elderly, little is known about their financing
and use of long-term care.[1]

Interest in the younger population with disabilities grew for two
distinct, but mutually reinforcing, reasons. First, the younger population with disabilities demanded recognition. Following the enactment in 1990 of the Americans with Disabilities Act (P.L. 101-336),
younger disabled persons made long-term care reform a major priority and pushed themselves into the political process.[2] Second, to
counter arguments that public spending for long-term care was gen-
erationally unfair to younger people, advocacy groups for elderly
Americans promoted long-term care as a problem that affected all age
groups, not just older people.[3]

In this chapter we synthesize the limited research available on
long-term care for the younger disabled population to shed light on
four important policy issues. First, what is the size of the younger
population with disabilities? Second, what do younger persons with
disabilities want from the long-term care system? In particular, what
are the philosophical underpinnings of the disability movement?[4]
Third, how should the service delivery system be organized? And

Additional financial support for this research was provided by the Alcoa
Foundation. John Burklow provided important information on persons with
mental illness and mental retardation.

fourth, what are the options to finance needed services? Special emphasis is placed on comparisons between the older and younger disabled populations. We conclude by suggesting several avenues for further research.

DISABLED PERSONS UNDER AGE 65

A critical element in developing policies for younger people with disabilities is estimating the size of the population. Although fundamental to policymaking, these estimates also have enormous and conflicting political implications. On the one hand, if the population is large, then its needs demand attention. On the other hand, the bigger the population at risk, the greater the expenditures required to solve its problems and the less willing public officials may be to commit the necessary resources.

Unfortunately, a wide range of estimates has been made of the number of persons under age 65 with disabilities. For 1995 the estimated number of noninstitutionalized younger persons with disabilities varied from 20 million to 33 million (table 12-1), with 1 million to 14 million having substantial disabilities (table 12-2).[5] Depending on the estimates used, nonelderly persons with disabilities account for from one-third to nearly three-quarters of the noninstitutionalized population with disabilities. In addition, approximately 1 million persons under age 65 with disabilities are homeless, incarcerated, or reside in institutions, such as nursing homes, mental hospitals, and other long-term care facilities (table 12-3).

Several factors contribute to the range of estimates, including differing measures of disability and the statistical difficulty of precisely estimating relatively rare events such as impairment in the younger population. In addition, considerations of social stigma and self-perception are important components of whether individuals consider themselves disabled.[6] Estimates are especially imprecise for a number of groups because they are especially uncommon or difficult to measure. These groups of younger people include children with disabilities, persons with developmental disabilities or mental retardation, and persons with severe mental illness.

TABLE 12-1. *Disability Prevalence Estimates for the Civilian Noninstitutionalized U.S. Population, 1995*

	Number of persons (millions)		Population group (percent)		Population with disabilities (percent)	
Age group	National Health Interview Survey	Survey of Income and Program Participation	National Health Interview Survey	Survey of Income and Program Participation	National Health Interview Survey	Survey of Income and Program Participation
Under 65	20.0	33.0	8.9	14.7	73.0	66.0
Over 65	7.3	17.0	22.9	53.9	27.0	34.0
Total	27.3	50.0	10.6	19.4	100.0	100.0

Sources: Authors' calculations based on population projections in Jennifer Cheeseman Day, "Population Projections of the United States by Age, Sex, Race, and Hispanic Origin: 1993 to 2050," *Current Population Reports, Household Economic Studies,* series P-25, no. 1104 (Department of Commerce, Bureau of the Census, 1993); Veronica Benson and Marie A. Marano, "Current Estimates from the National Health Insurance Survey, 1993," *Vital and Health Statistics,* series 10, no. 190 (Hyattsville, Md.: Department of Health and Human Services, Public Health Service, National Center for Health Statistics, December 1994), table 67, p. 106; and John M. McNeil, "Americans with Disabilities: 1991–92, Data from the Survey of Income and Program Participation," *Current Population Reports, Household Economic Studies,* series P-70, no. 33 (Department of Commerce, Bureau of the Census, 1993), table A, p. 5.

Note: The civilian noninstitutional population numbered 258 million in 1995. Estimates derived from the National Health Interview Survey included persons limited, as a result of a chronic condition, in their major, age-appropriate activity: play (under age 5), school (ages 5 to 17), work and keeping house (ages 18 to 69), and basic life activities (age 70 and above). Estimates derived from the Survey of Income and Program Participation included persons meeting at least one of twelve disability indicators subdivided by age group: For persons 15 years old and over, use of mobility aids, sensory and physical functional activities (for example, walking up a flight of stairs), activities of daily living (ADLs), instrumental activities of daily living (IADLs), specific conditions (for example, mental retardation); 16 to 67 years old, work limitation; and 16 years old and older, housework limitation. Parents were asked about limitations in usual activities for their children (under age 6); receipt of therapy or diagnostic services for developmental needs (under age 6); school work limitations (ages 6 to 21); and any long-lasting condition limiting the child's ability to walk, run, or climb stairs (ages 3 to 14). In addition, any person receiving medicare or supplemental security income on the basis of his or her disability status was included.

Even basic demographic information on the younger population with disabilities is relatively scarce. Limited information indicates that the younger population with disabilities is less educated and more likely to be unemployed and to live in low-income households than the younger population without disabilities.[7]

TABLE 12-2. Estimates of the Civilian Noninstitutionalized U.S. Population with Substantial Disabilities, 1995

Age group	Number of persons (millions)			Population group (percent)			Population with disabilities (percent)		
	Survey of Income and Program Participation	National Medical Expenditure Survey	Office of Disability, Aging, and Long-Term Care Policy	Survey of Income and Program Participation	National Medical Expenditure Survey	Office of Disability, Aging, and Long-Term Care Policy	Survey of Income and Program Participation	National Medical Expenditure Survey	Office of Disability, Aging, and Long-Term Care Policy
Under 65	14.1	4.1	1.0	6.2	1.9	0.4	57.0	40.0	32.0
Over 65	10.7	6.2	2.1	34.0	20.1	6.7	43.0	60.0	68.0
Total	24.8	10.3	3.1	9.6	4.0	1.2	100.0	100.0	100.0

Sources: Authors' calculations based on population projections in Day, "Population Projections of the United States by Age, Sex, Race, and Hispanic Origin: 1993 to 2050"; McNeil, "Americans with Disabilities: 1991–92, Data from the Survey of Income and Program Participation"; Mitchell P. LaPlante and Karen S. Miller, "People with Disabilities in Basic Life Activities in the U.S.," *Disability Statistics Abstract*, no. 3 (Department of Education, National Institute on Disability and Rehabilitation Research, April 1992), table 1, p. 2; and Office of the Assistant Secretary for Planning and Evaluation, Office of Disability, Aging, and Long-Term Care Policy, *Cost Estimates for the Long-Term Care Provisions under the Health Security Act* (Department of Health and Human Services, March 1994), table 8, p. 11.

Note: The civilian noninstitutional population numbered 258 million in 1995. The severe disability measure used by the Survey of Income and Program Participation was based on six categories subdivided by age group; for example, inability to perform one or more functions or activities, had one or more specific conditions, or used mobility equipment. Estimates from the National Medical Expenditure Survey were based on 1987 data on persons who reported difficulties with basic life activities, which included a combination of activities of daily living (ADLs) and instrumental activities of daily living (IADLs). The Office of Disability, Aging, and Long-Term Care Policy based its estimates on multiple data sources. The disability measure was persons with three or more ADL limitations, severe or profound mental retardation or developmental disabilities, or a similar level of mental or cognitive impairment.

TABLE 12-3. *Disability Prevalence Estimates for Selected Groups in the Younger Population, 1995*

Group	Disability measure	Prevalence estimate	Number in group (millions)	Limitations of data
Children with disabilities	Children with activity limitations based on age-appropriate criteria	1.4 to 5.8 percent of children under age 18	0.9–3.9	Excludes children in institutions
Persons with severe mental illness	Adults who reported one or more psychiatric disorders within the past year that seriously interfered with one or more aspects of daily life	1.4 to 1.8 percent of the younger adult population ages 18 to 64	2.2–2.8	Excludes children, persons living in institutions, and homeless persons
Persons in institutions	Resident of long-term care facility, homeless shelter, or prison	0.4 percent of total population under 65	1.0	No information on level of disability among persons in institutions; multiple data sources
Persons with mental retardation or developmental disabilities	Legislative definition based on a condition acquired before age 22 causing lifelong and substantial impairment	0.8 to 2.9 percent of population ages 18 to 64	1.3–4.8	Excludes children, persons living in institutions, and persons who developed a disability as adults

Sources: Authors' calculations based on population projections in Day, "Population Projections of the United States by Age, Sex, Race, and Hispanic Origin: 1993 to 2050"; McNeil, "Americans with Disabilities: 1991–92, Data from the Survey of Income and Program Participation"; Peggy R. Barker and others, "Serious Mental Illness and Disability in the Adult Household Population: United States, 1989," *Advance Data from Vital and Health Statistics*, no. 218 (Department of Health and Human Services, Public Health Service, National Center for Health Statistics, September 16, 1992); Michele Adler, "Population Estimates of Disability and Long-Term Care," *ASPE Research Note* (Department of Health and Human Services, Office of Assistant Secretary for Planning and Evaluation, Office of Disability, Aging, and Long-Term Care Policy, February 1995); and Craig Thornton, *Characteristics of Persons with Developmental Disabilities: Evidence from the Survey of Income and Program Participation*, contract no. HHS 100-88-0035 (Department of Health and Human Services, Office of Assistant Secretary for Planning and Evaluation, January 1990).

PHILOSOPHICAL UNDERPINNINGS OF THE
DISABILITY MOVEMENT

Probably the greatest impact of the disability movement has been to force a rethinking of the goals of long-term care, which generally have been limited to little more than keeping older persons safe, clean, and well fed. Advocates for the younger population with disabilities reject these goals as far too circumscribed. For this group, the aims should be to maximize independence and self-sufficiency.[8] Ideas about personal autonomy shared by advocates of the independent living movement for persons with physical disabilities, proponents of community support and the emerging recovery movement for persons with mental illnesses, and supporters of normalization and community integration for persons with mental retardation and developmental disabilities suggest a philosophical commonality across disability subgroups.[9] This emphasis on personal autonomy and empowerment implies a radical change in how long-term care should be organized and financed.[10]

While highly intertwined, the philosophy has five basic tenets. First, younger persons with disabilities reject the notion that a disability somehow makes any one of them less of a person than someone without a disability. The fundamental premise is that persons with disabilities are handicapped by societal attitudes and barriers in the environment, not by their impairment.[11] Thus the goal of the service system should be to provide access to the same freedoms and life enjoyed by nondisabled persons, including the right to live separately, autonomously, and independently; work at paying jobs; marry and have a family; and generally realize their potential as human beings.

As part of the notion that disabled individuals should lead normal lives, the philosophy holds that those individuals should be integrated into community life. For example, one definition of *normalization* insists that services "must recognize and reflect that individual's dignity as a person, his/her natural membership in a native society and community, and his/her right to live as closely as possible in the manner of the culture."[12] Not surprisingly, advocates strongly dislike institutions because they separate the individual from the rest of society. Because the population with disabilities seeks to live as normal a life as possible, it follows that assistance should be provided wherever the disabled person wants to go—to work, to the shopping center, or to the movies. Likewise, to lead an independent life, persons with disabilities will assume multiple roles throughout their lives—as parents, employees, and community activists—and should have the assistance they need to fulfill these roles. Thus the emphasis is on community services, not home care.[13]

Second, this philosophy insists that disabled persons are capable of making decisions about their lives. For persons with mental retardation and mental illness, the scope of decisionmakers is usually expanded to include family and friends, although not always. Adherents of this philosophy oppose medical models of long-term care, professional case management, and all institutions (including nursing homes, mental hospitals, and intermediate care facilities for mentally retarded persons), because decisionmaking authority resides in someone other than the disabled person. Instead, they support consumer-directed services—that is, when the disabled person hires, fires, and directs the long-term care service worker.[14]

Third, because each person is different, the philosophy holds that services should be tailored to the individual needs and desires of each disabled person. Inevitably, each individual has different wants and needs. As a result, the range of services provided must be much broader than the homemaker and personal care services that dominate noninstitutional services for the elderly disabled population and should include anything that maximizes the independence and life of the individual.[15] Many advocates urge provision of cash benefits or tax credits instead of services, thus giving disabled persons complete freedom to choose whatever services they like from whatever provider they want.[16] The emphasis on a broad range of services blurs the boundaries between long-term care and other services (such as vocational training).

A traditional goal of long-term care for elderly persons has been to create a seamless continuum of care (including personal care, home health, congregate housing, and nursing homes) along which the aging individual would move as his or her needs changed. Rejecting this model as too narrow, advocates support systems in which services follow the individual and are provided regardless of where the individual lives. People should not have to move from place to place as their needs and desires change.

Fourth, if disabled persons are capable of living normal lives and making their own decisions, then they should receive services as a matter of right, not as a result of charity. In one striking contrast with the elderly population, unpaid, informal care from family and friends is considered an undesirable substitute for paid care because it leaves persons with disabilities vulnerable to the whims of their caregivers.

To replace the existing system, advocates for people with disabili- ᵥ ties have proposed a more unified financing system that would provide a broader range of mechanisms for persons with disabilities to finance their personal needs. The basic premise of the financing system would be the individual's need for personal assistance, not their financial circumstances. Thus, while limited cost-sharing provisions could be acceptable for higher-income persons with disabilities, no one would be turned away from services.[17] Underlying this proposed financing system is the idea that people with disabilities have a right to economic parity with the nondisabled population; they should not be forced to impoverish themselves or their families to obtain services.[18]

DELIVERY SYSTEM ORGANIZATION

Although the use of institutions by the younger population with disabilities is declining, they still play a significant role in the delivery of long-term care services for this population, especially those with mental retardation or developmental disabilities. In 1987, younger persons with disabilities accounted for approximately 40 percent of the population with severe disabilities living in the community, but they made up only 10 percent of the nursing home and personal care home population.[19]

Although nursing homes never played a major role in providing services to younger persons with disabilities, intermediate care facilities for persons with mental retardation (ICF/MRs) and mental hospitals historically have been at the center of services for their target populations. As of 1993, 147,729 persons, most under age 65, were residents of medicaid-certified ICF/MRs.[20] As a result of policy changes and numerous court cases, the proportion of residents in large facilities has dropped dramatically since 1977.[21]

Inpatient hospital mental health services are provided by state and county governments, private organizations, general hospitals, and the Department of Veterans Affairs. An estimated 197,277 nonelderly adults were residents of such institutions in 1990.[22] Similar to services for mentally retarded and developmentally disabled persons, the role of mental hospitals, especially those run by the states, has declined significantly over the years.[23]

For persons with disabilities who live at home, the existing delivery system relies heavily on informal care. In 1986 an estimated 87 percent of noninstitutionalized persons ages 15 to 64 who reported needing help with personal care, getting around the house, preparing meals, doing housework, or managing their money received help from family members.[24]

Paid services account for a small, but significant, share of home care. Of the nearly 6 million users of formal home care in 1987, about half were under age 65.[25] Consumer-directed personal assistance services (PAS) have emerged at the heart of efforts by advocates for the younger disabled population to expand community-based long-term care services for the physically disabled population. The World Institute on Disability defined PAS as "assistance, under maximum feasible user control, with tasks aimed at maintaining well-being, personal appearance, comfort, safety, and interactions within the community and society as a whole."[26] This definition could be broadened to encompass the special needs of persons with cognitive impairment, including assistance with planning and managing daily life.[27]

Policy Issues

The focus of the disability community on flexible, consumer-directed home and community-based services raises several questions related to the role of institutions, broadened flexibility of services, the impact of managed care, and the barriers to consumer-directed personal assistance services.

Replacing institutional care. A strong dividing line between younger and older persons with disabilities relates to the role of institutions in the long-term care delivery system. Advocates for the younger population with disabilities view institutions as the antithesis of almost everything that the delivery system should be—little personal autonomy and empowerment, segregation from the community, professional domination, and standardized services that do not meet the needs of individuals—and want to see their role radically reduced.[28]

Using litigation to require treatment in the least restrictive alternative, advocates for mentally ill persons and persons with mental retardation or developmental disabilities sued to transfer clients out of institutions and lobbied for increased funding for community-based services, with varying success.[29] In contrast, while elderly persons seek to avoid nursing home placement, there is a general acceptance of a major role for institutions for severely disabled older persons, especially for those without family support.[30]

A key question for policymakers is whether the advocates' goal of radically reducing institutional services and replacing them with home and community-based care is practical and affordable.[31] As states reduced the number of people in large state mental hospitals and ICF/MRs, they generally moved the least disabled persons first, leaving the population with the most severe disabilities in institutions.[32] By and large, the population remaining in institutions is very severely disabled and requires constant supervision and intensive services.[33]

Although virtually everyone could be served in the community if enough resources were available, the question is how much does it cost to do so for very severely disabled persons, especially those with cognitive impairment. A traditional justification of institutions has been that economies of scale allow services to be provided on a less costly basis. As discussed by Korbin Liu, Jean Hanson, and Teresa Coughlin in chapter 9, providing home and community-based services to severely disabled elderly persons could exceed the cost of nursing home care, especially for persons without strong informal supports.

However, ICF/MRs are so expensive that community-based services are commonly less costly on a per person basis. The cost per person in ICF/MRs averaged $62,180 in 1993, while the cost per person under the medicaid home and community-based waiver program averaged $25,176.[34] ICF/MRs are expensive because they serve a dwindling population of highly disabled persons, must meet strict regulatory standards, employ staff with relatively high salaries, and commonly have physical plants with high fixed costs.[35]

Although per person costs remain an issue, what traditionally bedevils home and community-based care is the increased number of persons who might use a broad range of community-based services if they were available. Extensive research suggests that, in demonstration projects offering expanded home care to elderly persons, total costs rose rather than declined.[36] Large increases in home care use more than offset relatively small reductions in nursing home use. Similar dynamics could work for the younger population, although it is not certain. Many countries attempt to force a substitution of home care for institutional services for elderly persons by having a conscious policy of constraining the growth in institutional services.[37]

Of particular concern to budgeteers is that the broader and more inclusive the range of services provided, the more likely that disabled persons will find something on the menu of services that they want, further increasing the number of persons receiving services or monetary benefits. What disabled person would not want additional cash, especially if it could be spent on anything he or she wants? Advocates for the younger disabled population argue that, given a choice, the consumer would choose lower cost and a lesser volume of services than would be authorized by professionals.[38] They also suggest that untapped efficiencies associated with the use of assistive technology and environmental modifications are available that the traditional service model largely ignores.[39]

Flexibility and scope of services. The broader range of consumer-directed services advocated by the disability community implies a reconsideration of issues associated with accountability for public funds. In particular, what is the responsibility of taxpayers to the disabled population? Is the public's responsibility only to help disabled persons meet certain basic, minimal needs, or is it to truly help people with disabilities realize their potential and live life as nondisabled persons do? Providing disabled persons with help getting dressed or going to the bathroom is one thing, but if a disabled person maximizes his or her independence by going bungee jumping or to the beach, is that an acceptable use of public dollars? And who decides? Individuals using private funds can do whatever they want, but the limits, if any, on the use of public funds are not clearly delineated.

A major issue for the nonelderly disabled population is the extent to which the existing long-term care delivery system could be adapted to encourage greater work force participation. Although less than one-quarter of the working-age population with disabilities is employed, most unemployed disabled adults say they would like to work.[40] Advocates view real employment, as opposed to sheltered workshops that pay substandard wages, as the key to financial independence for adults with disabilities.[41] They suggest greater emphasis be placed on helping persons with disabilities find and keep a job—for example, by providing training and on-the-job support in the form of job coaches for persons with mental retardation, and through use of assistive technology or personal care assistance for persons with physical disabilities. This strategy requires a rethinking of existing income support programs that encourage dependency by limiting eligibility to persons who are unable to work, while raising questions about the extent to which public funding should be used to subsidize private-sector employment of persons with disabilities.

Managed care. As with the elderly population, increasing policy interest is evident in integrating acute and long-term care services, principally through the use of health maintenance organizations (HMOs) and other forms of managed care.[42] Several initiatives are either under way or being developed to use managed care with the younger disabled population.[43] A major concern of advocates for disabled persons is that long-term care will become overmedicalized and less consumer directed in integrated settings. Some argue that the essence of managed care is the shift in the balance of power from the client and his or her chosen provider to HMOs, insurance companies, or other administrative entities.[44] Managed care need not, however, mean a loss of consumer empowerment. If consumer-directed services and self-help strategies cost less than agency-directed services, then using these approaches would be in the financial interest of managed care organizations.

Personal assistance services. Although few would dispute that personal assistance is a key component of long-term care for people with severe disabilities, a more controversial issue is whether services should be agency or consumer directed. Most personal assistance service programs are agency based, meaning that a third party is responsible for hiring, firing, and directing workers.[45] Proponents of agency-directed models contend that this structure enhances accountability; ensures adequate supervision of staff; improves efficiency of personnel allocation; guarantees compliance with requirements for payment of social security, unemployment, and other taxes; and assures quality of care.

Rejecting these arguments, advocates of a consumer-directed model argue that persons who use the services should be in direct control of their delivery.[46] The person with disabilities should have the authority to hire, train, supervise, direct, and, if necessary, fire the attendant.[47] This power gives the disabled individual greater flexibility in scheduling and assigning tasks to be performed. Almost by definition, the worker does what the client wants done.

The use of consumer-directed PAS raises at least five issues. First and foremost is whether disabled individuals are able to perform the necessary functions. Arguably, the model consumer for the younger disability movement is a person with an advanced degree who is disabled because of a car accident that left him or her with quadriplegia. Although managing one's source of care can be extremely demanding, few would dispute that the cognitively intact population with physical disabilities are intellectually capable of performing these functions. More controversial, however, is the applicability of this model to persons with severe mental illness, profound mental retardation, or advanced Alzheimer's disease. In these cases, the decisionmaker is not the person with disabilities, but a family member or personal advocate of some kind. In these circumstances, conflicts sometimes emerge among surrogate decisionmakers.[48] In other cases, surrogate decisionmakers are not available.

No research has been done on who is likely to have the individual management capacities necessary to handle the responsibilities of consumer-directed services, but the World Institute on Disability compared the skills required to manage an attendant to those required to run a small business.[49] Thus some advocates of consumer-driven services stress the importance of providing information and counseling to aid the disabled person in finding and assessing services.[50] Advocates for persons with developmental disabilities sometimes refer to a circle of friends to describe the type of informal structures based on individualized relationships among people in a community (a church group, for example) that provide a natural environment in which adults with disabilities could find support in managing their service needs.[51]

Closely related to the issue of whether an individual has the capacity to manage his or her services is whether everyone with disabilities wants to do so. In a pilot survey of fifty-four users of home care in Minnesota, Nancy N. Eustis and Lucy Rose Fischer found that younger persons were more likely to make their own decisions about home care.[52] In general, they found older clients relied more on family and paid medical professionals (home care agencies and others). The authors observed that distinctions between older and younger clients "seemed to reflect differences in health status, the availability of family members and regulations regarding the reimbursement of service providers as well as differences in client age."[53]

Second, the presumption of consumer-directed advocates is that the market for personal assistance workers functions relatively well. But during the late 1980s shortages of nurses and home health aides were reported in many parts of the country.[54] Personal assistance workers tend to be poorly educated, low-skilled, and poorly paid workers with high levels of turnover.[55] Moreover, given the difficulty of hiring workers, disabled persons may put up with unsatisfactory employees because they do not want to go through the effort of finding a replacement, could be unable to survive with a break in service, or could fear retribution from the fired service worker.[56] Finally, without agency backup, disabled persons could be especially vulnerable when an attendant does not show up for work.

Third, one of the most contentious issues between agency providers of home care and advocates of consumer-directed services concerns quality assurance. At the very least, defining what services a personal care attendant may provide raises questions of potential conflict with state nurse practice laws. Most states prohibit paid unlicensed providers from performing nursing functions, such as giving injections and catheter assistance, but some states have made exceptions for personal assistance services. Disability advocacy groups tend to be dismissive of the question of how quality of care is to be assured, but there is a long history of providers exploiting disabled elderly persons.[57]

Fourth, although persons with disabilities are free to enter into contracts for the provision of services on a private basis, the nature of the employment contract is problematic for publicly financed personal assistance service programs. A threshold issue is whether attendants are employees of the disabled person or independent contractors. Employers have certain normal financial responsibilities for their employees—including payment of salary, social security, and unemployment compensation taxes and withholding of federal, state, and local income taxes—and must assume some degree of liability for the actions of their workers. Severely disabled persons, especially those with mental illness, mental retardation, or cognitive impairment, could find these responsibilities difficult to perform, but government payers would rather not assume them.

Fifth, one of the attractions to policymakers of personal assistance services is the potential of providing services at lower per unit cost. Lance Egley concluded that independent providers of personal care services, who on average earned just slightly above the federal minimum wage, cost about half of what agencies charged in 1989.[58] Lower wages and benefits and lower administrative expenses each accounted for about half of the price differential.[59] Deborah A. Stone and others questioned the equity of depending on a low-wage work force with few benefits and little or no job security.[60] In addition, advocates of agency services contend that the administrative expenses represent valuable supervision of workers, quality assurance, and more efficient scheduling of workers.

LONG-TERM CARE FINANCING

Long-term care services for the younger population with disabilities are financed by a bewildering array of sources, including a large number of public programs at the federal and state level (mainly medicaid and medicare), out-of-pocket payments, and private insurance.[61] Public programs dominate the financing of long-term care for the younger population (table 12-4). Advocates for younger disabled persons consider the existing financing system flawed. In addition to overall spending levels being inadequate, funding is mostly limited to institutions and to a narrow set of home and community-based services. Furthermore, the reliance on medicaid excludes large numbers of persons who are not poor but who cannot afford to pay for services out of pocket. In addition, strong work disincentives are endemic to the medicaid program as a result of efforts to limit eligibility to persons unable to work. Finally, private long-term care insurance, which holds some promise for elderly persons, is unlikely to work for the younger population.

TABLE 12-4. *Public and Private Long-Term Care Expenditures, 1993*

Billions of dollars

Age group	Institutional services	Home and community-based services	Total
Under 65			
Public			
Medicare	0.2	0.7	0.9
Medicaid	12.8	3.6	16.4
Federal	7.3	2.0	9.2
State	5.5	1.6	7.1
Other	2.2	4.0	6.2
Federal	0.3	0.0	0.3
State	1.9	4.0	5.9
Total public	15.2	8.3	23.5
Private			
Out of pocket and other	1.4	3.7	5.1
Long-term care insurance	0.0	0.0	0.0
Total private	1.4	3.7	5.1
Total under 65	16.6	12.0	28.6
Over 65			
Public			
Medicare	5.5	9.4	14.9
Medicaid	23.5	3.8	27.3
Federal	13.3	2.1	15.4
State	10.2	1.7	11.9
Other	1.3	2.1	3.4
Federal	0.7	1.6	2.3
State	0.6	0.5	1.1
Total public	30.3	15.3	45.6
Private			
Out of pocket and other	28.2	5.2	33.4
Long-term care insurance	0.1	0.1	0.2
Total private	28.3	5.3	33.6
Total over 65	58.6	20.6	79.2
Total all ages	75.2	32.6	107.8

Source: Office of the Assistant Secretary for Planning and Evaluation, *Cost Estimates for the Long-Term Care Provisions under the Health Security Act*, tables 2–4, pp. 5–6.

Note: Based on data about elderly persons, physically disabled persons, and persons with mental retardation or developmental disabilities. Funding for mentally ill persons was not included. Totals may not be exact because of rounding.

Public Sources of Financing

Medicaid, the federal-state health care program for poor Americans, covers care in nursing facilities, ICF/MRs, mental hospitals for persons under age 22 or age 65 and over, home health care, personal care, and a variety of other home and community-based services. Program eligibility for younger persons with disabilities is limited to low-income persons with few assets and is largely linked to receipt of cash assistance through the supplemental security income (SSI) program. Excluding mental health services, medicaid spent approximately $44 billion on long-term care in 1993, of which an estimated 38 percent was for the nonelderly population. Medicaid accounted for a significantly larger proportion of long-term care financing for the younger population with disabilities than for elderly persons.

Medicaid is an especially important source of financing for institutional long-term care services. Total medicaid nursing home and ICF/MR expenditures were $36.3 million in 1993, of which approximately 35 percent was spent on the nonelderly population.[62] Although relatively few younger people are in nursing homes, the nonelderly population is far more dependent on medicaid to finance their care than is the elderly population.[63] The vast majority of residents of ICF/MRs are under age 65, and virtually all are medicaid eligible.[64] Medicaid plays a somewhat smaller role in financing institutional mental health services than might be expected because federal law specifically excludes coverage for persons ages 22 to 64 in "institutions for mental disease."[65] However, medicaid pays for inpatient mental health services in general hospitals for persons of all ages.[66]

Medicaid also plays an important role in financing noninstitutional long-term care services for younger persons with disabilities. Total medicaid noninstitutional long-term care expenditures were $7.4 billion in 1993, of which an estimated 49 percent was spent on the nonelderly population.[67]

Coverage for personal care and waiver services varied by state. As of 1994, thirty states and the District of Columbia offered personal care services as an option to at least some medicaid beneficiaries.[68] New York accounted for two-thirds of national medicaid personal care expenditures.[69]

Under Section 2176 of the Omnibus Budget Reconciliation Act of 1981 (P.L. 97-35), states can request a waiver of medicaid rules to provide a wide range of noninstitutional long-term care services. In addition, the waiver authority allows states to limit the number of participants and to more tightly target services than is allowed under the medicaid personal care program. Most states have at least one waiver, although many target only a small number of persons.[70] In 1992 spending for persons with mental retardation and developmental disabilities accounted for about two-thirds of the expenditures under medicaid's home and community-based waiver program.[71] Recent changes in federal regulations eased the waiver approval criteria somewhat, but the target population remains persons who would be institutionalized without home-based services.[72]

Disabled persons who receive social security disability insurance (SSDI) for twenty-four months are eligible for medicare. Medicare plays a modest role in financing long-term care for elderly persons, accounting for about 20 percent of nursing home and home care expenditures in 1993.[73] In contrast, medicare paid for just 3 percent of total long-term care expenditures for the younger population with disabilities in 1993.

State funding accounts for a substantially greater proportion of long-term care spending for the nonelderly population than for older people. Excluding medicaid matching payments, the states contributed 20 percent of the total long-term care expenditures for the nonelderly population compared with just 1 percent for the elderly population in 1993. This dramatic difference was likely explained by several factors, including advocacy at the state level for persons with developmental disabilities and mental retardation.[74]

Policy Issues

The existing system of financing raises at least five major issues. First, as with services, financing for the younger population is mostly available for institutional rather than noninstitutional services. In 1993 an estimated 58 percent of total long-term care expenditures for the younger disabled population was for nursing homes and ICF/MRs. Disability advocates argue that vast sums are wasted on unwanted institutional care.[75] For example, American Disabled for Attendant Programs Today (ADAPT) demands that 25 percent of federal nursing home expenditures be redirected to personal attendant services.[76]

Second, a fundamental conflict exists between open-ended entitlement programs, such as medicaid, and the government financing of a very broad range of services. An entitlement is a legal obligation of the government to provide services to individuals who meet established criteria regardless of the aggregate cost. As we discussed in the section on services, the basic dilemma is that the more flexible the set of services provided, the more difficult it is to keep expenditures within a preestablished amount. The broader the range of available services, the more likely persons will use them, raising overall expenditures. Thus programs that provide a very wide range of services often have capped funding and no legal entitlement. In such programs, the number of persons receiving services can be controlled, largely eliminating the problem of induced demand. However, a major risk of capped programs is that funding may not increase over time to compensate for inflation and increasing numbers of persons with disabilities.[77]

Third, eligibility rules for medicare and medicaid encourage dependence, not independence. Specifically, to qualify for medicaid or medicare as a disabled person, applicants must meet the requirements for eligibility for SSDI or SSI cash benefit programs, which are based on an inability to work.[78] In addition, SSDI and SSI regulations require applicants to demonstrate that their disability would likely last for at least a year or result in death and meets established medical criteria. SSDI applicants must have previously been employed (or be a disabled widow or child of someone eligible for social security coverage) and must demonstrate that their current earnings are less than $500 per month, a level of income determined to represent "substantial gainful activity."[79] SSI eligibility rules do not require a work history, but applicants must meet their state's means-test for substantial gainful activity (generally less than $446 per month in income) and have no more than $2,000 in assets.[80] Severely disabled persons whose earnings exceed the substantial gainful activity criteria are ineligible for medicaid and medicare, even if they may need services. In 1994 a total of 7.2 million persons under age 65 received SSDI or SSI benefits based on disability.[81]

As a result of the linkage of medicaid eligibility to an inability to work, disabled persons are presented with a difficult dilemma: They can work and lose not only income support, but also health and long-term care coverage, or they can remain unemployed and continue to receive benefits but give up the opportunity for financial and personal independence. Ironically, the long-term care benefits that enable an individual to work will be withdrawn precisely because the person is working. Under the existing system, few disabled beneficiaries leave the rolls of either SSDI or SSI.[82] Initiatives designed to lessen the work disincentive by allowing more employed disabled persons to retain medicaid coverage have not resulted in increased levels of employment among persons in the SSI program.[83] Nor does it appear that the Americans with Disabilities Act has increased the labor force participation of persons with disabilities.[84]

A closely related problem is that the important sources of long-term care financing are means tested. Compared with more universalistic approaches, means-tested programs often have lower political support, stigmatize beneficiaries, and provide inferior access to services that are sometimes of lesser quality.[85] Moreover, although many severely disabled persons have low incomes and meet the income and asset tests of medicaid, others who work are likely to make too much money to qualify for benefits. Medicare is not a means-tested program, but it does not cover much in the way of long-term care services.

A major disadvantage of all universalistic approaches to long-term care is their expense. The Clinton administration's proposals for a home care program for persons with severe disabilities of all ages would have cost an additional $34 billion in 2003, when fully phased in.[86] The combination of an intractable federal budget deficit and resistance to new taxes makes this a formidable barrier.

Finally, with growing resistance to the expansion of public programs, there is increasing interest in private long-term care insurance as a means of financing services. Unfortunately, its role in financing long-term care is limited by problems of affordability and marketability. Most studies found that only a relatively small minority of the elderly population—generally 10 to 20 percent—could afford private long-term care insurance.[87] Other studies found the percentage of elderly persons who could afford private insurance to be higher, but they assumed that policies with limited coverage were purchased, expected that elderly persons would use their assets as well as income to pay premiums, or excluded a large proportion of elderly individuals from the pool of people considered interested in purchasing insurance.[88]

Although the purchase of individual policies by the nonelderly population could largely solve the affordability problem, most younger persons are not interested in buying policies.[89] Moreover, because all individually sold policies are medically underwritten, the younger disabled population is excluded from purchasing policies. Although long-term care policies sold through the employer-group market often do not require medical underwriting for active employees, this segment of the market is still small and labor force participation by working-age persons with disabilities is low.[90]

A RESEARCH AGENDA FOR THE FUTURE

Our synthesis of policy issues and research concerning the younger disabled population's need for, use of, and financing of long-term care services began with the premise that, although not much is known about the nonelderly population with disabilities, they are an increasingly important force in the policy arena. Any future policy initiatives in long-term care will almost certainly include the younger as well as the older disabled population.

This review of policy-oriented research pointed to two major gaps in the literature. First, existing national survey data are inadequate in providing useful information about the younger population with disabilities. In large part because of small sample sizes in most surveys, even something as basic as the prevalence of disability cannot be estimated with any precision. Small sample sizes also prevent the use of multivariate statistical techniques. Current data on persons with mental illness, mental retardation, and children with disabilities are especially weak. Longitudinal data in particular are lacking. As a result, data limitations inhibit policy development. The 1994–95 disability supplement to the National Health Interview Survey represents a major step forward because of its large sample of younger persons with disabilities.[91]

The second major gap concerns research on differences between consumer-directed and agency-directed services for the disabled population. Although advocates for the younger population with disabilities are nearly unanimous in their support for consumer-directed service approaches, virtually no empirical research has been done on the cost, effectiveness, and quality of service provided through this strategy. Potential areas for research relate to the level of self-directedness feasible for different subpopulations; the functioning of the market for consumer-directed personal assistance services; and the use, cost, quality, and outcomes of services. Research on the use of personal care assistance services should also include an examination of the role of informal caregiving among younger persons with disabilities.

The pure model of consumer-directed services assumes a cognitively intact individual who has the energy, determination, and intelligence to take on the responsibilities of hiring, training, directing, and firing workers. Not all disabled persons want these responsibilities or are cognitively capable of performing these tasks on their own. Even admitting that the answer varies with differing levels of awareness, the question is what role do disabled persons want in directing their services and how does that change across subpopulations? For example, what do consumer-directed services mean for a person with severe mental retardation?

Consumer-directed services generally assume the efficiency and effectiveness of an extremely well-functioning free market. Especially for personal assistance services, this raises a variety of questions, including: How easy is hiring workers? What kind of training do workers need? What kind of employer-employee problems evolve and how are they resolved? How is poor quality performance addressed?

A major premise of consumer-directed services is that persons with disabilities use different kinds and amounts of services than they would in an agency-directed system. Is that accurate and if so, in what ways? This is a question particularly for programs that provide disabled persons with great flexibility in the choice of services. In programs with a great deal of flexibility, a key consideration is whether money would be spent on services that are somehow deemed inappropriate from a public policy perspective.

Advocates for persons with disabilities contend that consumer-directed services are less costly than agency-directed services because persons with disabilities will choose cheaper services and use less of them than they would under more traditional approaches. With the availability of an extremely broad range of services, skeptics worry that everybody would find some service that he or she wants. As a result, overall levels of program participation, utilization, and costs would be much higher than under a system with fewer choices. Which vision is accurate, and why? If consumer-directed services are less expensive, is it because workers are paid lower wages and have fewer benefits, or is it because of lower administrative overhead? What, if anything, is lost from not having that level of management?

Defenders of agency-directed services argue that quality of care is lower with consumer-directed services and that chances of abuse are higher because workers are not supervised by professionals accountable for the services provided. Accepting the fact that measuring quality of care is extremely difficult and that definitions of quality could differ between consumers and professionals, is this assertion accurate? If so, are there quality assurance mechanisms that could be used successfully with consumer-directed approaches?

A variety of policy initiatives would increase the use of managed care to provide acute and, sometimes, long-term care services to younger persons with disabilities, but there is little experience or research on managed care with this population. These managed care organizations may do better at controlling health care spending and could provide more coordinated care. Yet access to potentially beneficial but costly services could be reduced. The impact of managed care on costs, utilization, and quality for younger persons with disabilities is an especially critical issue about which little is known. Also of great importance is whether or not managed care is consistent with consumer-directed services.

Finally, overlaying all of these research topics is the question of whether the elderly and younger disabled populations are fundamentally different. One possibility is that the divergence between the elderly and younger populations with disabilities is an historical artifact that will fade over time as the baby boom generation ages. Persons of all ages who have disabilities want more choices in meeting their long-term care needs. The alternate possibility is that differences are more deep-seated and would persist. Does a single financing and delivery system for persons of all ages with disabilities make sense, or should there be separate systems for the younger and older populations? Within the younger disabled population, are there major distinctions that mean program designs should be different?

NOTES

1. Estimates of the nonelderly population with disabilities varied in part because of the use of several different definitions of disability. For example, based on the 1993 National Health Interview Survey, 73 percent of the civilian noninstitutionalized population who reported they were limited in their major

activity because of a chronic condition were under age 65. An individual's major life activity was defined by age-appropriate activities: ordinary play for children under age 5; attending school for ages 5 to 17; working or keeping house for ages 18 to 69, and living independently (without need of assistance from another person to perform activities of daily living [ADLs]) for ages 70 and above. Authors' calculations based on data in Veronica Benson and Marie A. Marano, "Current Estimates from the National Health Interview Survey, 1993," *Vital and Health Statistics,* series 10, no. 190 (Hyattsville, Md.: Department of Health and Human Services, Public Health Service, National Center for Health Statistics, December 1994), table 68, p. 108. Studies of the prevalence of disability in the U.S. population that focused primarily on limitations in the ability to perform basic ADLs judged the proportion of the population with disabilities who were under age 65 to be from 33 to 42 percent. See, for example, Mitchell P. LaPlante, *Disability in Basic Life Activities Across the Life Span,* Disability Statistics Report 1 (Department of Education, National Institute on Disability and Rehabilitation Research, 1991), pp. 2–3; Office of the Assistant Secretary for Planning and Evaluation, Office of Disability, Aging, and Long-Term Care Policy, *Cost Estimates for the Long-Term Care Provisions under the Health Security Act* (Department of Health and Human Services, March 1994), table 8, p. 11; General Accounting Office, *Long-Term Care: Diverse, Growing Population Includes Millions of Americans of All Ages,* GAO/HEHS-95-26 (November 1994), p. 4; and Michele Adler, "Population Estimates of Disability and Long-Term Care," *ASPE Research Note* (Department of Health and Human Services, Assistant Secretary for Planning and Evaluation, Office of Disability, Aging, and Long-Term Care Policy, February 1995).

2. Not all policy decisions that concern people with disabilities are related to long-term care. On other issues—income support, for example—there has been a long-standing interest among policymakers in the working-age population with disabilities. Deborah A. Stone, *The Disabled State* (Temple University Press, 1984); and President's Committee on Employment of People with Disabilities' 1993 Teleconference Project, "Operation People First: Toward a National Disability Policy," *Journal of Disability Policy Studies,* vol. 5, no. 2 (1994), pp. 81–106.

3. Joshua Wiener and Laurel Hixon Illston, "Health Care Reform in the 1990s: Where Does Long-Term Care Fit In?," *Gerontologist,* vol. 34 (June 1994), pp. 402–408.

4. Throughout this chapter, the term *disability movement* is used to denote the varied organizations that represent persons with disabilities while recognizing that these groups do not speak with a single voice. The intent is not to minimize differences, but to highlight the commonalities among individuals and advocacy organizations that share the broad goal of achieving greater independence for persons with disabilities in all aspects of their lives. Similarly,

the terms *younger persons with disabilities* and *disabled persons* describe a heterogeneous population of individuals. In the context of this discussion, disability encompasses both biological and social dimensions.

5. Mitchell P. LaPlante estimated that up to one-half of the adult population could be defined as disabled if the definition included all persons with chronic conditions. Mitchell P. LaPlante, "Demographics of Disability," *Milbank Quarterly*, vol. 69, supplements 1 and 2 (1991), pp. 64–65.

6. Ibid., p. 64. LaPlante found that a significant percentage of persons who reported they could not perform their major activity did not identify themselves as disabled.

7. John M. McNeil, "Americans with Disabilities: 1991–92, Data from the Survey of Income and Program Participation," *Current Population Reports, Household Economic Studies*, series P-70, no. 33 (Department of Commerce, Bureau of the Census, 1993).

8. Gerben DeJong, "Independent Living: From Social Movement to Analytic Paradigm," *Archives of Physical Medicine and Rehabilitation*, vol. 60 (1979), pp. 435–46.

9. Andrew I. Batavia, Gerben DeJong, and Louise Bouscaren McKnew, "Toward a National Personal Assistance Program: The Independent Living Model of Long-Term Care for Persons with Disabilities," *Journal of Health Politics, Policy, and Law*, vol. 16, no. 3 (Fall 1991), pp. 523–45; William A. Anthony, "Recovery from Mental Illness: The Guiding Visions of the Mental Health Service System in the 1990s," *Psychosocial Rehabilitation Journal*, vol. 16, no. 4 (April 1993), pp. 11–23; Patricia E. Deegan, "The Independent Living Movement and People with Psychiatric Disabilities: Taking Back Control of Our Own Lives," *Psychosocial Rehabilitation Journal*, vol. 15, no. 3 (January 1992), pp. 3–19; Julie Ann Racino and Judith E. Heumann, "Independent Living and Community Life: Building Coalitions among Elders, People with Disabilities, and Our Allies," in Edward F. Ansello and Nancy N. Eustis, eds., *Aging and Disabilities: Seeking Common Ground* (Amityville, N.Y.: Baywood, 1992), pp. 79–90; and Elizabeth Monroe Boggs, "Benchmarks of Change in the Field of Developmental Disabilities," in Valerie J. Bradley, John W. Ashbaugh, and Bruce C. Blaney, eds., *Creating Individual Supports for People with Developmental Disabilities: A Mandate for Change at Many Levels* (Baltimore: Brookes, 1994), pp. 46–54.

10. Lori Simon-Rusinowitz and Brian F. Hofland, "Adopting a Disability Approach to Home Care Services for Older Adults," *Gerontologist*, vol. 33, no. 2 (1993), pp. 159–67.

11. DeJong, "Independent Living"; and David Pfeiffer, "Overview of the Disability Movement: History, Legislative Record, and Political Implications," *Policy Studies Journal*, vol. 21, no. 4 (1993), pp. 724–34.

12. K. Charlie Lakin and others, *Medicaid Services for Persons with Mental*

Retardation and Related Conditions (University of Minnesota, Institute on Community Integration, 1989), pp. 7–8.

13. Simon-Rusinowitz and Hofland, "Adopting a Disability Approach to Home Care Services for Older Adults."

14. Simi Litvak, Hale Zukas, and Judith E. Heumann, *Attending to America: Personal Assistance for Independent Living* (Oakland, Calif.: World Institute on Disability, April 1987).

15. Evidence from the home care demonstration projects and the medicaid Home and Community-Based Waiver Programs targeted to older people indicated that about 75 percent of the home care dollars were allocated to personal care, home health aide care, or homemaker services. Peter Kemper, Robert Applebaum, and Margaret Harrigan, "Community Care Demonstrations: What Have We Learned?," *Health Care Financing Review,* vol. 8, no. 4 (Summer 1987), pp. 87–100; and Nancy A. Miller, "Medicaid 2176 Home and Community-Based Waivers: The First Ten Years," *Health Affairs,* vol. 11, no. 4 (Winter 1992), pp. 162–71. For example, Julie Ann Racino and Pamela Walker suggested the following as a partial list of services that should be available to support persons with disabilities in the community: "live-in roommate; support from a neighbor; personal assistance; peer support; coordination; adaptive equipment; emergency back-up systems; meals on wheels; home-making and related tasks; creating a family; health care; basic academic skills; facilitation of decisionmaking and communication; work-related assistance; appliances, home furnishings, and other goods; income subsidy; housing related assistance; community connections, relationships, and social interactions." Julie Ann Racino and Pamela Walker, "Being with People: Support and Support Strategies," in Julie Ann Racino and others, eds., *Housing, Support, and Community: Choices and Strategies for Adults with Disabilities* (Baltimore: Brookes, 1994), p. 89.

16. Kathleen A. Cameron and James P. Firman, "International and Domestic Programs Using 'Cash and Counseling' Strategies to Pay for Long-Term Care," National Council on the Aging, March 1995; William Scanlon, "Possible Reforms for Financing Long-Term Care," *Journal of Economic Perspectives,* vol. 6 (Summer 1992), pp. 43–58; Litvak and others, *Attending to America*; and Charles Brecher and James Knickman, "A Reconsideration of Long-Term Care Policy," *Journal of Health Politics, Policy, and Law,* vol. 10 (Summer 1985), pp. 245–73.

17. See, for example, Consortium for Citizens with Disabilities, "Recommended Federal Policy Directions on Personal Assistance Services for Americans with Disabilities," November 1992; and Simi Litvak, "Financing Personal Assistance Services: Federal and State Legislative and Revenue Enhancing Options," *Journal of Disability Policy Studies,* vol. 20, no. 3 (1992), pp. 93–106.

18. Margaret A. Nosek and Carol A. Howland, "Personal Assistance Services: The Hub of the Policy Wheel for Community Integration of People with Severe Physical Disabilities," *Policy Studies Journal*, vol. 21, no. 4 (1993), pp. 789–800.

19. Mitchell P. Laplante and Karen S. Miller, "People with Disabilities in Basic Life Activities in the U.S.," *Disability Statistics Abstract*, no. 3 (Department of Education, National Institute on Disability and Rehabilitation Research, April 1992); and Tamra Lair, *A Profile of Nursing Home Users under Age 65*, AHCPR Pub. No. 92-006, National Medical Expenditure Survey, Research Findings 13, Agency for Health Care Policy and Research (Rockville, Md.: Department of Health and Human Services, Public Health Service, August 1992).

20. Troy Mangan and others, *Residential Services for Persons with Mental Retardation and Related Conditions: Status and Trends through 1993* (University of Minnesota, Institute on Community Integration, Research and Training Center on Residential Services and Community Living, June 1994); and Sheryl A. Larson and K. Charlie Lakin, *Status and Changes in Medicaid's Intermediate Care Facility for the Mentally Retarded (ICF-MR) Program: Results from Analysis of the Online Survey Certification and Reporting System* (University of Minnesota, Center on Residential Services and Community Living, Institute on Community Integration, 1995).

21. David Braddock and others, *The State of the States in Developmental Disabilities: Fourth National Study of Public Spending for Mental Retardation and Development Disabilities* (University of Illinois at Chicago, Institute on Disability and Human Development, October 1994), p. 7.

22. Joanne E. Atay, Michael J. Witkin, and Ronald W. Manderscheid, "Data Highlights on Utilization of Mental Health Organizations by Elderly Persons," *Mental Health Statistical Note*, no. 214 (February 1995), table 1.

23. Richard W. Redick and others, "Specialty Mental Health System Characteristics," in Ronald W. Manderscheid and Mary Anne Sonnenshein, eds., *Mental Health, United States, 1992* (Rockville, Md.: Department of Health and Human Services, Public Health Service, Center for Mental Health Services and National Institute of Mental Health, 1992), pp. 1–162.

24. Cynthia J. Harpine, John M. McNeil, and Enrique J. Lamas, "The Need for Personal Assistance with Everyday Activities: Recipients and Caregivers," *Current Population Reports, Household Economic Studies*, series P-70, no. 19 (Department of Commerce, Bureau of the Census, 1990).

25. Barbara M. Altman and Daniel C. Walden, "Home Health Care: Use, Expenditures, and Sources of Payment," AHCPR Pub. No. 93-0040, National Medical Expenditure Survey, Research Findings 15, Agency for Health Care Policy and Research (Rockville, Md.: Department of Health and Human Services, Public Health Service, April 1993).

26. Tasks include "1) personal maintenance and hygiene activities such as dressing, grooming, feeding, bathing, respiration, and toilet functions, including bowel, bladder, catheter and menstrual tasks; 2) mobility tasks (getting into and out of bed, wheelchair or tub); 3) infant and child-related tasks such as bathing, diapering and feeding; 4) household maintenance tasks such as cleaning, shopping, meal preparation, laundering, and long-term heavy cleaning and repairs; 5) cognitive or life management activities, money management, planning, and decisionmaking; 6) security-related services, such as daily monitoring by phone; and 7) communication services, such as interpreting for people with hearing or speech disabilities and reading for people with visual disabilities." Litvak and others, *Attending to America*, p. 1.

27. For a discussion of the range of tasks included for persons with cognitive impairment, see Julie Ann Racino, "Personal Assistance and Personal Support Services for/by/with Adults, Youth, and Children with Disabilities," revised paper prepared for the 1994 annual meeting of the American Public Health Association.

28. Joseph P. Shapiro, "Forcing the Young into Nursing Homes," *APF Reporter*, vol. 14, no. 1 (Winter 1991), pp. 11–15; and Joseph P. Shapiro, "A Life Worse than Death," *Washington Post*, April 15, 1990, p. D1.

29. Robert M. Gettings, "The Link between Public Financing and Systemic Change," in Valerie J. Bradley and others, eds., *Creating Individual Supports for People with Developmental Disabilities: A Mandate for Change at Many Levels* (Baltimore: Brookes, 1994), chapter 9; David Mechanic, "Mental Health Services in the Context of Health Insurance Reform," *Milbank Quarterly*, vol. 71, no. 3 (1993), pp. 349–64; and Theodore R. Marmor and Karyn C. Gill, "The Political and Economic Context of Mental Health Care in the United States," *Journal of Health Politics, Policy and Law*, vol. 14, no. 3 (Fall 1989), pp. 459–75.

30. Fully 95 percent of chronically disabled elderly persons living at home in 1982 said they would prefer to stay out of a nursing home as long as possible. Alice M. Rivlin and Joshua M. Wiener, with Raymond J. Hanley and Denise A. Spence, *Caring for the Disabled Elderly: Who Will Pay?* (Brookings, 1988), p. 15.

31. Gary A. Smith and Robert M. Gettings, *The HCB Waiver and CSLA Programs: An Update on Medicaid's Role in Supporting People with Developmental Disabilities in the Community* (Alexandria, Va.: National Association of State Directors of Developmental Disabilities Services, October 1994), p. 102.

32. Robert W. Prouty and K. Charlie Lakin, *A Summary of States' Efforts to Positively Affect the Quality of Medicaid Home and Community-Based Services for Persons with Mental Retardation and Related Conditions* (University of Minnesota, Institute on Community Integration, Center for Residential and Community Services, June 1991); and William R. Shadish, Jr., Arthur J. Lurigio, and Dan A.

Lewis, "After Deinstitutionalization: The Present and Future of Mental Health Long-Term Care Policy," *Journal of Social Issues*, vol. 45, no. 3 (1989), pp. 1–15.

33. Peter W. Shaughnessy and Andrew M. Kramer, "The Increased Needs of Patients in Nursing Homes and Patients Receiving Home Health Care," *New England Journal of Medicine*, vol. 322 (January 4, 1990), pp. 21–27; Larson and Lakin, *Status and Changes in Medicaid's Intermediate Care Facility for the Mentally Retarded (ICF-MR) Program*; and William H. Fisher and Barbara F. Phillips, "Modeling the Growth of Long-Term Populations in Public Mental Health Hospitals," *Social Science and Medicine*, vol. 30, no. 12 (1990), pp. 1341–47.

34. Mangan and others, *Residential Services for Persons with Mental Retardation and Related Conditions*, pp. 65–68.

35. Braddock and others, *The State of the States in Developmental Disabilities*; Mangan and others, *Residential Services for Persons with Mental Retardation and Related Conditions*; and Thomas Nerney and Ronald W. Conley, "A Policy Analysis of Community Costs for Persons with Severe Disabilities," *Journal of Disability Policy Studies*, vol. 3, no. 2 (1992), pp. 31–52.

36. Joshua M. Wiener and Raymond J. Hanley, "Caring for the Disabled Elderly: There's No Place Like Home," in Stephen M. Shortell and Uwe E. Reinhardt, eds., *Improving Health Policy and Management: Nine Critical Research Issues for the 1990s* (Ann Arbor, Mich.: Health Administration Press, 1992), pp. 75–110.

37. General Accounting Office, *Long-Term Care: Other Countries Tighten Budgets While Seeking Better Access*, GAO/HEHS-94-154 (August 1994).

38. Gary Smith, "Paying for Supports: Dollars, Payments, and the New Paradigm," in Valerie Bradley, John Ashbaugh, and Bruce Blaney, eds., *Creating Individual Supports for People with Developmental Disabilities: A Mandate for Change at Many Levels* (Baltimore: Brookes, 1994), pp. 481–90.

39. An evaluation funded by the Robert Wood Johnson Foundation of the New Hampshire Self-Determination Project, which provides funding to persons with disabilities, will explore the issue of whether cost savings could be achieved through a flexible budgeting system in which individuals and their advocates decide what to purchase. Budgets are based on a percentage of the costs of what the state was previously paying to provide assistance to that individual. One hypothesis to be tested is that allowing individuals with disabilities to make one-time investments in equipment or services would discourage long-term reliance on public funding and thus reduce costs over time. Cameron and Firman, "International and Domestic Programs Using 'Cash and Counseling' Strategies to Pay for Long-Term Care."

40. Louis Harris and Associates, *National Organization on Disability, Harris Survey of Americans with Disabilities* (Washington, 1994).

41. Kristin Magis-Agosta, "Organizational Transformations: Moving from

Facilities to Community Inclusive Employment," in Valerie Bradley, John Ashbaugh, and Bruce Blaney, eds., *Creating Individual Supports for People with Developmental Disabilities: A Mandate for Change at Many Levels* (Baltimore: Brookes, 1994), pp. 255–79.

42. Joshua M. Wiener and Jason Skaggs, *The Integration of Acute and Long-Term Care Financing and Services: A Policy Synthesis* (Washington: American Association of Retired Persons, forthcoming).

43. Ibid.

44. Mark Schlesinger and David Mechanic, "Challenges for Managed Competition from Chronic Illness," *Health Affairs,* supplement (1993), pp. 123–37.

45. Charles Sabatino and Simi Litvak, "Consumer-Directed Home Care: What Makes It Possible," in Edward F. Ansello and Nancy N. Eustis, eds., *Aging and Disabilities: Seeking Common Ground* (Amityville, N.Y.: Baywood, 1992), pp. 99–109.

46. Irving K. Zola, "Policies and Programs Concerning Aging and Disability: Toward a Unified Agenda," in Sean Sullivan and Marion Ein Lewin, eds., *The Economics and Ethics of Long-Term Care and Disability* (Washington: American Enterprise Institute for Public Policy Research, 1988), pp. 90–130; and Batavia and others, "Toward a National Personal Assistance Program."

47. Litvak and others, *Attending to America;* and Batavia and others, "Toward a National Personal Assistance Program."

48. See, for example, Jonathan Rabinovitz, "Future Plight of Retarded Adults Tied to School's Uncertain Fate," *New York Times,* March 13, 1995, pp. A1, B6.

49. "Activities of daily living and instrumental activities of daily living have become household concepts in long-term care, but a scale for 'activities of service management' is still a foreign notion." Sabatino and Litvak, "Consumer-Directed Homecare," p. 105; and Litvak and others, *Attending to America,* p. 109.

50. Cameron and Firman, "International and Domestic Programs Using 'Cash and Counseling' Strategies to Pay for Long-Term Care"; Racino, "Personal Assistance and Support Services for/by/with Adults, Youth, and Children with Disabilities"; and Margaret A. Nosek, "Personal Assistance for Persons with Mental Disability," Baylor College of Medicine, 1990.

51. See, for example, Racino and Walker, "Being with People," pp. 81–106.

52. Nancy N. Eustis and Lucy Rose Fischer, "Common Needs, Different Solutions? Younger and Older Homecare Clients," in Edward R. Ansello and Nancy N. Eustis, eds., *Aging and Disabilities: Seeking Common Ground* (Amityville, N.Y.: Baywood, 1992), pp. 25–37.

53. Eustis and Fischer, "Common Needs, Different Solutions?," p. 33.

54. *Long-Term Care Personnel: Incentives for Training and Career Development,* Hearings before the House Select Committee on Aging, 102 Cong. 1 sess. (Government Printing Office, March 4, 1991).

55. Anthony J. "Tony" Young, on behalf of the Consortium for Citizens with Disabilities Long-Term Services and Supports Task Force, testimony on H.R. 3600 submitted to Subcommittee on Health and the Environment of the House Energy and Commerce Committee, 103 Cong. 2 sess., February 3, 1994; and Batavia and others, "Toward a National Personal Assistance Program," p. 530.

56. Margaret A. Nosek, "Personal Assistance Services: A Review of the Literature and Analysis of Policy Implications," *Journal of Disability Policy Studies,* vol. 2, no. 2 (1992), pp. 1–17.

57. Bruce C. Vladeck, *Unloving Care: The Nursing Home Tragedy* (Basic Books, 1980); and Institute of Medicine, *Improving the Quality of Care in Nursing Homes* (Washington: National Academy Press, 1986).

58. Lance Egley, *Program Models Providing Personal Assistant Services (PAS) for Independent Living* (Oakland, Calif.: World Institute on Disability, May 1994).

59. Ibid.

60. Deborah A. Stone, "Caring Work in a Liberal Polity," *Journal of Health Politics, Policy, and Law,* vol. 16 (Fall 1991), pp. 547–52; Sabatino and Litvak, "Consumer-Directed Homecare," p. 103; and Pamela Doty and others, "Consumer Choice and the Frontline Worker," *Generations,* vol. 18, no. 3 (Fall 1994), pp. 65–70.

61. The National Academy of State Health Policy counted more than one hundred federal programs, including medicare and medicaid, that support people with disabilities. These include the following, which specifically target long-term care services: Social Services Block Grant (Title XX of the Social Services Act); Older Americans Act; Community Mental Health Services Block Grant; Department of Veterans Affairs (disabled veterans programs); U.S. Department of Education, Rehabilitation Act (Centers for Independent Living, Vocational Rehabilitative Services, Individuals with Disabilities Education Act); and Title V of the Social Security Act (Maternal and Child Health Block Grant programs for Children with Special Health Care Needs). See National Academy for State Health Policy, *A Guide to Federal Programs for People with Disabilities* (Portland, Maine, December 1994); and National Academy of Social Insurance, *Preliminary Status Report of the Disability Policy Panel* (Washington, March 1994), appendix C.

62. Teresa A. Coughlin, Leighton Ku, and John Holahan, *Medicaid Since 1980: Costs, Coverage, and the Shifting Alliance Between the Federal Government and the States* (Washington: Urban Institute Press, 1994).

63. Office of Assistant Secretary for Planning and Evaluation, Office of Disability, Aging, and Long-Term Care Policy, "Cost Estimates for the Long-Term Care Provisions under the Health Security Act."

64. Congressional Research Service, *Medicaid Source Book: Background Data and Analysis,* Committee Print, prepared for the Subcommittee on Health and the Environment of the House Energy and Commerce Committee, 103 Cong. 1 sess. (GPO, January 1993), p. 878.

65. Coughlin and others, *Medicaid since 1980,* p. 109.

66. Richard W. Redick and others, "Highlights of Organized Mental Health Services in 1990 and Major National and State Trends," in Ronald W. Manderscheid and Mary Anne Sonnenshein, eds., *Mental Health, United States, 1994* (GPO, 1994), pp. 77–125.

67. Office of Assistant Secretary for Planning and Evaluation, Office of Disability, Aging, and Long-Term Care Policy, "Cost Estimates for the Long Term Care Provisions of the Health Security Act," tables 2–4, pp. 5–6.

68. Brian Burwell, "Medicaid Long-Term Care Expenditures in FY 1994," SysteMetrics/MEDSTAT, Cambridge, Mass., April 14, 1995, appendix C.

69. Ibid.

70. Charlene Harrington and Richard DuNah, "The Medicaid Home and Community-Based Waiver Program in the States in 1992," University of California at San Francisco, Department of Social and Behavioral Sciences, November 1994.

71. Harrington and DuNah, "The Medicaid Home and Community-Based Waiver Program in the States in 1992," table 1.

72. Smith and Gettings, *The HCB Waiver and CSLA Programs.*

73. Joshua M. Wiener, Laurel Hixon Illston, and Raymond J. Hanley, *Sharing the Burden: Strategies for Public and Private Long-Term Care Insurance* (Brookings, 1994), table 2-3, p. 40.

74. David Braddock, "Community Mental Health and Mental Retardation Services in the United States: A Comparative Study of Resource Allocation," *American Journal of Psychiatry,* vol. 149 (February 1992), pp. 175–83.

75. Braddock and others, *The State of the States in Developmental Disabilities,* p. 9; and Nosek and Howland, "Personal Assistance Services."

76. "ADAPT Puts On a Las Vegas Show at AHCA Meeting," *McKnight's Long-Term Care News,* December 1994, pp. 8–9.

77. Rivlin and Wiener, with Hanley and Spence, *Caring for the Disabled Elderly;* Wiener and others, *Sharing the Burden; and* General Accounting Office, *Block Grants: Characteristics, Experience, and Lessons Learned,* GAO/HEHS-95-74 (February 1995).

78. The large majority of persons who reported some type of work limitations (80 percent) also said that they were able, without the assistance of another person, to perform ADLs and instrumental activities of daily living (IADLs). Conversely, a smaller number of individuals reported no work limitation but needed assistance with ADLs and IADLs. Mitchell P. LaPlante, unpublished data from the 1990 National Health Interview Survey, cited in

National Academy of Social Insurance, *Preliminary Status Report of the Disability Policy Panel.*

79. National Academy of Social Insurance, *Preliminary Status Report of the Disability Policy Panel,* chapter 2.

80. The income and asset limits were 50 percent higher for couples.

81. General Accounting Office, "Social Security: Federal Disability Programs Face Major Issues," GAO/T-HEHS-95-97 (March 2, 1995).

82. General Accounting Office, "Social Security."

83. Section 1619(b) of P.L. 99-643 was designed to provide work incentives to supplemental security income (SSI) beneficiaries, in part by enabling disabled SSI beneficiaries who worked to maintain their medicaid coverage. However, an evaluation completed in 1986 on an earlier version of the law (P.L. 98-460) found that few persons returned to work as a result of the program. "Implementation and Analysis of Public Law 98-460—Section 1619 (The Social Security Disability Benefits Reform Act of 1984)," *Social Security Bulletin,* vol. 49 (November 1986), pp. 11–45.

84. Jay Mathews, "Disabilities Act Failing to Achieve Workplace Goals: Landmark Law Rarely Helps Disabled People Seeking Jobs," *Washington Post,* April 16, 1995, pp. A1, A18.

85. Wiener and others, *Sharing the Burden.*

86. Office of the Assistant Secretary for Planning and Evaluation, Office of Disability, Aging, and Long-Term Care Policy, "Cost Estimates for the Long-Term Care Provisions of the Health Security Act," table 5, p. 8.

87. Wiener and others, *Sharing the Burden;* Rivlin and Wiener, with Hanley and Spence, *Caring for the Disabled Elderly;* Robert B. Friedland, *Facing the Costs of Long-Term Care* (Washington: Employee Benefits Research Institute, 1990); Families USA Foundation, *Nursing Home Insurance: Who Can Afford It?* (Washington, February 1993); Sheila Rafferty Zedlewski and Timothy D. McBride, "The Changing Profile of the Elderly: Effects on Future Long-Term Care Needs and Financing," *Milbank Quarterly,* vol. 70, no. 2 (1992), pp. 247–75; and William H. Crown, John Capitman, and Walter N. Leutz, "Economic Rationality, the Affordability of Private Long-Term Care Insurance, and the Role for Public Policy," *Gerontologist,* vol. 32, no. 4 (August 1992), pp. 478–85.

88. Marc A. Cohen and others, "The Financial Capacity of the Elderly to Insure for Long-Term Care," *Gerontologist,* vol. 27 (August 1987), pp. 494–502; Marc A. Cohen and others,"Financing Long-Term Care: A Practical Mix of Public and Private," *Journal of Health Politics, Policy, and Law,* vol. 17 (Fall 1992), pp. 403–23; and Ronald D. Hagen, testimony, *Long-Term Care Insurance,* Hearings before the Subcommittee on Oversight and Investigations of the House Committee on Energy and Commerce, 101 Cong. 2 sess. (GPO, May 2, 1990), pp. 180–207.

89. Wiener and others, *Sharing the Burden.*

90. Susan Coronel and Diane Fulton, *Managed Care and Insurance Operation Report: Long-Term Care Insurance in 1993* (Washington: Health Insurance Association of America, March 1995); and McNeil, "Americans with Disabilities," pp. 11–13.

91. Lois M. Verbrugge, "The Disability Supplement to the 1994–95 National Health Interview Survey" (Hyattsville, Md.: Department of Health and Human Services, Public Health Service, National Center for Health Statistics, October 1994).